Structural Interventions for HIV Prevention

Structural Interventions for HIV Prevention

Optimizing Strategies for Reducing New Infections and Improving Care

Edited by

RICHARD A. CROSBY, Ph.D

and

RALPH J. DICLEMENTE, Ph.D

OXFORD
UNIVERSITY PRESS

OXFORD
UNIVERSITY PRESS

Oxford University Press is a department of the University of Oxford. It furthers
the University's objective of excellence in research, scholarship, and education
by publishing worldwide. Oxford is a registered trade mark of Oxford University
Press in the UK and certain other countries.

Published in the United States of America by Oxford University Press
198 Madison Avenue, New York, NY 10016, United States of America.

Library of Congress Cataloging-in-Publication Data
Names: Crosby, Richard A., 1959– editor. | DiClemente, Ralph J., editor.
Title: Structural interventions for HIV prevention /
[edited by] Richard A. Crosby, Ralph J. DiClemente.
Description: Oxford ; New York : Oxford University Press, [2019] |
Includes bibliographical references and index.
Identifiers: LCCN 2018022325 | ISBN 9780190675486 (hbk. : alk. paper)
Subjects: | MESH: HIV Infections—prevention & control | Acquired
Immunodeficiency Syndrome—prevention & control | Socioeconomic Factors |
Internationality | Social Medicine
Classification: LCC RA643.8 | NLM WC 503.6 | DDC 614.5/99392—dc23
LC record available at https://lccn.loc.gov/2018022325

9 8 7 6 5 4 3 2 1

Printed by Sheridan Books, Inc., United States of America

This volume is dedicated to Dr. Jonathan Mann. Isaac Newton once remarked that "he stood on the shoulders of giants." We in the field of HIV prevention have also benefitted from a "giant." Many of us have stood on the broad shoulders of Jonathan Mann. As a mentor to the field of HIV prevention, it was Mann who pioneered and championed the ethic that protecting human rights and dignity must be the foundational approach to all HIV prevention efforts. His guidance to the field lives on and continues to shape the structural-level approaches being used today.

It is also dedicated to Sir Elton John, a man whose dedication and passion to confronting the HIV epidemic on a global scale is exemplary. He has been in the forefront of the global response to HIV since its recognition. He has been tireless in his efforts on behalf of those infected with HIV and those vulnerable to HIV. His efforts to catalyze HIV prevention research and compassionate care have been instrumental on a global level. To him, we as a global society owe a heartfelt debt of gratitude.

Contents

Foreword

Greetings,

This new book of Dr. DiClemente and Dr. Crosby is timely. It provides a comprehensive examination of different structural-level intervention programs to prevent HIV transmission. In recent years we have seen large improvements in access to HIV treatments that have reduced mortality rates due to HIV/AIDS and secondarily reduced new HIV infections. However, major gaps still remain, and progress has been experienced inequitably across the globe and for certain key populations. There is still much work to be done in order to realize the UNAIDS stated goal: the end of AIDS as a pandemic.

The UNAIDS target calls for at least 90% of people living with HIV knowing their HIV status, 90% of them receiving sustained antiretroviral therapy, and 90% of them maintaining an undetectable viral load by 2020. Meeting the proposed target would ensure that at least 73% of all people living with HIV worldwide will be virally suppressed, and this in turn will be expected to lead to a 90% decrease in AIDS-related deaths and a 90% decrease in HIV transmission, thereby transforming the once raging AIDS pandemic into a low-level endemic disease by 2030. This is an ambitious goal, and while it is within reach, it will also require an unprecedented effort.

One critical and often overlooked aspect of this effort relates to the need to urgently address the structural inequities experienced by marginalized populations. These populations vary across and within countries. However, structural factors frequently impede their ability to access HIV testing, treatment, care, and support. Addressing these upstream social determinants and conditions will be not only be a key to our collective success in the control of HIV/AIDS, but far-reaching in terms of health and social benefits for these communities.

Canada has been an international leader in health promotion, especially around the social determinants of health. The Ottawa Charter for Health Promotion represents a landmark international agreement signed in 1986 in order to achieve health for all. The field of HIV prevention needs this new book to move us forward in theory and practice. To date, the prevention of HIV infections has largely relied on biomedical innovations and technology. While these developments and success are necessary to our HIV response, these are not sufficient. This book critically considers the structural factors and social conditions that limit the success of solely biomedical approaches. Of course, these must be done in tandem in order that structural interventions optimize the value and benefits of biomedical technologies.

The British Columbia Centre for Excellence in HIV/AIDS pioneered Treatment as Prevention®, first proposed in *The Lancet* in 2006. Since then, our experience has clearly demonstrated that expanding population coverage of highly active antiretroviral therapy (HAART) leads to inversely proportional changes in HIV/AIDS morbidity and mortality, as well as HIV new diagnoses. However, to be successful, Treatment as Prevention® has required a multifaceted intervention to shift health systems and structures. This includes removing barriers and increasing access to HIV testing, improving referral pathways to reduce the time to treatment initiation for those newly diagnosed, and universal access to HAART (free of cost). This has also included a focus on improving the social conditions for people living with and disproportionately affected by HIV. To name a few, urgent needs exist to work to reduce HIV stigma, improve access to good nutrition and housing, and create improved access to harm reduction and drug substitution programs, with concomitant concerted community mobilization. Further gains are anticipated with the addition of universal fully subsidized access to HIV post-exposure and pre-exposure prophylaxis programs.

This book is edited by two eminent scholars in health psychology, education, and promotion. Dr. DiClemente has focused on developing intervention packages that blend community and technology-based approaches that are designed to optimize program effectiveness and enhance programmatic sustainability. Dr. Crosby is a leader in the field of health promotion and HIV intervention research and has written several books on theory and methodology that have advanced our research and practice.

Dr. DiClemente and Dr. Crosby have gathered a rich and illustrious array of international contributors who provide key insights from their successes using a structural-level approach across diverse global settings. The book uses a case study approach, taking readers on a trip around the world. These include interventions focused on schooling and education, income, housing, and food security. The authors also discuss the importance and value of a key population focus and working with and helping to mobilize vulnerable communities to advance their health.

We hope that you enjoy and benefit from this new book. All the best in your ongoing work to prevent HIV transmission, end the AIDS pandemic, and ensure health for all!

Sincerely,
Nathan Lachowsky, PhD
Michael Smith Foundation for Health Research Scholar
Research Director of the Community-Based Research Centre for Gay Men's Health
Assistant Professor, University of Victoria

Julio Montaner, OC, OBC, MD, FRCPC, FCCP
Director, British Columbia Centre for Excellence in HIV/AIDS
Director and Physician Program Director for HIV/AIDS Providence Health Care
Killam Professor of Medicine, University of British Columbia

Contributors

Tessa Ahner-McHaffie, MPH
Department of Global Health
Milken Institute School of
    Public Health
George Washington University
Washington, DC

Angelina A. Aidala, PhD
Associate Research Scientist
Sociomedical Sciences
Columbia University Mailman
    School of Public Health
New York, NY

Sarah Baird, PhD
Associate Professor
Department of Global Health
Milken Institute School of
    Public Health
George Washington University
Washington, DC

Kim M. Blankenship, PhD
Professor
Department of Sociology
Codirector, Social and Behavioral
    Sciences Core, District of
    Columbia Center for AIDS
    Research
American University
Washington, DC

Richard A. Crosby, PhD
Endowed Professor of Public Health
University of Kentucky
Lexington, KY

Julia Dickson-Gomez, PhD
Professor of Psychiatry and
    Behavioral Medicine
Center for AIDS Intervention
    Research
Medical College of Wisconsin
Milwaukee, WI

Ralph J. DiClemente, PhD
Professor and Chair, Department
    of Social & Behavioral Sciences
Professor, Department of
    Epidemiology
Associate Dean, Public Health
    Innovation
College of Global Public Health
    New York University
New York, NY

Stefanie Dringus, PhD Candidate
Faculty of Public Health Policy
Department of Social Health
    Research
London School of Hygiene &
    Tropical Medicine
London, UK

Robyn Eakle, PhD
Assistant Professor
SaME, Department of Global
  Health and Development,
  LSHTM
London, UK

Nabila El-Bassel, PhD
Professor
Columbia University School of
  Social Work
The Willma and Albert Musher
  Professor of Social Work
Director of the Global Health
  Research Center of Central Asia
Director of the Social
  Intervention Group
New York, NY

Robert Fullilove, EdD
Associate Dean, Community and
  Minority Affairs
Professor, Clinical Sociomedical
  Sciences, Columbia University
  Medical Center
Codirector, Cities Research Group
Columbia University Mailman
  School of Public Health
New York, NY

Jonathan Garcia, PhD
Assistant Professor
Global Health
School of Biological and
  Population Health Sciences
College of Public Health and
  Human Sciences
Oregon State University
Corvallis, OR

Louisa Gilbert, PhD
Associate Professor
Codirector, Social
  Intervention Group
Columbia University School of
  Social Work
New York, NY

Dawn A. Goddard-Eckrich, EdD
Associate Research Scientist
Columbia University School of
  Social Work
New York, NY

James Hargreaves, BSc, MSc, PhD
Professor in Epidemiology and
  Evaluation
Director of the Centre for
  Evaluation
Public Health, Environments and
  Society
Faculty of Public Health
  and Policy
London School of Hygiene &
  Tropical Medicine
London, UK

Bernadette Hensen, BSc, MSc, PhD
Research Fellow,
  Epidemiology
London School of Hygiene &
  Tropical Medicine
London, UK

Timothy Hunt, PhD, MSW, LCSW-R
Associate Research Scientist
Associate Director
Social Intervention Group
Global Health Research Center of
  Central Asia
Principal Investigator, USWEEP
  Project in Uzbekistan (UNICEF)
Co-Principal Investigator,
  WORTH Transitions
  Implementation Project
  (SAMHSA)
Co-Investigator, BRIDGE
  Implementation Project, UNI,
  PACT, and E-WORTH (NIDA)
Director, CONNECT HIP CDC
  Dissemination Project (CDC)
(Former) Executive Director,
  CSSW Projects in Middle East
  and GCC
MINT Member
Columbia University School of
  Social Work
New York, NY

Kyle Hunter, MD Candidate
University of California,
  San Francisco
School of Medicine
San Francisco, CA

Deanna Kerrigan, MPH, PhD
Professor
Department of Sociology
American University
Washington, DC

Nathan Lachowsky, PhD
Michael Smith Foundation for
  Health Research Scholar
Research Director of the
  Community-Based Research
  Centre for Gay Men's Health
Assistant Professor
University of Victoria
Victoria, BC, Canada

Jennifer L. Leigh, MPH Candidate
Columbia University Mailman
  School of Public Health
New York, NY

Samuel Likindikoki, MD
Lecturer
Department of Psychiatry
Muhimbili University of Health
  and Allied Sciences
Dar es Salaam, Tanzania

Andrea Mantsios, MHS, PhD
Assistant Scientist
Department of Health, Behavior
  and Society
Johns Hopkins Bloomberg School
  of Public Health
Baltimore, MD

Phillip L. Marotta, PhD
Assistant Professor
School of Social Work
Social Intervention Group
Columbia University Population
  Research Center
New York, NY

Jessie Mbwambo, MD
Senior Lecturer
Department of Psychiatry
Muhimbili University of Health
    and Allied Sciences
Dar es Salaam, Tanzania

Julio Montaner, OC, OBC, MD,
FRCPC, FCCP
Director, British Columbia
    Centre for Excellence in
    HIV/AIDS
Director and Physician Program
    Director, HIV/AIDS Providence
    Health Care
Killam Professor of Medicine,
    University of British
    Columbia
Vancouver, BC, Canada

Miguel Muñoz-Laboy, DrPH
Associate Professor
School of Social Work
College of Public Health
Temple University
Philadelphia, PA

Laura Rebecca Murray, PhD
Postdoctoral Researcher
Department of Health Policy,
    Planning, and
    Administration
Institute of Social Medicine
State University of Rio de Janeiro
Rio de Janeiro, RJ, Brazil

Will Nutland, BSC, DrPH
Faculty of Public Health
    and Policy
London School of Hygiene &
    Tropical Medicine
London, UK

Berk Özler, PhD
Senior Economist
Development Economics
    Research Group
The World Bank
Washington, DC

Richard Parker, PhD
Senior Visiting Professor
Institute for the Study of
    Collective Health
Federal University of Rio de
    Janeiro
Professor Emeritus,
    Sociomedical Sciences and
    Anthropology
Member, Columbia University
    Committee on
    Global Thought
Columbia University,
    New York
Editor-in-Chief, Global
    Public Health
Executive Director,
    Brazilian Interdisciplinary
    AIDS Association
Rio de Janeiro, RJ, Brazil

Katherine Quinn, PhD
Assistant Professor
Psychiatry and Behavioral
    Medicine
Center for AIDS Intervention
    Research
Medical College of Wisconsin
Milwaukee, WI

Michelle Remme, PhD
Assistant Professor
Health Economics
Department of Global Health and
  Development
Faculty of Public
  Health and Policy
London School of Hygiene &
  Tropical Medicine
London, UK

Fernando Seffner, EeD
Associate Professor
Education Faculty
Federal University of Rio
  Grande do Sul
Campus Central da Universidade
  Federal do Rio Grande do Sul
Porto Alegre, RS, Brazil

Catherine Shembilu, PhD
Independent Consultant
Iringa, Tanzania

Susan Sherman, PhD, MPH
Professor
Health, Behavior and Society
Johns Hopkins Bloomberg School
  of Public Health
Baltimore, MD

Jacqueline P. Sims, PhD
Research Scientist
Boston University School of
  Education
Boston, MA

Sandra Springer, MD
Associate Professor
Yale School of Medicine
Section of Infectious
  Diseases
Yale AIDS Program
New Haven, CT

Elwin Wu, PhD
Associate Professor
Codirector, Social
  Intervention Group
Columbia University School of
  Social Work
New York, NY

Maiko Yomogida, MA
Senior Research Associate
Columbia University Mailman
  School of Public Health
New York, NY

1

Global Burden of HIV/AIDS

A DIVERSE PANDEMIC

Ralph J. DiClemente, Richard A. Crosby, and Jacqueline P. Sims

TRULY THE LARGEST and longest-lasting pandemic in the history of humankind, AIDS continues to claim lives around the world. As is so often the case with infectious diseases, people living in developing nations bear a vastly disproportionate burden of the pandemic. Within these developing nations, and even within developed nations, AIDS has disproportionately affected populations who are socially marginalized and those who are economically marginalized. Prevalence rates by region, or even country, only tell a very coarse story—one that misses the looming point that AIDS has a tendency to invade subpopulations within a nation that are the most marginalized.

As noted early in the pandemic, in a 1992 speech delivered by Nelson Mandela, the rapid spread of AIDS was fueled by inequities in employment, women's rights, housing; poverty; and overcrowding.[1] In nearly every conceivable way, the AIDS virus has exploited social and economic disparities—in all areas of the world—to progressively become a disease of the most disadvantaged populations on earth. The pandemic, then, can be viewed as being intimately linked with inequalities among humans. As noted by former US president Bill Clinton, "We live in a completely interdependent world, which simply means we can not escape each other. How we respond to AIDS depends, in part, on whether we understand this interdependence. It is not someone else's problem. This is everybody's problem."[2]

Rather than a summary of HIV incidence rates, AIDS prevalence rates, AIDS death rates, and so on, the goal of this chapter is to provide a contextual overview of the global epidemic through in-depth examinations of various national HIV/AIDS epidemics. Our aim is to characterize the vast differences that exist across the national HIV *epidemics* that comprise the global *pandemic*. To achieve this, we have selected five nations that have distinctly different epidemics. We begin with the nation of Lesotho.

HIV/AIDS in Lesotho

Surrounded by South Africa, the small nation of Lesotho (approximately 2 million people) has the second highest prevalence rate of HIV in the world. This translates to 25% of all adults living with HIV or AIDS.[3] This inordinately high prevalence creates ample opportunity for transmission given that *community viral load* is inevitably high in this nation where only 42% of the 330,000 people living with HIV/AIDS are taking antiretroviral therapy (ART; with the number being adherent and thus achieving viral suppression being unknown). The concept of community viral load is one that is easily illustrated using this nation as an example. In essence, the high prevalence rate coupled with low ART coverage engenders low rates of viral suppression—and thus heightened viral loads exist among many HIV-infected people. When aggregated up to the population level, these individual viral loads together reflect a higher community viral load and greater risk of ongoing HIV transmission. In other areas with greater ART coverage and lower prevalence rates, including some that we will discuss shortly, more HIV-infected persons achieving suppression translates into lower community viral loads and lesser risk of ongoing HIV transmission.[4]

Yet even in a high-burden nation such as Lesotho, a nationwide prevalence rate obscures the disproportionate share of the burden shouldered by particular subgroups of the population. As is the case in many other nations, women and girls experience heightened risk of HIV in Lesotho due to their unequal status in society.[5,6] Structural factors rooted in the country's patriarchal culture prevent many women from exerting full autonomy over their own medical and sexual decisions, leaving them disproportionately vulnerable to HIV's impact. Indeed, until recently, married women in Lesotho were legally required to obtain spousal consent in many decisions, including some related to sexual and reproductive health.[7] Social norms surrounding marriage and sexual relationships carry on this patriarchal legacy today, with the majority of men reporting that it is acceptable for husbands to threaten their spouse if she refuses to have sex with him and smaller but substantial portions of both men and women stating that a woman is never justified in refusing sex with her husband.[8] These attitudes and norms toward gender relations are linked with Lesotho's high prevalence of gender-based violence, which increases HIV risk among women.

These vulnerabilities that women and girls face make them a priority population for HIV prevention treatment such as increased access to healthcare and oral pre-exposure prophylaxis (PrEP).[9] Given the low ART coverage in Lesotho, though, it comes as no surprise that PrEP services are also lacking in the country.[10] This low coverage serves to perpetuate the vicious cycle of HIV transmission across the general population but particularly among groups experiencing heightened risk: prevalence increased more rapidly among women than men between 2004 and 2014.[5] For these reasons, women and girls represent over one half of the roughly 24,000 beneficiaries that PEPFAR aims to provide PrEP services to in 2018.[10]

HIV/AIDS in the United Kingdom

We will now consider the United Kingdom's HIV epidemic, which provides an interesting juxtaposition to that of Lesotho's. The United Kingdom, comprised of England, Scotland, Wales, and Northern Ireland, has a relatively low prevalence rate of HIV: roughly 0.16% of all adults are living with HIV or AIDS.[11] Along with this stark difference in prevalence, the United Kingdom and Lesotho are notably dissimilar in their availability of treatment services. In the United Kingdom, the vast majority of adults living with HIV or AIDS are on HIV treatment: 96% of those who are aware of their HIV status are receiving treatment.[12] This stellar coverage, made possible by the free and universally available testing and treatment available throughout the United Kingdom, drives a 94% viral suppression rate among those receiving treatment and suggests particularly low community viral load.

Despite the United Kingdom's low prevalence rate, there is substantial heterogeneity within the United Kingdom in the severity of the HIV epidemic. Men who have sex with men (MSM) experience exponentially heightened risk of HIV compared to the general population in the United Kingdom: 5% of MSM are living with the virus compared to the 0.16% seen among the general population.[13] A host of factors—social, biological, and behavioral—contribute to this high vulnerability among MSM, with research emphasizing the pivotal role that social factors play in heightened risk.[14] Exposure to and experiences of homophobia, in particular, have been linked with a variety of behaviors that further increases risk for HIV infection, ranging from substance abuse and risky sexual behaviors to difficulty maintaining long-term same-sex relationships.[15-18] Acutely problematic for attempts to curb the epidemic, homophobia and sexual stigma—and the mental health burden associated with them—interfere with treatment uptake and adherence among members of this marginalized group.[19,20]

Given the far-reaching and deleterious effects of homophobia, it is unsurprising that rates of new diagnoses among MSM rose steadily in the United Kingdom for years. However, recent reports reflect the first-ever drop in new diagnoses among MSM in London, and it is a newsworthy accomplishment: 5 of London's leading sexual health clinics reported a downturn of 32% in new diagnoses.[21] Practitioners and researchers have attributed this incredible achievement to myriad factors including the high volume of HIV testing in London, the rapid treatment following diagnosis, and—albeit to a lesser extent at this point—the use of PrEP among high-risk MSM.[22] As the provision of PrEP services increases across the United Kingdom—both England and Wales have recently begun large-scale trial rollouts alongside Scotland's widely available provision of PrEP through sexual health clinics[22-25]—officials are hopeful that the downturn seen in London can be scaled up across the United Kingdom and across other vulnerable groups. The significant drop in new diagnoses undoubtedly provides promising insights into the potential for targeted HIV prevention and treatment services in ending the region's epidemic.

HIV/AIDS in Ukraine

We next consider Ukraine's HIV epidemic, where we find 1 of the highest prevalence rates in Eastern Europe and Central Asia. Despite its smaller population, Ukraine has notably more adults living with HIV or AIDS than the United Kingdom: HIV prevalence was estimated at 0.9%, or about 240,000 people, in 2016. Yet, among people who inject drugs (PWID), who comprise one of the most vulnerable groups to HIV infection around the globe, HIV prevalence in Ukraine is a staggering 21.9%.[26] The course of the country's epidemic, both within the injection drug use community and among the generalized population, nicely illustrates the profound ways that social and political forces shape disease burden.

Prior to 1994, diagnoses of HIV infection in Ukraine were uncommon, but the following few years brought rapid transmission through injection drug use. By 1996, there were an estimated 25,000 diagnoses of HIV in the country, with 7% of registered PWID in Ukraine living with HIV.[27] Healthcare services at this time posed significant barriers to HIV prevention for this group, as PWID faced criminal prosecution and were required to register as drug users upon admission of drug use to a healthcare provider.[28] This criminalization and marginalization fostered mistrust of the healthcare sector and perpetuated the rapid transmission of HIV throughout the injection drug use community. For over a decade, injection drug use continued as the primary driver of the increasingly widespread epidemic: by 2006, 1.7% of the population was living with HIV.[29]

Amidst increasing prevalence rates, Ukraine formulated a more proactive response to the epidemic that included no-cost opioid substitution therapy to help stem transmission in the injection drug use community as well as initiate free HIV testing and treatment services.[30] Even with the provision of these services, though, rates of treatment today are not nearly as high as they are in the United Kingdom due to the country's fragile economy as well as insufficient linkages between nongovernmental organizations and health services.[30] Just over one-half of adults living with HIV or AIDS in Ukraine are aware of their status, and 66% of those are receiving treatment, with only 60% of those receiving treatment achieving viral suppression.[26] Given the high community viral load and likelihood of transmission, sexual transmission overtook injection drug use as the primary driver of the Ukrainian HIV epidemic in 2008, as partners of PWID increasingly became HIV positive.[30] Nonetheless, recent data suggest a slowed infection rate in 2014 and 2015, pointing to the promise and importance of ongoing efforts to maintain and bolster treatment and prevention services.[31]

Yet, a variety of factors jeopardize these efforts. Despite the increasingly generalized epidemic in the country, PrEP-related services for vulnerable people are virtually nonexistent in the Ukraine. An nongovernmental organization-spearheaded initiative recently secured approval to provide the first PrEP services in Ukraine, but only to a targeted group of 100 people.[32] Military actions in the area also threaten the progress being made. It is estimated that nearly one fourth of Ukraine's new HIV infections in 2014 occurred in conflict-affected areas,[33] and the unfolding sociopolitical context is particularly hostile to prevention efforts among PWID. As Russian control in the area expands, Russian health policies are spreading throughout the region: access to opioid substitution therapies, which are banned in Russia for medical purposes, have markedly diminished in the area over the last 3 years.[34] The proliferation of these policies poses grave risks not only for those being stripped of their services but also for the future of the fight against HIV in Eastern Europe as a whole.

HIV/AIDS in Thailand

We now depart Europe to consider the HIV epidemic in Thailand, where roughly 450,000 people were living with HIV in 2016. This translates to just over 1% of the population living with HIV, 91% of whom are aware of their status.[26] Prevalence rates are notably higher among *key affected populations* such as sex workers: 2014 prevalence was nearly 12% and 2% among male and female sex workers, respectively.[35] Such heightened prevalence rates among sex workers, in Thailand and around the globe, are driven by the legal, social, and economic marginalization that this population faces. Punitive laws, including Thailand's prohibition on prostitution,[36] not only foster stigma toward sex workers but also complicate attempts to regulate health practices and protect workers from violence on the job—even in countries with well-established sex industries such as Thailand. Economic disenfranchisement also places sex workers at heightened risk of HIV infection, given the potential economic disincentives to promote and practice safe sex. Sex workers and establishment owners who insist on condom usage face the potential of losing clients—and money—to those who do not. These potential ramifications are particularly salient for sex workers, many of who were initially propelled into the profession by poverty and economic disadvantage.[37]

Thailand's 100% condom program in the early 1990s aimed to regulate and require condom usage in sex work, thereby ameliorating the economic disincentives to condom usage.[38] The program is largely recognized as a public health success, with rates of condom usage spiking in the sex industry and millions of infections averted over time.[39] But decades after the condom program's rollout, the work to slow the disproportionate rate of new HIV infections seen among sex workers is still ongoing. One problematic issue is Thailand's shift to indirect sex work over time. It is notably more difficult to reach and regulate indirect sex workers, or those who work in settings such as clubs and bars (as opposed to direct sex workers, who may work in brothels or sex bars),[40] highlighting the need for adaptive strategies to reach vulnerable populations.

An existing area of innovation and adaptation in the fight against HIV in Thailand is in the provision of PrEP. PrEP coverage in Thailand is somewhat limited but has been available through targeted trials in Bangkok since

2014 and through pilot programs in 4 other high-prevalence provinces since 2015.[41,42] Despite this limited scope, the rollouts have seen successes among key populations in Thailand by drawing on social networks to recruit and retain clients through online-to-offline models. Initial evidence suggests that these innovative approaches, which have included relevant social media apps, such as Grindr, have successfully translated online outreach to offline uptake of PrEP services.[43,44]

HIV/AIDS in India

We remain in South Asia for our final stop on this journey, India, where the national HIV prevalence rate of 0.3% is concentrated in many of the key affected populations that we have already considered in the context of other countries.[26] In addition to high rates among MSM (4.3%) and female sex workers (2.2%), HIV prevalence rates in India are even higher in the transgender community: an estimated 7.2% of transgender people in India were living with HIV in 2015.[26,45] Commonly referred to as identifying with a "third gender" in India, members of this vulnerable group are roughly 49 times more at risk of HIV compared to the general population around the world.[42]

The heightened vulnerability experienced in transgender communities is linked with histories of stigma, discrimination, exclusion, violence, and—often as a function of these experiences—poverty, given that educational and workplace discrimination result in unemployment and underemployment in the transgender community.[46] This marginalization extends to healthcare settings and poses particularly problematic barriers to HIV prevention. Transgender people not only receive inadequate care as a function of limited access to transgender-specific care but many also report experiencing hostile or humiliating care from providers.[47] These experiences not only exasperate the mental health burden but also have the potential to push transgender people to obtain care from unqualified and unregulated providers for medical procedures such as silicone injections.[47] Such unregulated care may include unsafe needle injection practices that heighten the risk for HIV.

Given that India did not legally recognize the third gender until 2014, when transgender people were formally granted the opportunity to be recognized outside the gender binary, it is not surprising that the mental health burden in transgender communities is poorly addressed in the country's current HIV programs and guidelines.[48,49] Legal recognition, however, carries with it the requirement for the government to formulate targeted programs to support transgender communities. As India works to improve its HIV programming (only 49% of people living with HIV in India are receiving treatment, despite the provision of free treatment since 2004[26]), it is hopeful that such programming will also begin to incorporate approaches that reduce stigma against transgender people and begin to address and support the mental health ramifications of that stigma.

In addition to these gaps in care, India lacks a national policy regarding PrEP, leaving key affected populations such as those that identify as a third gender particularly vulnerable. Initial feasibility and demonstration projects are underway in the country, and preliminary results suggest high interest in PrEP services in India. Nonetheless, there are concerns that the current projects may lack the scope and diversity to yield adequate evidence for the national or state AIDS control programs to make PrEP sufficiently available, pointing to the need for additional projects that span diverse regions and key populations in the country.[50,51]

Conclusion

The HIV/AIDS pandemic is diverse in nature; a singular set of drivers and corresponding solutions will not be effective. Instead, each nation must constantly monitor and evaluate its epidemic, with the goal always being to identify populations most at risk of acquisition and most at risk of transmission. The subsequent goal of evaluation involves ongoing identification of the socio-structural drivers that can best be altered to foster positive change. Although the commitment to the prevention and control of each national epidemic may be uniformly high, the actual policy-level and resource-allocation needs will greatly vary from one nation to another. Within each affected nation, political courage will be vital to truly leverage the structural changes needed to stem the epidemic.

References

1. Bosely S. How Nelson Mandela changed the AIDS agenda in South Africa. *The Guardian*. December 6, 2013. Available at: https://www.theguardian.com/world/2013/dec/06/nelson-mandela-aids-south-africa
2. Silva C. National youth HIV, AIDS awareness day quotes: 10 inspirational sayings for 2016 annual observance. *International Business Times*. April 10, 2016. Available at: http://www.ibtimes.com/national-youth-hiv-aids-awareness-day-quotes-10-inspirational-sayings-2016-annual-2350869

3. AVERTing HIV and AIDS. HIV and AIDS in Lesotho. Available at: https://www.avert.org/professionals/hiv-around-world/sub-saharan-africa/lesotho

4. Castel AD, Befus M, Willis S, et al. Use of the community viral load as a population-based biomarker of HIV burden. *AIDS*. 2012;26:345–353.

5. Ministry of Health (Lesotho) and ICF International. *Lesotho Demographic and Health Survey 2014*. 2016. Available at: https://dhsprogram.com/pubs/pdf/FR309/FR309.pdf

6. UNAIDS. *The Gap Report*. 2014. Available at: http://www.unaids.org/en/resources/campaigns/2014/2014gapreport/gapreport

7. Lesotho National AIDS Commission. *Lesotho: HIV Prevention Response and Modes of Transmission Analysis*. 2009. Available at: http://documents.worldbank.org/curated/en/802971468331880614/pdf/483570SR0P11131010sameobox101PUBLIC1.pdf

8. Lesotho Ministry of Health. *Lesotho Global AIDS Response Country Progress Report*. 2012. Available at: http://www.unaids.org/sites/default/files/country/documents//file,68395,fr..pdf

9. World Health Organization. *Policy Brief: WHO Expands Recommendation on Oral Pre-Exposure Prophylaxis of HIV Infection (PrEP)*. 2015. Available at: http://apps.who.int/iris/bitstream/10665/197906/1/WHO_HIV_2015.48_eng.pdf

10. PEPFAR. *Lesotho Country Operational Plan (COP/ROP) 2017*. 2017. Available at: https://www.pepfar.gov/documents/organization/272218.pdf

11. AVERTing HIV and AIDS. HIV and AIDS in the United Kingdom (UK). Available at: https://www.avert.org/professionals/hiv-around-world/western-central-europe-north-america/uk

12. Public Health England. *HIV in the UK*. 2016. Available at: https://www.gov.uk/government/uploads/system/uploads/attachment_data/file/602942/HIV_in_the_UK_report.pdf

13. Public Health England. *HIV in the UK—Situation Report 2015. Incidence, Prevalence and Prevention*. 2015. Available at: https://www.gov.uk/government/uploads/system/uploads/attachment_data/file/477702/HIV_in_the_UK_2015_report.pdf

14. AVERTing HIV and AIDS. *Homophobia and HIV*. Available at: https://www.avert.org/professionals/hiv-social-issues/homophobia#footnote6_f73u144

15. Mayer KH, Bradford JB, Makadon HJ, Stall R, Goldhammer H. Sexual and gender minority health: what we know and what needs to be done. *Am J Public Health*. 2008;98:989–995.

16. Halkitis PN, Fischgrund BN, Parsons JT. Explanations for methamphetamine use among gay and bisexual men in New York City. *Subst Use Misuse*. 2005;40:1–15.

17. Wolitski RJ, Stall R, Valdiserri RO, eds. *Unequal Opportunity: Health Disparities Affecting Gay and Bisexual Men in the United States*. Oxford: Oxford University Press; 2008.

18. Diaz RM, Ayala G, Bein E, Henne J, Marin BV. The impact of homophobia, poverty, and racism on the mental health of gay and bisexual Latino men: Findings from 3 U.S. cities. *Am J Public Health.* 2001;91:927–932.

19. World Health Organization. *Prevention and Treatment of HIV and Other Sexually Transmitted Infections among Men Who Have Sex with Men and Transgender People.* 2011. Available at: http://www.who.int/hiv/pub/guidelines/msm_guidelines2011/en/

20. Ayala G, Santos GM. Will the global HIV response fail gay and bisexual men and other men who have sex with men? *J Int AIDS Soc.* 2016;19(1):21098.

21. Brown AE, Mohammed H, Ogaz D, et al. Fall in new HIV diagnoses among men who have sex with men (MSM) at selected London sexual health clinics since early 2015: testing or treatment or pre-exposure prophylaxis (PrEP)? *Euro Surveill.* 2017;22(25):30553.

22. Developing HIV Literacy, HIV Scotland, and PrEPster. *Know about PrEP.* 2017. Available at: https://prepscot.files.wordpress.com/2017/08/prep-a5-booklet-web.pdf

23. Public Health Wales. *PrEPARED in Wales.* 2017. Available at: http://friskywales.org/wales-prep-project.html

24. McCormack S, Dunn DT, Desai M, et al. Pre-exposure prophylaxis to prevent the acquisition of HIV-1 infection (PROUD): effectiveness results from the pilot phase of a pragmatic open-label randomised trial. *Lancet.* 2016;387(10013):53–60.

25. National Health Service England. *Update on Commissioning and Provision of Pre Exposure Prophylaxis (PREP) for HIV Prevention.* March 21, 2016. Available at: https://www.england.nhs.uk/2016/03/prep/

26. UNAIDS. *Data 2017.* 2017. Available at: http://www.unaids.org/en/resources/documents/2017/2017_data_book

27. Dehne KL, Khodakevich L, Hamers FF, Schwarländer B. The HIV/AIDS epidemic in eastern Europe: recent patterns and trends and their implications for policy-making. *AIDS.* 1999;13(7):741–749.

28. Amon JJ. The HIV/AIDS epidemic in Ukraine: stable or still exploding? *Sex Transm Infect.* 2003;79:263–264.

29. Hankivsky O. The challenges of HIV/AIDS in Ukraine. In: Pope C, White RT, Malow R, eds. *HIV/AIDS: Global Frontiers in Prevention/Intervention.* New York: Routledge; 2009.

30. World Health Organisation Europe. *Good Practices in Europe: HIV Prevention for People Who Inject Drugs Implemented by the International HIV/AIDS Alliance in Ukraine.* July 2014. Available at: http://www.euro.who.int/__data/assets/pdf_file/0003/254352/FINAL-Ukraine-Good-Practice-July-2014-with-covers.pdf

31. European Centre for Disease Prevention and Control and World Health Organization. *Surveillance Report: HIV/AIDS Surveillance in Europe 2015.* 2016.

Available at: http://www.euro.who.int/__data/assets/pdf_file/0019/324370/HIV-AIDS-surveillance-Europe-2015.pdf?ua=1

32. Alliance Global. *Pre-Exposure Prophylaxis PrEP Soon Available in Ukraine.* Available at: http://ga.net.ua/language/en/news-en/pre-exposure-prophylaxis-prep-soon-in-ukraine/

33. European Centre for Disease Prevention and Control and World Health Organization. *Surveillance Report: HIV/AIDS Surveillance in Europe 2015.* 2016. Available at: http://www.unaids.org/sites/default/files/country/documents/UKR_narrative_report_2015.pdf

34. Mackey TK, Strathdee SA. Responding to the public health consequences of the Ukraine crisis: an opportunity for global health diplomacy. *J Int AIDS Soc.* 2015;18(1):19410.

35. National AIDS Committee. *Thailand AIDS Response Progress Report. Reporting Period: Fiscal Year of 2014.* 2015. Available at: http://www.unaids.org/sites/default/files/country/documents/THA_narrative_report_2015.pdf

36. United Nations Action for Cooperation against Trafficking in Persons. *Thailand's Prevention and Suppression of Prostitution Act (1996).* Available at: http://un-act.org/publication/thailands-prevention-and-suppression-of-prostitution-act-1996/

37. Centers for Disease Control and Prevention. *HIV Risk among Persons Who Exchange Sex for Money or Nonmonetary Items.* September 26, 2016. Available at: https://www.cdc.gov/hiv/group/sexworkers.html

38. UNAIDS, AIDS Division, Ministry of Public Health, Thailand. *Evalaution of the 100% Condom Programme in Thailand.* July 2000. Available at: http://data.unaids.org/publications/irc-pub01/jc275-100pcondom_en.pdf

39. Siraprapasiri T, Ongwangdee S, Benjarattanaporn P, Peerapatanapokin W, Sharma M. The impact of Thailand's public health response to the HIV epidemic 1984-2015: understanding the ingredients of success. 2016. *J Virus Erad.* 2016;2(Suppl 4):7–14.

40. United Nations Development Programme. *Thailand's Response to HIV/AIDS: Progress and Challenges.* 2004. Available at: http://www.hivpolicy.org/Library/HPP000242.pdf

41. UNAIDS. *Countries in Asia Start to Roll Out PrEP.* November 2, 2016. Available at: urces/presscentre/featurestories/2016/november/20161102_asia

42. UNAIDS. *Prevention Gap Report.* 2016. Available at: http://www.unaids.org/sites/default/files/media_asset/2016-prevention-gap-report_en.pdf

43. United States Agency for International Development, President's Emergency Plan for AIDS Relief, LINKAGES. Linkages across the Continuum of HIV Services for Key Populations Affected by HIV (LINKAGES) Project. July 31, 2017. *Thailand Quarterly Progress Report: April 1–June 30, 2017.* Available at: http://pdf.usaid.gov/pdf_docs/PA00MWR9.pdf

44. Anand T, Nitpolprasert C, Trachunthong, D. A novel online-to-offline (O2O) model for pre-exposure prophylaxis and HIV testing scale up. *J Int AIDS Soc*. 2017;20(1):21326.

45. National AIDS Control Organisation. *National Integrated Biological and Behavioural Surveillance (IBBS) 2014-15: High Risk Groups*. Available at http://www.aidsdatahub.org/sites/default/files/highlight-reference/document/India_IBBS_report_2014-15.pdf

46. Winter S, Diamond M, Green J, et al. Transgender people: health at the margins of society. *Lancet*. 2016;388:390–400.

47. WHO Western Pacific Region. *Regional Assessment of HIV, STI and Other Health Needs of Transgender People in Asia and the Pacific*. 2013. Available at: http://www.who.int/hiv/pub/transgender/tg_needs_regional/en/

48. Pandey G. India court recognizes transgender people as third gender. *BBC News*. April 15, 2014. Available at: http://www.bbc.com/news/world-asia-india-27031180

49. United Nations Development Programme, India. *Hijras/Transgender Women in India: HIV, Human Rights and Social Exclusion*. December 2010. Available at: http://www.undp.org/content/dam/india/docs/hijras_transgender_in_india_hiv_human_rights_and_social_exclusion.pdf

50. Mayer KH, Chandhiok N, Thomas B. Antiretroviral pre-exposure prophylaxis: a new opportunity to slow HIV in India. *Indian J Med Res*. 2016:143;125–128.

51. Reza-Paul S, Lazarus L, Doshi M, et al. Prioritizing risk in preparation for a demonstration project: A mixed methods feasibility study of oral pre-exposure prophylaxis (PrEP) among female sex workers in South India. *PLoS One*. 2016;23(11):e0166889.

2

Applying Behavioral and Social Science Theory to HIV Prevention

THE NEED FOR STRUCTURAL-LEVEL APPROACHES

Richard A. Crosby and Ralph J. DiClemente

Overview

Nearly 40 years into the AIDS pandemic, a critical question concerns the role of the behavioral and social sciences in preventing new infections and controlling the viral load in people living with HIV/AIDS. Early in the pandemic, behavioral interventions (defined as organized and manualized programs designed to promote safer sex behaviors) were the mainstay of HIV prevention and control efforts. One universal aspect of safer sex programs has been the promotion of consistent and correct condom use. A litany of safer sex programs found to have prevention value is maintained by the Centers for Disease Control and Prevention. At approximately the turn of the millennium, it became increasingly clear that the social sciences (including the study of socio-sexual networks, the role of social capital, the role of poverty and gender-based power imbalances) had a tremendous role to play in mitigating the pandemic.

Early in the new millennium, antiretroviral medications (ARVs) became increasingly used as a staple to control the transmission of HIV. At a population level, a primary goal of widespread antiretroviral therapy (ART) use is to decrease the amount of viral replication occurring in people living with HIV thereby leading to a decline in what is termed *community viral load*. In turn, low levels of community viral load offer passive protection against HIV acquisition as the odds of the virus being transmitted to easily drop in a dramatic fashion. Following the widespread initiatives to lower community viral load (a global form of intervention known as Treatment as Prevention [TasP]), a second type of ARV (pre-exposure prophylaxis [PrEP]) became widely embraced as a method of averting HIV acquisition. PrEP works by creating cellular conditions that do not favor the attachment of HIV to the receptor sites of cells in the person who is not yet infected.

By approximately 2015 it became clear that ARV use (for TasP and in the form of PrEP) required a tremendous level of support from the behavioral and social sciences. In full recognition that this support should occur in parallel with safer sex promotion efforts, the term *high impact prevention* (HIP) was created to represent a synthesis of these three interlocking forms of averting further growth of the pandemic. This chapter will provide a summary of how the behavioral and social sciences have contributed to refining HIP programs. Moreover, this chapter will introduce the concept of structural-level intervention in the context of achieving HIP-associated goals that have not materialized using only the behavioral and social sciences as a framework.

This chapter will address five basic objectives. First, it will provide an understanding regarding the value and limitations of applying behavioral and social science theories to individual-level changes designed to reduce HIV acquisition and transmission risk. Next, it will identify emerging, structural-level approaches to achieving population-level HIV prevention in developing and developed countries. Subsequently the chapter will distinguish structural-level interventions from multilevel interventions. Finally, it will describe strengths and weaknesses of structural-level approaches to HIP.

The Value and Limitations of Behavioral Science Theories

The emergence of HIV in the early 1980s was first addressed by a structural-level change. Known as the blood donor screening and deferral program, this structural-level change created systems for persons giving their blood to self-defer or to have the blood labeled "not for transfusion."[1] This program did result in safer blood supplies in countries adopting the corresponding practices. Other structural-level changes were not implemented for several years. Instead, the behavioral sciences became the cornerstone of the global prevention response.

At first, many countries began vigorous awareness campaigns designed to promote individual-level behavior change in three forms: (i) limiting the number of sex partners, preferably to only one; (ii) "knowing" the sex history and of partners before having sex with them; and (iii) using condoms consistently and correctly during every act of sex. These three suggested protective responses were highly promoted in the United States through the *Surgeon General's Report to the American Public on HIV Infection and AIDS*.[2] In October of 1986 a brochure from this report was mailed to every household in that country. Although admirable at the time, these types of information-based and advice-based approaches were not shown to be effective, and it has been argued that advice such as "know your partner" may actually have done more harm than good in that people felt that "knowing" a partner's sex history was grounds for unprotected sex.[3]

Fortunately, subsequent behavioral attempts to protect against the spread of HIV became grounded in theory. Specifically, initial efforts were based on theories developed in the discipline of psychology—thus giving rise to a paradigm of using individual-level approaches to combat the pandemic. Box 2.1 provides an overview of one example of a theory-based HIV prevention program.

BOX 2.1

Example of a Behavioral Theory-Based Program

¡Cuídate! (Take Care of Yourself) is a small-group, culturally based intervention to reduce HIV sexual risk among Latino youth.[4] The intervention consists of six 60-minute modules delivered to small, mixed-gender groups. *¡Cuídate!* incorporates salient aspects of Latino culture, including familialism (i.e., the importance of family) and gender-role expectations (i.e., *machismo*, which is described as the man's responsibility in caring for and protecting one's partner and family). These cultural beliefs are used to frame abstinence and condom use as culturally accepted and effective ways to prevent sexually transmitted diseases, including HIV. Through the use of role plays, videos, music, interactive games, and hands-on practice, *¡Cuídate!* addresses the building of HIV knowledge, understanding vulnerability to HIV infection, identifying attitudes and beliefs about HIV and safe sex and increasing self-efficacy and skills for correct condom use, negotiating abstinence, and negotiating safer sex practices. The intervention curriculum is available in English and Spanish.

As shown in Box 2.1, this program is an example of a group-based approach to intervention. At first, it may thus appear that a program such as a *¡Cuídate!* functions beyond the individual level. This is not the case because the "target" of the program remains each individual comprising the group. Thus, a critical principle is that any program specifically designed to change behavior through the use of personal mediators (e.g., knowledge, attitude, values, skills) is considered an individual-level intervention. Mediators are best thought of as the "bridge" between program content and the desired behavior change. A thorough discussion of mediators in the context of behavioral theory-based interventions has been described elsewhere.[5]

A second example of using behavioral approaches to promote the adoption of HIV-protective behavior is the ABC approach as described by the United States President's Emergency Plan for AIDS Relief (PEPFAR).[6] This is targeted approach designed to provide people with a hierarchical set of options, ranging from most effective (A = abstinence) to the next most effective (B = be faithful to one partner), to one that can be highly effective but may be difficult to achieve and maintain (C = condom use). In countless countries, this approach has been the basis for the creation of behavioral theory-based programs that work through identification and alteration of individual-level mediators. Thus, again, because these programs work through personal mediators, they are considered individual-level interventions.

Regardless of the behavioral approach (e.g., ABC, small group interventions), it is important to understand that behavioral theory is the basis of changing the personal mediators. Perhaps the best example is a behavioral theory (more appropriately termed a model—the term *model* is used when theories have been combined) that was specifically designed in response to the AIDS pandemic. Known as the Information–Motivation–Behavioral Skills (IMB), this model has been successfully applied to HIV prevention efforts since the 1990s.[7] As implied by its name, the IMB designates three general classes of mediators: HIV-prevention relevant information, beliefs about positive outcomes when adopting HIV protective behaviors (thus enhancing motivation), and a combination of self-efficacy and skill needed to adopt and maintain HIV protective behaviors. The IMB model provides a foundation for organized behavior change programs. For example, it is the theoretical basis for a brief, clinic-based HIV prevention program known as Focus on the Future—a Centers for Disease Control and Prevention–designated evidence-based intervention (see Box 2.2).[8] Because of its sole focus on

---

BOX 2.2

Example of an Individual-Level Intervention

Focus on the Future (FOF) is a peer-delivered, clinic-based, single-session, individual-level behavioral intervention. FOF aims to educate and motivate clients to use condoms correctly and consistently in order to reduce the spread of HIV and other sexually transmitted diseases (STDs).

FOF is based on the IMB model, which states that people need information, motivation, and practice with a behavior to properly learn that behavior. It is also based on Bandura's[9] social learning theory, which states that people learn new behaviors through observational learning, imitation, and modeling.

Target Population: African American men, who have sex with women, ages 18 to 29 who are seeking care in an STD clinic due to reported symptoms of an STD or who have received an STD diagnosis, who have used a condom in the last three months, and who are not knowingly HIV-positive.

Source. Crosby RA, DiClemente RJ, Charnigo R, et al. A brief, clinic-based, safer sex intervention for African American men at-risk of HIV acquisition: A randomized controlled trial. *Am J Public Health.* 2009;99:S96–S103.

---

promoting consistent and correct condom use by sexualizing condoms, this IMB-based program is an example of an individual-level approach to preventing HIV.

Although intuitively attractive, theory-based individual-level behavior change programs have several pragmatic issues that limit their value relative to resolving the pandemic. In addition to issues with rapid decay of program effects,[10] the primary limitation of empirically tested, behavioral theory-based interventions is that they have not been widely disseminated, thereby making population-level change unlikely.[11,12] Further, they have not been implemented with fidelity to the program as tested in the original efficacy trial.[13] These issues are ubiquitous, and their corresponding limitations apply to a new generation of HIV prevention programs that promote PrEP as well as programs dedicated to the global effort of promoting the uptake of, and adherence to, ART for the suppression of HIV among those living with the virus. Indeed, the application of the behavioral sciences to the very powerful tools of PrEP and ART has only begun, with most studies focusing on adherence to ART. Ultimately, efforts to promote PrEP and ART may follow more of a structural-level approach rather than a primary reliance on the behavioral and social sciences.

The Value and Limitations of Social Science Theories

Unlike purely behavioral theories, those drawn from the social sciences provide insight into the factors that determine behaviors for entire populations. That behavior is a social phenomenon, rather than simply self-determined, has been the subject of numerous textbooks and journal articles. Perhaps one of the first applications of a social science theory to HIV prevention occurred through the use of a program known as Mpowerment.[14] Since the initial publication of this approach to risk reduction for young men who have sex with men, Mpowerment has been used in numerous countries. The operating principle of this program is that popular opinion leaders (POLs) can influence large numbers of their peers, and the recipients of that influence will then influence other peers as this peer-to-peer adoption of a protective behaviors spreads through social networks and sexual networks. The use of POLs to change behavior across entire populations is part of a long-standing theory in public health practice, known as diffusion of innovations (DOI).[15] DOI explains how, why, and at what rate new ideas and technology spread through cultures. DOI has also been used widely in prevention studies.[16–24]

A second genre of social sciences theories of great importance to HIV prevention involves the density and connections among members of sexual networks and the interconnections between sexual networks. Figure 2.1 displays an example of sexual network. As shown, diagrams like this typically indicate the presence of core transmitters (people who are connected with relatively larger numbers of sex partners). The utility of sexual network analysis lies in its ability to predict the spread of HIV through a network once it is first introduced. When used in conjunction with geospatial mapping techniques, social network analysis also provides the basis for identifying approximate locations of core transmitters, thus informing the use of targeted, individual-level interventions designed to foster safer sex of those most likely to be spreading HIV to others. Sexual network analysis can also be used in

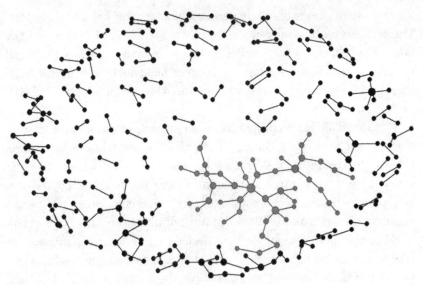

FIGURE 2.1 An example of a sexual network

conjunction with similar analyses relative to drug-use networks and social networks.

An example of using network theories in combination with DOI theory accentuates a critical principle: theories are meant to be used "as needed," and they may have greater impact in a combined form. For example, Latkin and colleagues[25] applied network analysis to people at risk of HIV acquisition/transmission through injection drug use and sexual risk behaviors. They identified likely core transmitters, who then became change agents for their networks. Compared to a control condition, this form of "natural intervention" produced large reductions in risky injection practices and large increases in condom use with casual partners. This is a variant of the POL aspect of DOI theory.[26]

Yet another approach commonly applied to HIV prevention is known as social marketing. Social marketing has been widely practiced throughout developed and developing countries as a primary method of promoting safer sex and harm reduction practices for people who inject drugs. Not a theory per se, social marketing is a common approach to health promotion for large populations.[27] It is predicated on the initial step known as audience segmentation, which "divides" the population into identifiable subpopulations thereby enabling tailoring of HIV prevention messages based on demographic and key behavioral factors. The HIV prevention messages may be focused around one or two key protective behaviors. The implicit goal is to favorably improve the social norms surrounding the adoption of these behaviors. In turn, these favorable norms influence and support the widespread adoption of HIV prevention behaviors.

Condom distribution programs are an example of social marketing applied to HIV prevention. Globally, the scale of these programs is massive. In 1996, for instance, the World Bank coordinated the distribution (along with education) of 783 million condoms in 50 countries.[28] Much like marketing promotes the sale of condoms, social marketing promotes the use of condoms (which may be offered at very nominal prices) by people at risk of HIV acquisition (i.e., an HIV-uninfected person becoming infected) or HIV transmission (i.e., an HIV-infected person passing the virus to a previously uninfected person). As an example, the Botswana Social Marketing Programme created the "Tsa Banana Project"—a youth-friendly approach to marketing condoms. A banana was used as a logo, thereby allowing youth to easily spot locations involved in the project. The project offered the condoms to youth in the larger context of education delivered in a nonjudgmental manner.[29] It is this type of change in the socio-contextual environment that ultimately precedes the larger concept of structural-level approaches. An eloquent advantage of structural-level approaches is that they transcend limitations of individual-level, and social-level, theories (see Box 2.3).

BOX 2.3

Insight

Social science theories ultimately rely on a self-directed change in HIV-risk behavior. Although the social sciences theories provide a broad scope for interventions to impact large populations, they nonetheless ultimately rely on a change in cognition, motivation, or confidence to bring about behavior change. Thus, neither the behavioral nor the social science theories target changes in structures (e.g., policy, economics, laws) that may be much more effective catalysts of change.

Promising Approaches to Achieving Population-Level HIV Prevention

In this fourth decade of the pandemic, it is now exceedingly clear that using the behavioral and social sciences in the absence of structural-level change will not be the answer to the global quest to end AIDS. Practitioners around the world have learned that structural-level supports for change must be implemented to have a prevention impact on entire populations. Perhaps the best way to describe this concept is through the "No Condom—No Sex" campaign that began in Thailand and was subsequently implemented in eight Asian countries.[30] This was a government-supported variant of social marketing that was developed in response to the network-based observation that HIV was being spread primarily through sex work. Rather than being only a message-oriented form of social marketing to sex workers, the campaign included self-help groups for sex workers, peer-to-peer education among sex workers, massive use of radio and television to broadcast "anti-AIDS" messages, and the distribution of free condoms to all sex workers.

With the exception of the distribution of free condoms, the aspects of the campaign as described in the previous paragraph are not structural level in nature. Further, the distribution of free condoms is a somewhat modest example of a structural-level intervention. The structural-level changes that may have been the most instrumental in the success of this campaign involved requirements to use condoms for all customers, and local laws that would revoke the licensure of brothels found to be in violation.[30,31] In the Thailand implementation, the number of sex workers using condoms consistently increased from 25% to 90% in three years and the incidence of HIV infections dropped dramatically.

Yet another example of great value comes from Brazil. In this very large, developed country the epidemic was dramatically reduced (by more than 50%) through aggressive government-sponsored actions, including a government-supported social marketing campaign, universal free access to HIV testing and ART, and a host of policy and economic supports.[32] Between 1996 and 2004, the estimated savings in hospitalization costs alone came to a total of approximately $2.2 billion. Hailed as a model for other countries, a cornerstone of the past Brazilian approach is an egalitarian basis for the prevention of new infections and the control of existing infections. Through government-sponsored economic supports, health advocacy organizations had a strong voice in how Brazil would overcome the epidemic. These organizations represented gay men, injection drug users, and other populations that would be considered marginalized in less egalitarian societies.

The past success of the Brazil campaign against AIDS can be credited to the use of behavioral science, social science, and, perhaps most important, the bold structural-level changes made relative to policy and economics. The behavioral science contribution took the form of government-sponsored brochures being distributed at postal offices and government-sponsored condom promotion campaigns that included the slogan "Use It and Trust It" as well the single word phrase *camisinha*, which means "little shirt" and was commonly used at the time as a way for people to refer to condoms. The social science contribution took the form of the social marketing campaign that was firmly grounded in egalitarian principles and large enough in scope and effectiveness to create new social norms surrounding HIV testing, condom use, and treatment of HIV. Yet, it can be argued that the most impactful program features involved policy and economics—making structural-level change the indispensable component of this multilevel approach to prevention and control. The phrase *multilevel* applies here because more than one paradigm (i.e., behavioral science, social science, and structural-level change) was employed.

The Brazilian success occurred at a time that predated PrEP. It also occurred prior to the completion of the research initiative known as HPTN 052 (testing TasP).[33,34] HPTN is the HIV Prevention Trials Network, and this was formed to unify prevention efforts and thus magnify their collective value.

Although far from a reality at the time of writing this chapter, perhaps the most ambitious plan to end AIDS is embodied by the UNAIDS goal of 90–90–90. This related set of objectives for the year 2020 targets HIV testing, treatment for those living with HIV, and *durable viral suppression* for those being treated for HIV. In each case, the target is 90%.[35] Reaching the first target will require a great deal of attention to resolving barriers that keep people most likely to be HIV-infected from presenting themselves for testing. Structural-level changes regarding locations, operating hours, clinic protocols, payment policies, protections of confidentiality, and so on will all become important relative to this goal. Similarly, reaching the second target will require structural-level changes in the way clinics provide services to persons testing positive for HIV. These changes may include the development and testing of home-based service delivery programs that allow ongoing HIV care to occur in the absence of the traditional clinical settings that may carry overwhelming levels of social stigma for people living with HIV. Care delivery in home-based settings may also be needed for people who cannot feasibly travel to a city that offers a clinic providing HIV care. The greatest challenge, however, for the 90–90–90 goals most likely pertains to viral suppression, as this goal requires ongoing financial commitments from governments to subsidize ART medications for the lifetime of each HIV-infected person (a financial challenge that has not yet been fully realized in nations with low rates of viral suppression). This last example is a structural-level intervention, even though its substance is purely economic and political.

A critical principle of structural-level interventions is that they function independently from the cognitive, attitudinal, and skill levels of individuals. A commonly cited explanation of structural-level approaches to HIV prevention defines structural-level factors are those comprising the physical, social, cultural, organizational, community, economic, legal, or policy aspects of the environment that impede or facilitate HIV infection.[36]

Factors the impede HIV prevention have often been identified at a super-structural level, meaning the factors are highly ingrained in society. Examples include gender inequality, poverty, income inequality, lack of healthcare, and racial disparities. Facilitating factors, on the other hand, are not simply the absence of impeding factors.

A facilitating structural-level factor can be defined as any aspect of a person's environment that enables either the easy translation of intention into behavior or creates conditions that removes intention from the equation entirely. For example, the previously noted laws in Thailand and other countries that require condom use in brothels enable sex workers to easily insist that all customers must use condoms from start to finish of sex. Conversely, mandatory HIV testing of sex workers bypasses the concept of voluntary intention and thereby represents a structure that becomes a constant in the larger scheme of shifting behaviors that determine the degree of success realized for any given HIV prevention program. With this principle in mind, it becomes important then to understand that a structural-level change could constitute an entire HIV prevention program—one that does not employ behavioral or social science-based efforts to foster HIV prevention. One example of this is found in the highly successful effort of averting mother-to-child transmission of HIV through "mandatory" HIV testing early in gestation followed by the use of chemotherapeutics for pregnant HIV-infected women. Although some countries did not legislate mandatory HIV testing in early pregnancy, in actual practice women seeing their providers (e.g., ob/gyn) may nonetheless gain the impression that testing is not optional. The eloquence, of course, in this type of structural intervention lies in its nearly universal effect on an entire population. The drawback, however, involves questions pertaining to the violation of individual freedoms.

Returning for a moment to the concept of HIP (presented early in this chapter), the vast majority of HIV intervention efforts occurring worldwide do not involve stand-alone structural-level changes. Instead, programs predominately invoke a strategic combination of the behavioral and social science approaches in a form that integrates with structural changes. These programs are known as multilevel HIV prevention programs. Figure 2.2 provides a visualization of a typical multilevel model; these are also referred to ecological models.

A key theme of this textbook is that multilevel programs are evolving to increasingly feature outer layers of the multilevel model shown in Figure 2.2. This is not to say that the inner layers of Figure 2.2 are not important—they are vital to creating eventual success of the structural level changes. The focus on structural-level changes is, however, the mainstay of the multilevel approach. This is the case for three reasons:

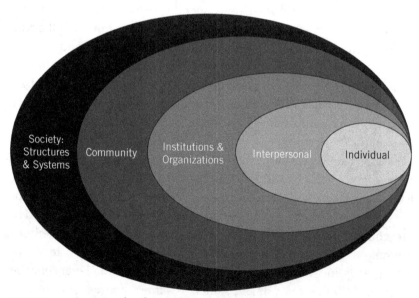

FIGURE 2.2 An example of an ecological model of influence

1. Structural changes are enduring—this leads to program sustainability.
2. Structural changes are universal for a given community or well-defined population—this leads to efficient implementations and dissemination.
3. Because of their universal nature, structural-level changes foster supportive social norms pertaining to their target—this has a positive effect on inner layers of the model shown in Figure 2.2.

Strengths and Weaknesses of Structural-Level Approaches to Achieving HIP

The use of structural-level approaches (either alone or in the context of multilevel interventions) to achieve HIP has several advantages in addition to those listed in the previous paragraph. Primary among these is a potentially high ratio of effectiveness to costs. Consider, for instance, the relatively straightforward intervention of engaging pharmacists in syringe exchange programs for injection drug users. By altering the legal/regulatory environment, this form of intervention has been demonstrated to work well in numerous settings.[37] This example is illustrative of a critical principle in that structural-level interventions do not have to be based on reversing those structures identified as being "drivers" of the HIV infection. Drivers are typically superstructural in nature, as noted previously (e.g., gender inequality, poverty, income inequality, lack of health care, racial disparities).[37] Although numerous journal articles have identified these (and similar) drivers of the HIV pandemic, it is a mistake to believe that changing the drivers is the only method of decreasing HIV incidence rates. Certainly, when the superstructures that promote HIV transmission can be changed, a tremendous number of benefits occur that go far beyond HIV/AIDS. As a long-term goal then, changing these superstructures is valuable to global health. In the interim, however, a valuable quest is to identify small to modest changes that can be reasonably made and that will have large impacts on the prevention and control of HIV. Consider, for example, the intervention concept of microenterprises on the HIV prevention behaviors of female sex workers. Evidence supports that practice of providing female sex workers with loans for the start-up of small businesses and providing them with skills needed to open and conduct a small business such as a making and selling jewelry.[38] Strong inverse associations between the success of the resulting small business operations and sex workers' HIV risk behavior have been observed.[37] These microenterprise programs serve as "outer layer" (referring to Figure 2.2) facilitating factors by providing female sex workers with an income that liberates them from having to sell sex to risky clients or to completely end their need to engage in sex work. In essence, public health efforts may not be able to end poverty among women, but targeted programs can alleviate poverty among at-risk subgroups of women.

The primary weakness of structural-level approaches is their reliance on community and government support relative to altering factors that impede and factors that facilitate HIV prevention. In communities and nations where HIV-related stigma and discrimination are common, the policy changes, financial support, and overall cultural norms may work against the implementation of structural-level approaches. In these circumstances increasingly more creativity is required to design and implement programs that will bolster facilitating factors—for example, allowing traditional birth attendants to conduct HIV testing of newly pregnant women, providing PrEP and ART to people in mutually agreeable community locations rather than asking people to attend a clinic, extending HIV clinic hours to include times when people are not working, and providing food to HIV-infected persons who are food insecure and thus may not fully benefit from ART.

A second weakness of structural-level interventions involves their lack of effectiveness across all communities and identified populations of persons at risk of HIV acquisition or transmission. As noted by Gupta and colleagues,[36] "When implementing a structural-level approach, there is no single blueprint that will work everywhere. Instead, strategy should be relevant to the particular needs of the population being served" (p. 766). The previously described microenterprise approach to HIV prevention is an example of this critical principle. In locations where poverty is extreme, the microfinanced small businesses may not thrive. Another example of a structural-level intervention being applicable in one culture but not another involves the facilitating factor of vaginal microbicides for women who cannot safely negotiate condom use with their male sex partners. Evidence suggests that male partners of some women in microbicides trials have reacted positively or in a neutral manner to the presence of the vaginal gel during intercourse; whereas others have reacted negatively, even to the point of being abusive.[39,40]

References

1. Leveton LB, Sox HC, Stoto MA. *Donor Screening and Deferral. In, HIV and the Blood Supply: An Analysis of Crisis Decision Making.* Washington, DC: National Academy Press; 1995.
2. Office of the Surgeon General. *Surgeon General's Report to the American Public on HIV Infection and AIDS.* Washington, DC: Public Health Service; 1986.
3. Metts S, Fitzpatrick MA. The risky business of "know your partner" advice. In Edgar T, Fitzpatrick MS, and Freimuth VS (Eds.) *AIDS: A Communication Perspective* (pp. 1–19). Hillsdale, NJ: Lawrence Erlbaum; 1992.
4. Complete Listing of Risk Reduction Evidence-based Behavioral Interventions. Centers for Disease Control and Prevention website. https://www.cdc.gov/hiv/research/interventionresearch/compendium/rr/complete.html. Updated February 6, 2018.
5. Crosby RA, DiClemente RJ, Salazar LF. Social cognitive theory applied to health behavior. In DiClemente RJ., Crosby RA., Salazar LF, eds. *Understanding and Changing Health Behavior: A Theory-Based Multidisciplinary Approach.* Burlington, MA: Jones & Bartlett Learning.
6. United States President's Emergency Plan for AIDS Relief. Defining the ABC approach. Available at: http://www.pepfar.gov/reports/guidance/75837.htm.
7. Fisher JD, Fisher WA, Shuper PA. The information-motivation-behavioral skills model of HIV preventive behavior. In: DiClemente RJ, Crosby RA, Kegler MC (eds.) *Emerging Theories in Health Promotion Practice and Research.* New York: Jossey-Bass; 2009:21–64.
8. Crosby RA, DiClemente RJ, Charnigo R, et al. A brief, clinic-based, safer sex intervention for African American men at-risk of HIV acquisition: a randomized controlled trial. *Am J Public Health.* 2009;99:S96–S103.
9. Bandura A, National Institute of Mental Health. *Prentice-Hall Series in social Learning Theory. Social Foundations of Thought and Action: A Social Cognitive Theory.* Englewood Cliffs, NJ: Prentice-Hall; 1986.
10. Choi KH, Coates TJ. Prevention of HIV infection. *AIDS.* 1994;8:1371–1389.
11. Rebchook GM, Kegeles SM, Hueber D. Translating research into practice: The dissemination and initial implementation of an evidence-based HIV prevention program. *AIDS Educ Behav.* 2006;18:119–136.
12. Glasgow RE, Eckstoin ET, Khair EM. Implementation science perspectives and opportunities for HIV/AIDS research: integrating science, practice, and policy. *JAIDS.* 2013;63:S26–S31.
13. Kelly JA, Heckman TG, Stevenson LY, et al. Transfer of research-based HIV prevention interventions to community service providers: Fidelity and adaptation. *AIDS Edu Prev.* 2000;12:87–98.

14. Kegeles SM, Hays RB, Coates TJ. The Mpowerment Project: A community-level HIV prevention intervention for young gay men. *Am J Public Health.* 1996;86:1129–1136.

15. Crosby RA, DiClemente RJ, Salazar LF. Diffusion of innovation theory. In DiClemente RJ., Crosby RA., Salazar LF, eds. *Understanding and Changing Health Behavior: A Theory-Based Multidisciplinary Approach.* Burlington, MA: Jones & Bartlett Learning; 2013.

16. Svenkerud PJ, Singhal A. Enhancing the effectiveness of HIV/AIDS prevention programs targeted to unique population groups in Thailand: lessons learned from applying concepts of diffusion of innovation and social marketing. *J Health Comm.* 1998;3(3):193–216.

17. Kelley RT, Hannans A, Kreps GL, Johnson K. The Community Liaison Program: a health education pilot program to increase minority awareness of HIV and acceptance of HIV vaccine trials. *Health Educ Res.* 2012;27(4):746–754.

18. Li L, Lin C, Guan J, Wu Z. Implementing a stigma reduction intervention in healthcare settings. *J Int AIDS Soc.* 2013;16(3 Suppl 2):18710.

19. Miller RL, Klotz D, Eckholdt HM. HIV prevention with male prostitutes and patrons of hustler bars: replication of an HIV preventive intervention. *Am J Commun Psychol.* 1998;26(1):97–131.

20. Anderson PL, Glidden DV, Liu A, et al. Emtricitabine-tenofovir concentrations and pre-exposure prophylaxis efficacy in men who have sex with men. *Sci Transl Med.* Sep 12 2012;4(151):151ra125.

21. Gengiah TN, Moosa A, Naidoo A, Mansoor LE. Adherence challenges with drugs for pre-exposure prophylaxis to prevent HIV infection. *Int J Clin Pharmacy.* Feb 2014;36(1):70–85.

22. Grant RM, Anderson PL, McMahan V, et al. Uptake of pre-exposure prophylaxis, sexual practices, and HIV incidence in men and transgender women who have sex with men: a cohort study. *Lancet Infect Dis.* Sep 2014;14(9):820–829.

23. Krakower DS, Mayer KH. The role of healthcare providers in the roll out of pre-exposure prophylaxis. *Curr Opin HIV AIDS.* Sep 28 2015;11:41–48.

24. The community popular opinion leader HIV prevention programme: conceptual basis and intervention procedures. AIDS 2007;21(Suppl 2):S59–S68.

25. Latkin CA, Sherman S, Knowlton A. HIV prevention among drug-users: Outcomes of a network-oreinted peer outreach intervention. *Health Psychol.* 2003;22:332–339.

26. Latkin CA. Outreach in natural settings: the use of peer leaders for HIV prevention among injection drug user's networks. *Public Health Rep.* 1998;113:151–159.

27. Salazar LF, Crosby RA, DiClemente RJ, Noar SM. Health communication theory. Social marketing, and tailoring. In DiClemente RJ, Salazar LF, Crosby RA, eds. *Health Behavior Theory for Public Health.* Burlington, MA: Jones and Bartlett Learning; 2013:187–210.

28. World Bank Policy Research Report, Appendix I: Socially Marketed Condom Sales in Developing Countries, 1991–1996, Confronting AIDS: Public Priorities in a Global Epidemic. Oxford: Oxford University Press; 1997.

29. Harris J, Meekers D, Stallworthy G. *Changing Adolescents' Belief About Protective Sexual Behavior: The Botswana Ta Banana Program.* PSI Research Division Working Paper No. 3. Washington, DC; 1997; Ahmed G, Meekers D, Molathegi TM. *Understanding Constraints to Adolescent Condom Procurement: The Case of Urban Botswana.* PSI Research Division Working Paper No. 12. Washington, DC; 1997.

30. Rojanapithayakorn W. The 100% condom use programme in Asia. *Reprod Health Matters.* 2006;14:41–52.

31. Anonymous. Thailand's new condom crusade. *Bull World Health Org.* 2010;88:401–480.

32. Okie S. Fighting HIV—lessons learned from Brazil. *New Eng J Med.* 2006;354:1977–1981.

33. Hammer SM. Antiretroviral treatment as prevention. *N Engl J Med.* 2011;365(6):561–562. doi:10.1056/NEJMe1107487

34. Cohen J. HIV treatment as prevention. *Science.* 2011;334(6063):1628. doi:10.1126/science.334.6063.1628. ISSN 0036-8075. PMID 22194547

35. UNAIDS. 90-90-90: An Ambitious Treatment Target to Help End the AIDS Epidemic. Available at: http://www.unaids.org/sites/default/files/media_asset/90-90-90_en_0.pdf

36. Sumartojo E, Doll L, Holtgrave D, et al. Enriching the mix: incorporating structural factors into HIV prevention. *AIDS.* 2000;14(Suppl 1):S1.

37. Gupta GR, Parkhurst JO, Ogden JA, Aggleton P, Mahla A. Structural approaches to HIV prevention. *Lancet.* 2008;372:764–775.

38. Cui RR, Lee R, Thirumurthy H, et al. Microenterprise development interventions for sexual risk reduction: a systematic review. *AIDS Behav.* 2013;17:2864–2877.

39. Green G, Pool R, Harrison S, et al. Female control of sexuality: illusion or reality? Use of vaginal products in southwest Uganda. *Soc Sci Med.* 2001;52:585–598.

40. Smith R, Magnet S. The introduction of vaginal microbicides must also target men. *J Men's Health Gender.* 2007;4:81–84.

3

Can Interventions to Increase Schooling and Incomes Reduce HIV Incidence Among Young Women in Sub-Saharan Africa?

Sarah Baird, Tessa Ahner-McHaffie, and Berk Özler

INTERVENTIONS THAT IMPROVE the lives of young people are essential to support the expanding global youth population. This is particularly true in sub-Saharan Africa (SSA), where more than 40% of the population in Africa is under 15 and 20% are 15 to 24.[1] This "youth bulge" offers an economic opportunity to expand economic prosperity and invest in the next generation as this large population comes of age. However, it also poses a danger to stability if young people do not have opportunities to be productive members of society. In SSA, the potential of youth is still constrained by HIV/AIDS, where adolescent females and young women bear the brunt of the epidemic.

Eighty percent of the 15- to 24-year-old women living with HIV reside in SSA,[2] and these young women make up 72% of the population of young people living with HIV in SSA.[3] Young women are infected, on average, five to seven years earlier than their male counterparts.[4] Despite decreases in new HIV infections over the past decade—largely due to scale up of antiretroviral therapy coverage and other HIV services—young women ages 15 to 24 still have up to eight times the HIV incidence rate as their male peers.[5]

The HIV/AIDS epidemic among young women differs significantly at national and subnational levels. HIV prevalence for young women ranges from 0.1% in Senegal to 16.7% in Swaziland.[1] Factors influence the epidemic in diverse ways in different communities. Young women in SSA are more likely to have partners older than themselves and to participate in transactional sex.[6] A review of the literature suggests that young women participate in these relationships to gain access to basic needs, to improve their social status, and for material expressions of love.[5] This is not solely a health issue. HIV transmission to adolescent girls and young women is intricately linked with issues of poverty, lack of education, lack of opportunities, and traditional gender norms.

Further reducing new infections, and supporting the young women living with HIV/AIDS, will likely require more than just health interventions. Structural interventions address social, political, or economic structures that create disproportionate risk for targeted groups.[7] In this case, structural factors that specifically influence young women's vulnerability to HIV infection include social factors (stigma, gender inequality), legal factors (urban policy, regulation), cultural factors (religious norms), and economic and education factors.[8] In this chapter, we concentrate on the latter, as they constitute the most cogent structural risks for young women in SSA.

Education enrollment and attainment have made marked achievements globally over the past decades. In SSA, gross primary enrollment rates increased from 68% in 1970 to over 100% by 2010.[9] While school enrollment and attainment has been improving globally, SSA still lags behind the rest of the world—it is the only region where secondary school enrollment rates are still below 50%. Females are also disadvantaged in terms of primary school completion—with over 62 million females ages 6 to 15 out of school.[8,10]

The impetus for structural interventions for HIV prevention came from an observation that "current behavior change interventions, by themselves, have been limited in their ability to control HIV infection in women and girls in low- and middle income countries" (p. S-44).[11] Prior to the mid-2000s, causal evidence linking increased schooling or income to reduced risk of contracting HIV was nonexistent. For example, while education had been suggested as a "social vaccine" to prevent the spread of HIV,[12] almost all the existing evidence linking school attendance (or attainment) to the risk of HIV infection came from cross-sectional studies.[13,14] Furthermore, the role of income (especially that of women's poverty) had been hypothesized as a significant factor in the spread of HIV in SSA, but there was little credible evidence showing a causal link between increased income and reduced HIV risk. Although many were quick to assert that poverty was a determinant of HIV status for women because poor women are more likely to engage in risky sexual activities such as commercial or informal sex work,[15,16] have multiple partners,[17–19] or have riskier types of sex for money,[20] many of the same sources were puzzled to report evidence to the contrary.[14,21] The emergence of structural interventions designed for young women in SSA, complemented by rigorous evaluations, has begun to fill this evidence gap.

The remainder of this chapter is structured as follows. The next section provides more detail about the types of interventions that fall in this space and provides a summary of the existing evidence. The subsequent section provides a detailed description of two studies: the Schooling, Income and Health Risk (SIHR)[22] study in Malawi and the Empowerment and Livelihood (ELA) study in Uganda.[23] The final section provides recommendations for policy and future research.

Interventions and Evidence

Four main types of structural interventions are the focus of this chapter: cash transfers, educational support, savings and microcredit, and vocational training. These interventions form the majority of the evidence base for young women in SSA with HIV or HIV-related risk factors reported as outcomes. We start this section with a summary of our methodology, before providing a description of each type of intervention and briefly summarizing the existing evidence.

Methodology

Virtually all the evidence on the link between structural interventions in the financial/education space and HIV-related outcomes among young people comes from SSA. Although the definition of young women and adolescent women varies across disciplines and geographies, the standard is somewhere around ages 15 to 24.[24] This is by and large the same age group with a high incidence of HIV and the target of many of the interventions reviewed here.

The search strategy for this review used a review on household economic-strengthening interventions that address HIV compiled by the

United States Agency for International Development–funded ASPIRES project as the starting point (this was a comprehensive review of the literature as of 2016).[25] We then conducted searches in PubMed, Popline, Google Scholar, EconLit, and NBER to identify any other studies published since then. A further reference review was conducted on included articles and on identified systematic reviews. Table 3.1 provides an overview summary of the existing evidence. Although Table 3.1 includes all relevant literature on the topic found in our searches, including qualitative work, we focus our discussion of the evidence on the experimental and quasi-experimental studies.

Although the majority of studies reviewed in this chapter do not study individuals above 24, we included two studies of vocational training programs that target young people but also include persons ages up to 27 and 34. We also included two studies that include community and household members older than 25 to examine the community-wide impact of economic interventions for female-headed households that did not target young people specifically.[26,27] We excluded articles that include individuals in the 15 to 25 age group but did not specifically target adolescents (e.g., we included Adoho et al.[28] and Jewkes et al.[29] but excluded de Walque et al.[30]). Finally, we excluded studies that specifically targeted other at-risk populations (such as female sex workers, covered elsewhere in this collection; see Chapter 7).

Cash Transfers

Conditional cash transfers (CCTs) aim to eliminate economic barriers to education or access to health services by providing cash, conditional on certain actions by the beneficiaries, such as attending school or taking up various health services. Unconditional cash transfers (UCTs) increase incomes without requiring any behavior change on the part of the beneficiaries. In the absence of market failures and externalities, UCTs are always better than CCTs. When there are market failures—such as intra-household bargaining issues, misinformation about the value of, say, schooling, and so on—or externalities (e.g., when individuals don't internalize or take into account the costs/benefits of their behavior on others), then CCTs can address some of these failures.[31] When it comes to effects of these alternative schemes on HIV infection, the policy choice will depend on the relationship between income, schooling, and HIV risk. For example, while individuals may be underinvesting in education, CCTs

Table 3.1 Existing evidence pertaining to household economic-strengthening interventions

Publication	Location & Setting	Study Population	Intervention	Research Design	Outcomes	Results
Cash Transfers						
Abdool Karim Q, Leask K, Kharsany A, et al. Impact of conditional cash incentives on HSV-2 and HIV prevention in rural South African high school students: results of the CAPRISA 007 cluster randomized controlled trial. In: 8th IAS Conference on HIV Pathogenesis, Treatment & Prevention; Jul 19–22, 2015; Vancouver, Canada. Abstract TUAC0101LB.	South Africa: 2010–2014	Students in grade 9 and 10, both male and female	Cash transfer conditional on participation in a life skills program, passing grades, and accessing an HIV test. All schools (intervention and control) received HIV education program.	Cluster RCT: 3,217 students in 14 clusters with outcomes measured at baseline, 12 months, and 24 months	HIV incidence, HSV-2 incidence	» HIV incidence was smaller than projected in the intervention group, and no detectable difference in HIV incidence was found between control and intervention. » Intervention boys had a 40% lower rate of HSV-2 than controls; intervention girls had a 24% lower rate of HSV-2. » Only one-third of the conditions on average were met for the students in the intervention group (so significantly less money was disbursed than was originally available).

Table 3.1 Continued

Publication	Location & Setting	Study Population	Intervention	Research Design	Outcomes	Results
Baird S, Chirwa E, McIntosh C, Ozler B. The Short-Term Impacts of a Schooling Conditional Cash Transfer Program on the Sexual Behavior of Young Women. *Health Economics.* 2010;19:55–68.	Malawi: 2007–2009	Never married women ages 13–22, both in and out of school	Girls and their families received cash transfers, either conditional on school attendance or unconditional.	cluster RCT: 176 enumeration areas were randomized control, conditional cash transfer (school attendance required to receive payment) and unconditional cash transfer. These were further randomized to receive different values ot cash to parents and to children. 2,692 girls and women were surveyed at baseline and at 12 months.	School enrollment, marital status, pregnancy, never had sex, number of partners in past year, average condom use, sexually active at least once a week, share of partners at least one year older than individual	» One year after program initiation, probability of getting married declined by 40% for program girls who were already out of school, and probability of becoming pregnant declined by 30% for program girls who were already out of school (as compared to controls). » The onset of sexual intiation was 38% lower in the intervention group as compared to controls. Intervention girls in school were less likely to have sex on a weekly basis, and less likely to have a partner more than 1 year older than themselves.

| Baird S, Garfein RS, McIntosh CT, Ozler B. Effect of a cash transfer programme for schooling on prevalence of HIV and herpes simplex type 2 in Malawi: a cluster randomised trial. *Lancet.* 2012;379(9823):1320–1329. | Malawi: 2007–2009 | Never married women ages 13–22, both in and out of school | Girls and their families received cash transfers, either conditional on school attendance or uncontional. cluster RCT: 176 enumeration areas were randomized control, conditional cash transfer (school attendance required to receive payment) and unconditional cash transfer. These were further randomized to receive different values of cash to parents and to children. 1,706 girls and women were surveyed at baseline, 12 and 18 months. | HSV-2 prevalence, HIV prevalence, ever married, currently pregnant, sexual debut, had unprotected sex, had sex once per week, had a partner more than 25 years old, had an HIV tst, HIV knowledge, syphilis prevalence | » HIV and HSV-2 prevalence was significantly lower in cash transfer groups for school girls (HIV = 1.2%, HSV-2 = 0.7%) compared to control girls (HIV = 3%, HSV-2 = 3%).
» There was no effect for dropouts on prevalence for either arm.
» Both schoolgirls and dropouts reported lower rates of sexual intercourse at least once a week.
» Intervention schoolgirls were less likely to have a sexual partner 25 or older, as compared to control girls. |

(continued)

Table 3.1 Continued

Publication	Location & Setting	Study Population	Intervention	Research Design	Outcomes	Results
Baird S, Chirwa E, McIntosh C, Ozler B. What Happens Once the Intervention Ends? The Medium-Term Impacts of a Cash Transfer Programme in Malawi. New Delhi, India: Initiative for Impact Evaluation (3ie); 2015.	Malawi: 2007–2013	Never married women ages 13–22, both in and out of school	Girls and their families received cash transfers, either conditional on school attendance or unconitional. The cash transfers were provided for 2 years, and then stopped.	cluster RCT: 176 enumeration areas were randomized control, conditional cash transfer (school attendance required to receive payment) and unconditional cash transfer. These were further randomized to receive different values ot cash to parents and to children. 1,706 girls and women were surveyed at baseline, 12 months, 18 months, and 2 years after program ended (2012–2013).	Grade completion, highest qualification obtained, achievement test scores, ever married, ever pregnant, age at first live birth, total live births, age at first marriage, desired fertility, psychological wellbeing, number of meals last week that contained meat or fish or eggs, ever had sex, number of lifetime sexual partners, being sexually active in the past 12 months, age at first sex, condom use during the most recent sexual encounter	» Schoolgirls who received the intervention did not report improved rates of sexual behaviors (sexual debut, age at first sex, number of sexual partners, condom use, and age of sexual partners) as compared to the controls after 2 years. » Any significant difference in pregnancy, marriage, and meals consumed per week disappeared 2 years after program completion. » Among girls not in school at baseline, the results were more durable after 2 years. » There was an average increase of 0.6 years of schooling, they were 10.3 pp less likely to be ever married, and 3.8 pp less likely to be ever pregnant. » There was no significant difference in sexual behaviors for dropouts comparing intervention to control.

| Cluver LD, Boyes M, Orkin M, Pantelic M, Molwena T, Sherr L. Child-focused state cash transfers and adolescent risk of HIV infection in South Africa: a propensity-score-matched case-control study. *Lancet Glob Health.* 2013;1(6):e362–70. | South Africa: 2009–2012 | Youth ages 12–18, both male and female | Government provided child support grant ($35 USD per month) or foster child grant ($96 USD per month). | Case-control study: 3,401 youth were surveyed at baseline and 1 year later | Incidence in the past year and prevalence of transactional sex, age-disparate sex, unprotected sex, multiple partners, and sex while drunk or after taking drugs | » Receipt of household transfer was associated with reduced transactional sex for girls (incidence of 2.5% compared to 5.5% in control).
» Age-disparate sex was also lower for girls in households that received a transfer. It did not affect the rate of multiple partners or any other measures (and while there were positive trends for boys in households that recieved transfers, no significant results were found). |

(*continued*)

Table 3.1   Continued

Publication	Location & Setting	Study Population	Intervention	Research Design	Outcomes	Results
Cluver LD, Orkin FM, Boyes ME, Sherr L. Cash plus care: social protection cumulatively mitigates HIV-risk behaviour among adolescents in South Africa. *AIDS*. 2014;28(S3):S389–97.	South Africa: 2009–2012	Youth ages 12–18, both male and female	Examined social "cash" protections provided by the government including cash transfers, pension, free schooling and materials, school meals, food gardens, and food parcels, as well as "care" including positive parenting, good parental monitoring, and teacher social support.	Longitudinal study: 2,668 adolescents in 4 randomly chosen districts were interviewed at baseline and one year later	Sex using drugs or alcohol, inconsistent condom use, 2+ partners in the past year, transactional sex, age-disparate sex, past year sexual debut, casual sex, pregnancy, any sexual risk behavior (combined)	» Cash was associated with decreased HIV-risk behaviors for girls, and cash and care together were associated with a greater decrease of risk behaviors for girls and a decrease for boys. » 41.2% of girls with no support reported HIV-risk behaviors, as comapred to 24.5% for those with cash support and 15.4% for those with both cash and care support.

| Cluver LD, Orkin FM, Yakubovich AR, Sherr L. Combination Social Protection for Reducing HIV-Risk Behavior Among Adolescents in South Africa. JAIDS Journal of Acquired Immune Deficiency Syndromes. 2016;72(1):96–104. | South Africa: 2009–2012 | Youth ages 12–18, both male and female | Examined social "cash" protections provided by the government including cash transfers, free schooling, pension, free schooling and materials, school counselor, school meals, food gardens, and food parcels, as well as "care" including positive parenting, good parental monitoring, and teacher social support. | Longitudinal study: 2,668 adolescents in 4 randomly chosen districts were interviewed at baseline and one year later | Economically-driven sex, incautious sex, ever pregnant | » HIV-risk behavior was significantly reduced with child-focused grants, free schooling, school feeding, teacher support, and parental monitoring (independently). » Combination social protection also had a strong effect: boys with no protection had a past-year incidence of incautious sex of 18.7%, with one protection the incidence was 9.5% to 13.7%, with two protections the incidence was 5.1% to 7.5%, and with all three the incidence was 3.5. » Similar trends were seen for girls past-year incidence of incautious sex, economic sex, and pregnancy. |

(continued)

Table 3.1 Continued

Publication	Location & Setting	Study Population	Intervention	Research Design	Outcomes	Results
Cluver LD, Orkin FM, Meinck F, Boyes ME, Yakubovich AR, Sherr L. Can Social Protection Improve Sustainable Development Goals for Adolescent Health? *PLoS One.* 2016;11(10):e0164808.	South Africa: 2009–2012	Youth ages 12–18, both male and female	Examined social "cash" protections provided by the government including cash transfers, free schooling and materials, and school feeding, as well as "care" including positive parenting, good parental monitoring, and teacher social support.	Longitudinal study: 2,668 adolescents in 4 randomly chosen districts were interviewed at baseline and one year later	Hunger, unprotected sex, multiple sex partners, sex while using substances, early sexual debut, tuberculosis, mental health risk, substance and alcohol misuse, school enrolment, past-year sexual abuse, past-year rape, transactional sex, access to SRH services, pregnancy, childbirth, violence perpetration	» "Cash" social protection were associated with reduced HIV-risk behavior, reduced mental health disorders, reduced substance use, reduced school dropout, and reduced violence perpetration for boys. » "Care" social protection was associated with reduced hunger, reduced HIV-risk behavior, reduced substance use, and reduced violence perpetration. » No interactive effects were found, but additive effects of cash and care were found on reduced substance use, violence perpetration, and HIV-risk behavior.

» For girls, "cash" social protection was significantly associated with reduced HIV-risk behavior, reduced substance abuse, reduced school dropout, reduced sexual exploitation, and reduced pregnancy.

» "Care" social protection was significantly associated with reduced hunger, reduced HIV-risk behavior, reduced substance use, and reduced sexual exploitation.

» Additive effects were found for reduced substance use, reduced HIV-risk behaviors, and reduced sexual exploitation.

(continued)

Table 3.1 Continued

Publication	Location & Setting	Study Population	Intervention	Research Design	Outcomes	Results
Cluver LD, Orkin FM, Meinck F, Boyes ME, Sherr L. Structural drivers and social protection: mechanisms of HIV risk and HIV prevention for South African adolescents. *J Int AIDS Soc.* 2016;19(1):20646.	South Africa: 2009–2012	Youth ages 12–18, both male and female	Examined social "cash" protections provided by the government including cash transfers, free schooling and materials, and school feeding, as well as "care" including positive parenting, good parental monitoring, and teacher social support.	Longitudinal study: 2,668 adolescents in 4 randomly chosen districts were interviewed at baseline and one year later	Adolescent HIV risk behaviors (transactional sex, age-disparate sex, sexual debut, unprotected sex, multiple sexual partners, casual sexual partners, sex while using substances, pregnancy), structural drivers (food insecurity, formal/informal housing, AIDS-affected, community violence), alcohol and drug misuse, adolescent behavior problems, child abuse, mental health distress	» Structural drivers (poverty, AIDS-affected, community violence) were associated with HIV risk behavior. » Those increases in HIV risk behavior were mediated by both cash and care protections. » For adolescents experiencing more structural deprivation, social protection had the greatest effect on HIV risk prevention.

| Cluver LD, Toska E, Orkin M, et al. Achieving equity in HIV-treatment outcomes: can social protection improve adolescent ART-adherence in South Africa? AIDS CARE. 2016;28(S2):1–10. | South Africa: 2014–2015 | Youth ages 10–19 years old who had initiated ART, both male and female | Examined social "cash" protections provided by the government including cash transfers, food security, school fees and materials, school feeding, clothing, as well as "care" including HIV support groups, sports groups, choir/art groups, positive parenting, and parental supervision. | Cross sectional design: 1,059 youth were identified through health facilites, tracked, and then surveyed at one time point | Past-week adherence, opportunistic infections, viral load | » Food provision, HIV support groups, and high parental supervision was associated with reduced non-adherence.
» Combined social protection showed additive benefits: youth with no social protection had 54% non-adherence, youth with one protection had non-adherence of 39–41%, youth with two protections had non-adherence of 27–28%, and youth with all three protections had non-adherence of 18%. |

(continued)

Table 3.1 Continued

Publication	Location & Setting	Study Population	Intervention	Research Design	Outcomes	Results
Department of Social Development (DSD), South African Social Security (SASSA), United Nations Children's Fund (UNICEF). The South African Child Support Grant Impact Assessment: Evidence from a survey of children, adolescents and their households. Pretoria, South Africa: UNICEF South Africa; 2012.	South Africa: 2010–2011	Youth ages 15–17, both boys and girls, who are in a household receiving child support grants and matched controls	The South African government child support grants are cash transfers of $18 USD every month, provided to child caregivers in poor households.	Cross-sectional study: 1,726 adolescents were matched and surveyed at one time point	Access and use of preventive health and nutrition care, access to schooling, scores on academic tests, health status, time allocation of children, school enrollment absences, grade repetition, grade attainment, adolescent work, risk behavior (never had sex, number of partners, ever pregnant, alcohol use, drug use, criminal activity)	» Adolescents in householdst that received the child support grant were less likely to have ever had sex comapred to adolescents not in households who had received the grant. » Girls were less likely to have been pregnant, and both girls and boys were less likely to have multiple sex partners if they lived in a household that had recieved a grant. » Boys were also less likely to be absent from school if their household recieved the grant.

| Foster C, McDonald S, Frize G, Ayers S, Fidler S. "Payment by Results"- financial incentives and motivational interviewing, adherence interventions in young adults with perinatally acquired HIV-1 infection: a pilot program. *AIDS Patient Care and STDs*. 2014;28(1):28–32. | United Kingdom: 2010–2012 | PLHIV ages 16–25 years old with CD4 counts at or below 200 and off ART, who had transitioned from pediatric services to a young persons HIV clinic | Young persons HIV clinic provided motivational interviewing with financial incentives frequently when viral load was suppressed (contingent on attending interviewing as well). | Pilot observational study: 11 youth were enrolled and provided this program for a year, and measured at baseline and throughout a year, and then 24 months after baseline. | CD4 cell count, viral load, viral load suppression | » 9 of 11 achieved viral load suppression at one point, and 5 of 11 mainted the suppression throughout the year of intervention.
» 6 of 10 (one participant dropped out) were virally suppressed at 24 months.
» With the small sample size and no comparison group, the conclusions we can draw from this study are limited. |

(continued)

Table 3.1 Continued

Publication	Location & Setting	Study Population	Intervention	Research Design	Outcomes	Results
Goodman ML, Kaberia R, Morgan RO, Keiser PH. Health and livelihood outcomes associated with participation in a community-based empowerment program for orphan families in semirural Kenya: a cross-sectional study. Vulnerable Children and Youth Studies. 2014:9(4):365–376.	See vocational & entrepreneurial training section	See vocational & entrepreneurial training section	See vocational & entrepreneurial training section	See vocational & entrepreneurial training section	See vocational & entrepreneurial training section	See vocational & entrepreneurial training section
Goodman ML, Selwyn BJ, Morgan RO, et al. Sexual behavior among young carers in the context of a Kenyan empowerment program combinding cash-transfer, psychosocial support, and entrepreneurship. Journal of Sex Research. 2016:53(3):331–345.	See vocational & entrepreneurial training section	See vocational & entrepreneurial training section	See vocational & entrepreneurial training section	See vocational & entrepreneurial training section	See vocational & entrepreneurial training section	See vocational & entrepreneurial training section

| Handa S, Halpern CT, Pettifor A, Thirumurthy H. The government of Kenya's cash transfer program reduces the risk of sexual debut among young people age 15–25. *PLoS One.* 2014;9(1):e85473. | Kenya: 2007–2009 | Orphans and vulnerable children ages 15–25, both male and female | The Kenyan government's cash transfer for orphans and vulnerable children, which is an unconditional cash transfer of $20 USD per month to the household caring for an orphan or vulnerable child. | cluster RCT: 28 locations were randomly assigned to intervention and control and provided cash transfer from 2007 to 2009, and then in 2014 2,210 adolescents were surveyed on sexual risk behaviors (reported here) | Sexual debut, condom use at last sex, number of partners, transactional sex, 2 or more partners in the past year, unprotected sex in the past 3 months | » The program reduced the odds of sexual debut by 31% (38% debuted in the intervention group, as compared to 44% in the control). » No other statistically significant effect was found for sexual risk behavior. |

(continued)

Table 3.1 Continued

Publication	Location & Setting	Study Population	Intervention	Research Design	Outcomes	Results
Heinrich CJ, Brill R. Stopped in the Name of the Law: Administrative Burden and its Implications for Cash Transfer Program Effectiveness. *World Development.* 2015;72:277–295.	South Africa: 2010–2011	Youth ages 15–17, both boys and girls, who are in a household receiving child support grants and matched controls	The South African government child support grants are cash transfers of $18 USD every month, provided to child caregivers in poor households.	Cross-sectional study: 1,726 adolescents were matched and surveyed at one time point	Never had sex, number of sex partners, ever pregnant, never drank alcohol, age at first alcohol use, never used drugs, no criminal activity, highest grade completed, program engagement	» Disconnection and interruption in recipt of cash transfer is associated with lower likelihood of abstaining from sexual activity, a higher number of sexual partners for both boys and girls. » For girls, disconnection and interruption of cash transfer is associated with lower educational attainment and higher likelihood of criminal activity. » For boys, disconnection and interruption is associated with lower likelihood of refraining from alcohol and younger age at drinking initiation.

| Heinrich CJ, Hoddinott J, Samson M. Reducing Adolescent Risky Behaviors in a High-Risk Context: The Effects of Unconditional Cash Transfers in South Africa. Chicago, United States of America: University of Chicago Press; 2017. | South Africa: 2010–2011 | Youth ages 15–17, both boys and girls, who are in a household receiving child support grants and matched controls | The South African government child support grants are cash transfers of $18 USD every month, provided to child caregivers in poor households. | Cross-sectional study: 1,726 adolescents were matched and surveyed at one time point | Sexual debut, use of drugs, use of alcohol, age at first alcohol use, involvement in criminal activity, involvement in gang activity, number of sex partners, ever pregnant, highest grade attained | » As months of the transfer increase, there is a decline in the number of sexual partners adolescents report for males and females.
» For females, the probability that they have made their sexual debut is significantly higher as months of the transfer increase.
» There was an association between receipt of cash transfer and engagement in selling drugs by adolescent males (no other associations with alcohol or drugs were statistically significant).
» If females received the grant in adolescent, they were 11pp less likely to make their sexual debut and the number of sexual partners they have is lowered by one-third.
» Receiving the grant in adolescence also decreases the probabiliy of pregnancy by 10.5pp.
» For males, recieving the grant in adolescence increases the likelihood that they will refrain from alcohol use. |

(continued)

Table 3.1 Continued

Publication	Location & Setting	Study Population	Intervention	Research Design	Outcomes	Results
MacPhail C, Khoza N, Selin A, et al. Cash transfers for HIV prevention: what do young women spend it on? Mixed methods findings from HPTN 068. *BMC Public Health.* 2018;18(10).	South Africa: 2011–2015	Young women ages 13–20 who were attending school at baseline	Provided young women and their parent or guardian with a monthly cash transfer conditional on 80% monthly school attendance.	RCT: 2,537 in-school adolescents were individually randomized, and data from the 1,214 adolescent in the intervention group is used here. Adolescents were surveyed annually until the program ended or until they graduated high school; a sub-sample of qualitative interviews were conducted twice annually with 39 young women	Primarily qualitative, but also measured how money was spent and what it was spent on.	» Seventy-eight percent of girls indicated that decisions on spending the money were their own. » Girls spend the money on toiletries, clothing, school uniforms and supplies, and other small items. » The interviews suggest that girls felt that they should spend the money responsibly, possibly because it was associated with school attendance. » About 10% said they had spent the money on condoms or birth control. » In the interviews, many adolescents speok about the significant role in independence and identity.

Citation	Country: Year	Population	Intervention	Study design	Measures	Results
Minnis AM, van Dommelen-Gonzalez E, Luecke E, Dow W, Bautista-Arredondo S, Padian NS. Yo Puedo–A Conditional Cash Transfer and Life Skills Intervention to Promote Adolescent Sexual Health: Results of a Randomized Feasibility Study in San Francisco. *Journal of Adolescent Health.* 2014;55(1):85–92.	United States of America: 2011–2012	Youth ages 16–21 who identified at Latino/a, both males and females	Life skills education and sexual health promotion are provided, youth identify performance goals on education, job training, and reproductive health and payments of $5–30 USD are provided upon completion of goals.	Cluster RCT: 162 youth were recruited and randomized into intervention and control, and then surveyed at baseline and 6 months	Friend risk profile, hanging out on corner frequently, frequent alohol use, frequent marijuana use, any sex in past 6 months, unprotected sex at last sex, contraceptive efficacy and motivation, accessed reproductive health services in past 6 months, enrolled in family planning care, STI test in past 6 months	» Participants had lower odds of hanging out on the street frequently, reporting that their close friends had been incarcerated, of reporting less regular alcohol use, and of having sex.

(continued)

Table 3.1 Continued

Publication	Location & Setting	Study Population	Intervention	Research Design	Outcomes	Results
Pettifor A, MacPhail C, Hughes JP, et al. The effect of a conditional cash transfer on HIV incidence in young women in rural South Africa (HPTN 068): a phase 3, randomised controlled trial. *The Lancet Global Health.* 2016;4(12):e978–e988.	South Africa: 2011–2015	Young women ages 13–20 who were attending school at baseline	Provided young women and their parent or guardian with a monthly cash transfer conditional on 80% monthly school attendance.	RCT: 2,537 in-school adolescents were individually randomized and surveyed annually until the program ended or until they graduated high school.	Attendance, food insecurity, HIV status, HSV-2 status, pregnant, ever had sex, early age of debut (less than 15 years old), lifetime sexual partners	» Cash transfer girls were less likely to experience partner violence in the past 12 months, to have had a sexual partner in the past 12 months, and to report engaging in unprotected sex in the past 3 months (as compared to the control). » There was no significant differences between groups on HIV or HSV-2 infection.

| Rosenberg M, Pettifor A, Thirumurthy H, Halpern CT, Handa S. The impact of a national poverty reduction program on the characteristics of sex partners among Kenyan adolescents. *AIDS Behav.* 2014;18(2):311–316. | Kenya: 2007–2009 | Youth ages 15–25 who are sexually active | The Kenyan government's cash transfer for orphans and vulnerable children, which is an unconditional cash transfer of $20 USD per month to the household caring for an orphan or vulnerable child. | cluster RCT: 28 locations were randomly assigned to intervention and control and provided cash transfer from 2007 to 2009, and then in 2014 2,210 adolescents were surveyed on sexual risk behaviors, and this analysis is restricted to those that had at least one sex partner in the past 2 years and had recieved the intervention for the two years (n=684). | Relative partner age, partner school status, transactional sex | » The program appeared to have no statistically significant impact on relative partner age, partner school status, or transactional sex, for either men or women. |

(continued)

Table 3.1 Continued

Publication	Location & Setting	Study Population	Intervention	Research Design	Outcomes	Results
Siaplay, M. The Impact of Social Cash Transfers on Young Adults' Labor Force Participation, Schooling, and Sexual Behaviors in South Africa [doctoral thesis]. Stillwater, United States of America: Graduate College of the Oklahoma State University; 2012.	South Africa: 2002–2006	Youth ages 14–22, both male and female	A government pension program that provides a monthly cash transfer of up to $75 USD to poor women more than 60 years old and poor men more than 65 years old.	Longitudinal study: data from a panel of 4,752 individuals was analyzed over 4 years, both from households that receive the pension and from households that do not receive the pension.	Sexual debut, number of multiple partners, condom use, marital status, labor force participation, school enrollment	» Recieving a pension was not associated with differences in the number of sexual partners or condom use by youth. » Recieving a pension was associated iwth a 16.8% reduction in sexual debut and a 19% lower probability of being married among girls in the household. » Both effects are larger when the pension recipient is a woman.

Cho H, Hallfors DD, Mbai I, et al. Keeping adolescent orphans in school to prevention Human Immunodeficiency Virus infection: evidence from a randomized controlled trial in Kenya. *Journal of Adolescent Health.* 2011;48:523–526.	Kenya: 2008–2009	Orphans ages 12–14, both male and female	School fees were paid, uniforms provided, and a "community visitor" monitored school attendance and helped to resolve problems that would cause dropout; all participants (including control) recieved mosquito nets, blankets, and food supplements	RCT: 105 youth were stratified and then randomzied to control and intervention and surveyed at baseline and one year later	Dropout, absenteeism, perception of caring adults, educational aspiration, future expectations, gender equity, acceptance of wife beating, sex attitudes, sexual debut	» Youth in the intervention group were less likely to drop out of school (4% drop-out as compared to 12% among control students), less likely to begin sexual intercourse (19% as compared to 33% in control), and less likely to report supporting early sex. » The youth in the intervention group were more likely to believe that adults cared about them and less liely to think that it is acceptable for a hustand to beat his wife.

(*continued*)

Table 3.1 Continued

Publication	Location & Setting	Study Population	Intervention	Research Design	Outcomes	Results
Cluver LD, Orkin FM, Yakubovich AR, Sherr L. Combination Social Protection for Reducing HIV-Risk Behavior Among Adolescents in South Africa. JAIDS Journal of Acquired Immune Deficiency Syndromes. 2016;72(1):96–104.	See cash transfer section	See cash transfer section	See cash transfer section	See cash transfer section	See cash transfer section	See cash transfer section
Cluver LD, Orkin FM, Meinck F, Boyes ME, Yakubovich AR, Sherr L. Can Social Protection Improve Sustainable Development Goals for Adolescent Health? PLoS One. 2016;11(10):e0164808.	See cash transfer section	See cash transfer section	See cash transfer section	See cash transfer section	See cash transfer section	See cash transfer section

Cluver LD, Orkin FM, Meinck F, Boyes ME, Sherr L. Structural drivers and social protection: mechanisms of HIV risk and HIV prevention for South African adolescents. J Int AIDS Soc. 2016;19(1):20646.	See cash transfer section	See cash transfer section	See cash transfer section	See cash transfer section	See cash transfer section
Cluver LD, Toska E, Orkin M, et al. Achieving equity in HIV-treatment outcomes: can social protection improve adolescent ART-adherence in South Africa? AIDS CARE. 2016;28(S2):1-10.	See cash transfer section	See cash transfer section	See cash transfer section	See cash transfer section	See cash transfer section

(continued)

Table 3.1 Continued

Publication	Location & Setting	Study Population	Intervention	Research Design	Outcomes	Results
Duflo E, Dupas P, Kremer M. Education, HIV, and early fertility: Experimental evidence from Kenya. *Am Econ Rev.* 2015;105(9):2757–2797.	Kenya: 2003–2010	Students in grade 6 at enrollment, both male and female	The education subsidy included free school uniforms, and HIV education included teacher training on HIV education.	cluster RCT: 328 schools were assigned to control, stand-alone education subsidy, stand-alone HIV education program, and integrated program, and 19,289 students were surveyed from 2003 to 2007, and then a follow-up study from 2009 to 2010.	Dropout, attendance rate, ever married, ever pregnant, reached 8th grate (follow-up study), grades completed (follow-up study), HIV (follow-up study), HSV-2 (follow-up study), HIV knowledge, condom use at last sex, ever had sex, reports abstinence, reports faithfulness,	» Girls with the education subsidy program were 3.1 percentage points less likely to drop out than the control girls (similar effect found in boys as well). » Education subsidy girls were 2.7 percentage points less likely to get pregnant (suggestive evidence that this is reduction at least primarily within-marriage). » HIV teacher educaiton did not change educational attainment, although girls in schools where teachers were trained were 1.4 pp less likely to get pregnant outside of wedlock (but may have increased marriage rates). » The combined program did not have the same effects as the standalone program in educational attainment and pregnant. » The joint program did find a reduction in paternity for the boys. » Overall, the prevalence of HIV in the group overall is low (less than 1% for girls and boysi nt he control), but no differences between groups can be measured. » The educational subsidy did not decrease HSV-2 infection, while the joint program decreased HSV-2 by 2-3 pp among girls.

Citation	Country: Year	Population	Intervention	Study design	Outcomes measured	Results
Hallfors DD, Cho H, Rusakaniko S, Iritani B, Mapfumo J, Halpern C. Supporting adolescent orphan girls to stay in school as HIV risk prevention: evidence from a randomized controlled trial in Zimbabwe. *Am J Public Health.* 2011;101(6):1082–1088.	Zimbabwe: 2007–2010	Orphaned adolescent girls, average age 12, grade 6–grade 10	Girls got school support including fees, uniforms, and school supplies. Female teachers were trained as helpers to monitor school attendance and help on absenteeism problems.	cluster RCT: 328 girls from 25 schools were randomly assigned by school to intervention and control and were surveyed at baselines and for 3 following years, control group got school fees the last year of the intervention	School dropout, marriage, prengnacy, school absense, percention that adults are caring, educational aspiration, future expectation, gender equity index, wife beatin endorsement, sexual behavior beliefs, sexual debut	» The intervention group had increased odds of staying in school and decreased odds of getting married. » The intervention group also had higher attendance.
Hallfors DD, Cho H, Mbai I, Milimo B, Itindi J. Process and Outcome Evaluation of a Community Intervention for Orphan Adolescents in Western Kenya. *Journal of Community Health.* 2012;37(5):1101–1109.	Kenya: 2011–2012	Orphan youth ages 11–14, both boys and girls	Intervention participants received school uniforms, school feeds, sanitary pads for girls, school fees, and a community visitor.	pilot RCT: 105 youth were randomized to intervention and control groups and measured at basline, 1 year, and 2 years	School absence, dropout, educational aspiration, future expectations, gender equity index, wife beating endorsement, perception on early sex, sexual debut, marital status, pregnancy status	» The intervention group did not show significant effects after 2 years. » There were issues with implementation including the small sample size and the dangers of conducting an RCT in a single community.

(continued)

Table 3.1 Continued

Publication	Location & Setting	Study Population	Intervention	Research Design	Outcomes	Results
Hallfors DD, Cho H, Rusakaniko S, et al. The impact of school subsidies on HIV-related outcomes among adolescent female orphans. *J Adolesc Health.* 2015;56(1):79–84.	Zimbabwe: 2007–2010	Orphaned adolescent girls, average age 12, grade 6–grade 10	Girls got school support including fees, uniforms, and school supplies. Female teachers were trained as helpers to monitor school attendance and help on absenteeism problems.	cluster RCT: 328 girls from 25 schools were randomly assigned by school to intervention and control and were surveyed at baselines and for 3 following years, control group got school fees the last year of the intervention	Sexual debut, married, pregnant, school dropout, years of schooling, meals per day, HIV, HSV-2	» No significant difference was found between intervention and control groups for HIV and HSV-2 prevalence. » Significantly less girls in the intervention group reported sexual debut, marriage, and pregnancy than the control girls. » The intervention also improved school retention and food security.
Hallfors DD, Cho H, Hartman S, Mbai I, Ouma CA, Halpern CT. Process evaluation of a clinical trial to test school support as HIV prevention among orphaned adolescents in Western Kenya. *Prev Sci.* 2017;18(8):955–963.	Kenya: 2012–2014	Adolescents ages 11–20, both males and females	Participants received school fees, uniforms, and nurse visits.	cluster RCT: 26 schools were randomized and 412 individuals were allocated to the intervention group and surveyed at baseline and throughout the study period, and a process evaluation is undertaken	HIV incidence, HSV-2 incidence, receipt of fees, receipt of uniforms, percent of nurse visits	» The original RCT found no effect on HIV/HSV-2 outcomes (although with around 400 participants it was underpowered to detect significant changes). » The intervention was implemented with fidelity above 90%, other than the nurse visits (although the requirements for those were changed during implemention because a monthly nursevisit was infeasible in the setting).

| Luseno W, Zhang L, Rusakaniko S, Cho H, Hallfors D. HIV infection and related risk behaviors: does school support level the playing field between orphans and nonorphans in Zimbabwe? AIDS Care. 2015;27(9):1191–1195. | Zimbabwe: 2007–2012 | Orphaned girls ages 15–21; Zimbabwe Demographic Health Survey (ZDHS) partipants were 15–17 girls, both orphans and nonorphans | Comprehensive school support including fees, uniforms, and school supplies | RCT with ZDHS with additional data: 25 primary schools (328 girls) were randomized into treatment and control in 2007, and three annual surveys were administered. In 2010, control students were offered school fees only, while the intervention group continued with full intervention for 2 years. A final survey was done in 2012, and the 2010–2011 ZDHS data from 464 girls was used as a comparison. | Ever married, ever pregnant, HIV status, ever had sex (sexual debut), school dropout, years of schooling, and socioeconomic status | » Intevention girls were less likely to be married, have gone through sexual debut, and dropped out of school as compared to the ZDHS nonorphans.
 » The delayed partial intervention were also less likely to have dropped out of school than the ZDHS nonorphans.
 » Both intervention and delayed partial intervention girls were less likely to be married, have gone through sexual debut, and dropped out of school as compared to ZDHS orphans.
 » Intervention girls were also less likely to be pregnant as compared to ZDHS orphans.
 » Intervention participants had higher socioeconomic and more schooling than all other groups, and the delayed intervention group had higher socioeconomic status than the ZDHS orphans.
 » No significant differences were found in HIV status (although the comparison was underpowered). |

(continued)

Table 3.1 Continued

Publication	Location & Setting	Study Population	Intervention	Research Design	Outcomes	Results
Miller T, Hallfors DD, Cho H, Lusenso W, Waehrer G. Cost-Effectiveness of School Support for Orphan Girls to Prevent HIV Infection in Zimbabwe. *Prev Sci.* 2013;14:503–512.	Zimbabwe: 2007–2010	Orphaned adolescent girls, average age 12, grade 6–grade 10	Girls got school support including fees, uniforms, and school supplies. Female teachers were trained as helpers to monitor school attendance and help on absenteeism problems.	cluster RCT: 328 girls from 25 schools were randomly assigned by school to intervention and control	Retention in school, early marriage, health-related quality of life	» Schooling support reduced early marriage, increased years of schooling, and increased QALY. » The cost-effectiveness analysis found that the intervention cost an average of $6 per QALY gained (making the intervention cost effective).

Citation	Location/Date	Population	Intervention	Study Design	Outcomes	Results
Toska E, Cluver LD, Boyes ME, Isaacsohn M, Hodes R, Sherr L. School, Supervision and Adolescent-Sensitive Clinic Care: Combination Social Protection and Reduced Unprotected Sex Among HIV-Positive Adolescents in South Africa. *AIDS Behav.* 2017;21(9):2746–2759.	South Africa: 2014–2015	Youth ages 10–19 years old who had initiated ART, both male and female	Examined social "cash" protections provided by the government including cash transfers, food security, school fees and materials, school feeding, clothing, as well as "care" including HIV support groups, sports groups, choir/art groups, positive parenting, and parental supervision.	Cross sectional design: 1,059 youth were identified through health facilites, tracked, and then surveyed at one time point	Unprotected sex at last sexual intercourse, STI symptomatic, pregnancy	» Adolescents that had access to school, parental supervision,a nd adolescent-sensitive clinic care were less likely to have unprotected sex. » More social protections were also more protective against unprotective sex for girls: 49% had unprotected sex with no protections, 13–38% of girls with 1–2 protections had unprotected sex, and 9% of girls with all 3 protections had unprotected sex.

(continued)

Table 3.1 Continued

Publication	Location & Setting	Study Population	Intervention	Research Design	Outcomes	Results
Visser M, Zungu N, Ndala-Magoro N. ISIBINDI, creating circles of care for orphans and vulnerable children in South Africa: post-programme outcomes. AIDS Care. 2015;27(8):1014–1019.	See vocational & entrepreneurial training section	See vocational & entrepreneurial training section	See vocational & entrepreneurial training section	See vocational & entrepreneurial training section	See vocational & entrepreneurial training section	See vocational & entrepreneurial training section

Savings & Microcredit——

Publication	Location & Setting	Study Population	Intervention	Research Design	Outcomes	Results
Austrian K, Muthengi E. Can Economic Assets Increase Girls' Risk of Sexual Harassment? Evaluation Results from a Social, Health and Economic Asset-Building Intervention for Vulnerable Adolescent Girls in Uganda. *Children and Youth Services Review.* 2014;42(2):168–175.	Uganda: 2009–2011	Girls primarily aged 10–19 (with about 5% 20–23)	Savings accounts, and groups that delivered financial education, social network and reproductive health information	Pre- and post- test with comparison group: an accident in implementation occurred where some girls allocated for intervention were only given the savings account and never told about the group services. So 1,064 girls, 451 with the entire intervention, 300 with just savings, and 313 comparison girls were surveyed at baseline and endline 1 year later.	Sexual harassment (touching, teasing), has a savings plan, has a budget, financial knowledge, has a mentor, has a place to meet outside the home, has someone to borrow money from, reproductive health knowledge, has had an HIV test	» Verbal harassment and indecent touching significantly increase among savings-only girls (19% to 25% and 9% to 15% respectively), while both indicators stayed constant among group girls. » There was no significant difference between the comparison group and the group girls. » Group girls had a greater improvement in savings than the savings-only girls, and both groups were two times as likely to have a budget as compared to the comparison group. » There was no significant differences in social assets between groups. » Group girls were significantly more likely to know HIV and contraceptive information, although no difference on knowledge of where to get an HIV test or having received an HIV test between group girls and comparison girls.

| Dunbar, MS, Maternowska MC, Kang MJ, Laver SM, Mudekunye-Mahaka I, Padian NS. Findings from SHAZ!: a feasibility study of a microcredit and life-skills HIV prevention intervention to reduce risk among adolescent female orphans in Zimbabwe. *Journal of Prevention & Intervention in the Community.* 2010;38(2):147–161. | Zimbabwe: 2004 | Girls ages 16–19 who are out-of-school orphans | Microcredit loans for business development, coupled with life skills HIV education and business training and mentorship. | Pre- and post-feasibility surveys: 50 girls surveyed at baseline and endline, 6 months later. | Sexual behavior, relationship power, experience of violence, HIV, HSV-2, pregnancy, HIV knowledge, income | » There was no significant change in condom use, and not powered to detect changes in HIV or HSV-2.
» Qualitative interviews reported increased exposure to physical harm, sexual abuse, and coercion (however, unable to compare baseline and endline data for violence since different measures were used).
» Significantly more girls reported having their own income (44%, up from 6% at baseline) and their own savings (88% up from 0% at baseline).
» HIV knowledge also significantly increased. There were significant macroeconomic challenges within Zimbabwe at the time, which affected girls' ability to succeed and repay loans. |

(continued)

Table 3.1 Continued

Publication	Location & Setting	Study Population	Intervention	Research Design	Outcomes	Results
Dunbar MS, Dufour MK, Lambdin B, Mudekunye-Mahaka I, Nhamo D, Padian NS. The SHAZ! Project: Results from a Pilot Randomized Trial of a Structural Intervention to Prevent HIV among Adolescent Women in Zimbabwe. PLoS ONE. 2014;9(11):1–1.	*See vocational & entrepreneurial training section*	*See vocational & entrepreneurial training section*	*See vocational & entrepreneurial training section*	*See vocational & entrepreneurial training section*	*See vocational & entrepreneurial training section*	*See vocational & entrepreneurial training section*

| Erulkar A, Chong E. Evaluation of a Savings & Micro-Credit Program for Vulnerable Young Women in Nairobi. New York, United States of America: The Population Council; 2005. | Kenya: 2002–2005 | Out-of-school girls aged 16–22 | Combined savings, microcredit, training in business and life skills, reproductive health education, and mentoring | Pre- and post-design: 222 girls and matched controls surveyed when they entered the program from 2002 through 2003 and as they dropped out mid-2003 to 2005. | Earnings, assets, savings, savings in a safe place, gender attitudes, reproductive health knowledge, condom use, negotiation of sexual behavior | » More than 90% of participants were exposed to training, savings, and mentors.
 » Only 54% took micro-loans. Many participants, particularly younger ones, were not interested in taking out loans and were more interested in only savings groups (which were established midway through implementation).
 » There was significant drop out in 2004 due to problems with implementation.
 » Still, intervention girls were more likely to have assets and were earning about 20% more than their matched controls.
 » They also had increased savings as compared to controls.
 » 80% of intervention girls felt able to refuse sex with their partner, as compared to 72% of controls.
 » Girls in the intervention group were significantly more likely to insist on condom use compared to controls (62% as compared to 49%).
 » Reproductive health knowledge increased for both groups indiscriminately. |

(continued)

Table 3.1 Continued

Publication	Location & Setting	Study Population	Intervention	Research Design	Outcomes	Results
Jennings L, Ssewamala FM, Nabunya P. Effect of savings-led economic empowerment on HIV preventive practices among orphaned adolescents in rural Uganda: results from the Suubi-Maka randomized experiment. *AIDS Care.* 2015;28(3):273–282.	Uganda, years not specified	Orphans enrolled in school ages 10–17, both male and female	Intervention group received usual orphan care plus mentoring, financial education, and matched savings accounts, comparison group received usual orphan care plus mentoring.	cluster RCT: 346 adolescents randomized to 1 year long intervention and control group and measured at baseline, 12 months, and 24 months (12 month post-intervention)	Savings, affirmative attitudes towards saving, affirmative attitudes towards HIV-preventive behaviors	» 92% of adolescents in intervention had savings at endline as compared to 43% in the control. » Intervention adolescents had a significantly larger increase in positive HIV-preventive attitudes (perceived risk of HIV, abstinence or sexual postponement, and condom use). » The intervention group also saw a significant increase in positive savings attitudes. » Cash saving and HIV-protective attitudes continued to increase after the intervention was finished.

Citation	Location/Year	Population	Intervention	Study design	Outcomes	Findings
Pronyk PM, Hargreaves JR, Kim JC, et al. Effect of a structural intervention for the prevention of intimate-partner violence and HIV in rural South Africa: a cluster randomised trial. *Lancet.* 2006;368(9551):1973–1983.	South Africa: 2001–2005	Women who receive intervention, people ages 14–35 living with those women, and people ages 14–35 living in intervention communities	Microfinance groups were started; groups received training on gender roles, cultural beliefs, relationships, communication, IPV, and HIV. After completion of training, key women were selected by groups for further leadership training and they worked with centers to mobilize around key issues.	Cluster RCT: 860 women directly receiving services and serving as controls, 1,835 people age 14–35 living with those women were surveyed at baseline and 2 years later; and 3,881 people age 14–35 living in intervention and control villages were surveyed at baseline and 3 years later	Physical IPV, Sexual IPV, unprotected sexual intercourse at last event, HIV incidence, household economic wellbeing, social capital, gender equity, HIV awareness, access to testing, sexual behavior	» The evaluation did not find an effect on the rate of unprotected sex among young people living in the houses of the intervention women or among young people in intervention communities. » The evaluation did not find differences between intervention and control communities on HIV incidence among young people.

(*continued*)

Table 3.1 Continued

Publication	Location & Setting	Study Population	Intervention	Research Design	Outcomes	Results
Pronyk PM, Kim JC, Abramsky T, et al. A combined microfinance and training intervention can reduce HIV risk behaviour in young female participants. *AIDS.* 2008;22(13):1659–1665.	South Africa: 2001–2005	Women ages 14–35	Microfinance groups were started; groups received training on gender roles, cultural beliefs, relationships, communication, IPV, and HIV. After completion of training, key women were selected by groups for further leadership training and they worked with centers to mobilize around key issues.	Secondary analysis of cluster RCT data: 220 women were surveyed at baseline and at 2 years	HIV-related knowledge and communication, access to HIV testing, more than one sexual partner in the past 12 months, unprotected sex at last occurrence	» Young women in the intervention group were significantly more likely to have gotten a test for HIV (29% in intervention and 18% in control). » Young women were significantly less likely to have unprotected sex at last encounter with a nonspousal partner in the intervention group (55%) as compared to the control (78%). » The evaluation did not find a difference between intervention and control on number of sexual partners.

Citation	Location: Year	Population	Intervention	Study design	Outcomes	Results
Spielberg F, Crookston BT, Chanani S, Kim J, Kline S, Gray BL. Leveraging microfinance to impact HIV and financial behaviors among adolescents and their mothers in West Bengal: a cluster randomized trial. *Int J Adolesc Med Health.* 2013;25(2):157–166.	India: 2007–2009	Girls who were self-help group members, or daughters or daughters-in-law of members, 10–19 years old	Self-help groups were given training on health and financial topics, control self-help groups were not given training	Cluster RCT: 55 villages were randomly assigned to either intervention or control, and 1,665 girls and women were surveyed at baseline, 6 months, and 12 months	Income, money owed, savings, food insecurity, plans for savings, satisfaction with savings, savings knowledge, HIV knowledge, sexually active in past 3 months, use of condoms during sex, confirmation of clean needle, had an HIV test	» The program resulted in significant gains in HIV knowledge and confirmation that safe needles were being used among intervention girls. » Knowledge of HIV testing resources significantly increased among intervention girls, and significantly more intervention girls advised others to use condoms to prevent HIV.
Ssewamala FM, Han C, Neilands TB, Ismayilova L, Sperber E. Effect of economic assets on sexual risk-taking intentions among orphaned adolescents in Uganda. *American Journal of Public Helath.* 2010;100(3):483–488.	Uganda: 2005–2008	AIDS-orphaned adolescents ages 12–17, both male and female	Intervention adolescents were provided child savings accounts, mentorship, and financial planning training, on top of standard care for orphans (which the control group had access to) of counseling and school support	Cluster RCT: 15 schools were randomly assigned to intervention and control and 260 students were surveyed at baseline and 10 months later	Intention to engage in sexual risk behaviors, parental communication about risk-taking behaviors	» Intervention adolescents had significantly lower intentions in engaging in risky sexual behaviors. » Boys were significantly more likely to report intention of engaging in risky sexual behaviors.

(continued)

Table 3.1 Continued

Publication	Location & Setting	Study Population	Intervention	Research Design	Outcomes	Results
Ssewamala FM, Alicea S, Bannon WM, Ismayilova L. A novel economic intervention to reduce HIV risk among school-going AIDS orphans in rural Uganda. *Journal of Adolescent Health*. 2008;42:102–104.	Uganda, years not specified	AIDS-orphaned adolescents in school with an average age of 13.6, both male and female	Usual care of AIDS orphans (peer conseling, health education, scholasitc materials) plus child/youth development account, 6 classes on career planning, career goals, microfinance, and financial well-being	cluster RCT: 7 schools randomized to treatment and control and 96 adolescents were surveyed at baseline and 12 months later	HIV prevention attitudes, education planning	» Adolescents in the treatment group significantly improved their HIV prevention attitudes, as compared to control group adolescents, whose prevention attitudes decreased. » There was a significant increase in educational plans for treatment adolescents from 88% to 96% having plans for secondary education. » The average participant was also able to save $26.55 monthly or US$318.60 per year with the matched savings.

Vocational & Entrepreneurial Training —

Adoho F, Chakravarty S, Korkoyah DT, Lundberg M, Tasneem A. The Impact of an Adolescent Girls Employment Program: The EPAG Project in Liberia. Washington, DC, United States of America: The World Bank Africa Region Poverty Reduction and Economic Management Unit & Human Development Network Social Protection and Labor Unit; 2014. Working Paper 6832.	Liberia: 2010–2011	Girls age 16–27 not enrolled in school	Provided 6 months of skills training (either in job skills or business development and including life skills) and then 6 months of follow-up support to link to IGA.	RCT. 1,960 girls individually randomized with baseline in 2010 and midline in 2011, 1 year later.	Engagement in IGA, ownership of assets, empowerment, sexual behaviors, fertility, food security	» The proportion of individuals in the treatment group engaged in IGA increased by 18pp; employment increased twice as much in the business development track as compared to the job skills track. » These effects were concentrated among the middle wealth quintile, missing the wealthiest and the poorest. » Savings also increased in the treatment group. » No significant effect was found on sexual risk behaviors or fertility. » There was evidence of improved food security and changing gender norm attitudes within households.

(continued)

Table 3.1 Continued

Publication	Location & Setting	Study Population	Intervention	Research Design	Outcomes	Results
Bandiera O, Buehren N, Burgess R, et al. Empowering Adolescent Girls: Evidence from a Randomized Control Trial in Uganda. Washington, DC: The World Bank; 2012.	Uganda: 2008–2010	Girls age 14–20 (some outside this range possible given difficulty verifying age)	Combined vocational skills training and life skills training	Cluster RCT: 4,888 girls in 150 clusters with baseline in 2008 and endline in 2010, 2 years later.	Risky behavior, fertility, condom use, HIV & SRH knowledge, engagement in income generating activities	» The treatment group documented condom use increase by 50%, unwilling sex decreased by 17.1pp, 26% decline in fertility, and engagement in income generating activity increased by 35%.
Boungou Bazika, JC. Effectiveness of small scale income generating activites in reducing risk of HIV in youth in the Republic of Congo. *AIDS Care.* 2007;19(S1):23–24.	Republic of the Congo: 2002–2006	Youth ages 15–24, both male and female	Small scale economic activities, mostly trade and craft apprenticeships that provided both income and training. Provided at the same time as HIV awareness campaign.	Cluster sampled cross-sectional survey: 372 youth surveyed in 2006, 4 years after the project was initially started.	Condom use with new partners, involvement in IGA, dependency, income	» This study finds that four years after the IGA program was begun, it had largely collapsed, and that only 24% of youth were still involved in IGA. » Those currently involved in an IGA were significantly more likely to use a condom with a new partner (although those involved in agriculture were significantly less likely than those not involved in IGA). » The youth did report that the are four possible avenues in which the activities could have reduced their susceptibility to HIV: the revenue earned, increased control/autonomy over their lives, the training and new skills, and the time commitment to useful activities.

| Buehren N, Goldstein M, Gulesci S, Sulaiman M, Yam V. Evaluation of an Adolescent Development Program for Girls in Tanzania. Washington, DC, United States of America: The World Bank Africa Region Office of the Chief Economist & Gender Cross Cutting Solution Area; 2017. Working Paper 7961. | Tanzania: 2009 – 2011 | Girls ages 13–19 (although participation was not restricted to those who were slightly older or younger, median age was 16) | Combined vocational skills training and life skills training | Cluster RCT: 150 communities were divided into two treatment groups and one control group. 50 communities received no intervetnion, 50 club and training only, and 50 club and training plus microfinance. 3,179 girls were surveyed at baseline about 2 years later. | Involvement in earning activity, income, plans for future activites, knowledge of safe sexual practices and productive health, fertility preferences, perception of gender roles, control over life | » As compared to the Ugandan implementation of the same model (Bandiera et al., 2012), this evaluation found no effect on social or economic outcomes.
 » The addition of microfinance did increase the take-up of services, from 19% in communities with microfinance, 13% for club-only communities, and 7% in the control communities.
 » There was also an increase in savings among the microfinance girls.
 » There were significant problems with implementation in Tanzania, including delay in rollout and staff turnover changing the original design, the meeting places for clubs was substandard as the program was relying on donated space, club materials could not be replaced when they were worn or broken, inadequate training of mentors, and lack of supervision of sites (among other issues). |

(continued)

Table 3.1 Continued

Publication	Location & Setting	Study Population	Intervention	Research Design	Outcomes	Results
Dunbar, MS, Maternowska MC, Kang MJ, Laver SM, Mudekunye-Mahaka I, Padian NS. Findings from SHAZ!: a feasibility study of a microcredit and life-skills HIV prevention intervention to reduce risk among adolescent female orphans in Zimbabwe. Journal of Prevention & Intervention in the Community. 2010;38(2):147–161.	*See savings & microcredit section*	*See savings & microcredit section*	*See savings & microcredit section*	*See savings & microcredit section*	*See savings & microcredit section*	*See savings & microcredit section*

| Dunbar MS, Dufour MK, Lambdin B, Mudekunye-Mahaka I, Nhamo D, Padian NS. The SHAZ! Project: Results from a Pilot Randomized Trial of a Structural Intervention to Prevent HIV among Adolescent Women in Zimbabwe. *PLoS ONE.* 2014;9(11):1-1. | Zimbabwe: 2006–2008 | Girls ages 16–19 who are out-of-school orphans | All participants received reproductive health services and life skills education and home-based care training. Intervention participants received financial literacy education and vocational training for 6 months, as well as guidance counselling. Once training was successfully completed, participants who developed business plans were supported in a microgrant for equipment, supplies, or additional training. | RCT: 315 girls individually randomized with baseline in 2006 and endline in 2008, with measures every 6 months until 2 years. HIV, HSV-2, physical/ sexual violence or rape, sexual behavior, transactional sex in last month, condom use with current partner, contraceptive use with current partner, unintended pregnancy, food insecurity, income | » For those within the intervention, 70% initiated vocational training, 63% passed, and 60% received a micro-grant.
» Girls who received vocational training were more likely to not be food insecure and to generate their own income.
» Intervention participants were less likely to participate in transactional sex, and were more likely to use a condom with their current partner (although this may be due to the girls getting older over the study period).
» The study was not powered to detect differences in HIV and HSV-2 outcomes.
» Unintended pregnancy did show a 40% reduction in the intervention group (which was marginally statistically significant, p = 0.06).
» There were some delays in implementation, so only 22% of the intervention participants finished their training before the 18-month visit (6 months before endline). |

(continued)

Table 3.1 Continued

Publication	Location & Setting	Study Population	Intervention	Research Design	Outcomes	Results
Erulkar A, Chong E. *Evaluation of a Savings & Micro-Credit Program for Vulnerable Young Women in Nairobi. New York, United States of America: The Population Council*; 2005.	*See savings & microcredit section*	*See savings & microcredit section*	*See savings & microcredit section*	*See savings & microcredit section*	*See savings & microcredit section*	*See savings & microcredit section*
Goodman ML, Kaberia R, Morgan RO, Keiser PH. Health and livelihood outcomes associated with participation in a community-based empowerment program for orphan families in semirural Kenya: a cross-sectional study. *Vulnerable Children and Youth Studies*. 2014;9(4):365–376.	Kenya: 2010–2012	OVC-headed households, OVCs aged 13–24, both male and female	Groups of 20–40 families meet weekly to get business, health, hygiene, and agricultural skills training. Groups collaborate on a joint venture, for which they receive both vocational training, a start-up kit, and recieve microgrants.	Cross-sectional survey of three cohorts with an intervention and control group: 707 OVC heads were interviewed either 4 months, 1 year and 4 months, or 2 years and 4 months after they had started the program	Income, savings, borrowing money, access to essential medical care, access to food, food source, water purification, number of sexual partners in past year, condom use at least occurrence	» Cohorts who had been in the program longer were more likely to be saving and have had access to needed medical care. » Women and girls in cohorts who had been in the program longer had fewer partners in the past year and were more likely to have used a condom at their last sexual encounter (these results were not found in men, although they only made up one-third of the sample).

Citation	Setting	Population	Intervention	Study design	Outcomes	Results
Goodman ML, Selwyn BJ, Morgan RO, et al. Sexual behavior among young carers in the context of a Kenyan empowerment program combining cash-transfer, psychosocial support, and entrepreneurship. *Journal of Sex Research.* 2016;53(3):331–345.	Kenya: 2012–2014	OVCs aged 14–24, both male and female	Groups of OVCs decide on shared entrepreneurial activities, allocate trainings and cash transfer, receive trainings on health topics. The groups have a shared bank account from which microgrants are dispersed.	Cross-sectional survey of three cohorts: 1,060 OVCs who had joined just before data collection, 1 year before data collection, or 2 years before data collection	Sexual initiation, unprotected last sex, multiple sex partners, food access, self-efficacy, resilience	» Girls in the longest serving cohort had half the odds of sexual initiation of those in the newest cohort. » Boys in the program for a year had twice the odds of sexual initiation as compared to the newest cohort. » Girls in the longest serving cohort had one-third the odds of unprotected last sex as compared to those in the newest cohort. » Boys in the program for a year had three times the odds of unprotected last sex compared to the newest cohort of boys. » Program participation was not associated with multiple sex partners in the past year for either boys or girls.

(continued)

Table 3.1 Continued

Publication	Location & Setting	Study Population	Intervention	Research Design	Outcomes	Results
Jewkes R, Gibbs A, Jama-Shai N, et al. Stepping Stones and Creating Futures intervention: shortened interrupted time series evaluation of a behavioural and structural health promotion and violence prevention intervention for young people in informal settlements in Durban, South Africa. *BMC Public Health.* 2014;14:1325.	South Africa, years not specified	Out-of-school youth aged 17–34, both male and female	Combination of a facilitated group economic empowerment intervention and a gender-sensitive participatory learning HIV and violence prevention program.	Interrupted time series design: 232 youth are measured twice before intervention and both 6 months and 1 year later.	Income, currently studying, work stress, financially supporting children, receiving a childhood grant, hungry, borrowing food or money, crime participation, access to money in an emergency, any club or group involvement, active in church, community cohesion score	» Men's mean earning increased by 247% and women's mean earnings increased by 278% from baseline to endline. » Women were more likely to be able to financially support their children. » Men and women were both more likely to be able to raise money in an emergency. » There was no change in perpetration of violence by men, but women experienced a significant reduction in physical and/or sexual IPV. » There was a significant reduction for men in suicidal thoughts and depressive symptoms. » Men were also significantly more likely to have had an HIV test: the proportion who had one increased from 57.3% to 69.1%.

Citation	Location/Years	Population	Intervention	Study design	Outcomes measured	Results
Rotheram-Borus MJ, Lightfoot M, Kasirye R, Desmond K. Vocational training with HIV prevention for Ugandan youth. *AIDS and Behavior.* 2012;16(5):1133–1137.	Uganda: 2005–2008	Youth ages 13–24, both male and female	Vocational training program through apprenticeships with local artisans added to 'Street Smart' – a program built for Ugandan youth on life skills.	Pre- and post-design: 100 youth were measured at baseline, 4 and 24 months later	Employment, number of sexual partners, sex acts, sex acts with condoms, alcohol use, drug use, mental health symptoms, delinquent acts, quality of life, social support	» Employment for the treatment group increased from 48% ever having a job, to 86% employed for the previous three months at endline. » Number of reported sexual partners decreased while condom use increased. » Decreases were also measured in mental health symptoms, delinquent acts, and drug use.
Visser M, Zungu N, Ndala-Magoro N. ISIBINDI, creating circles of care for orphans and vulnerable children in South Africa: post-programme outcomes. *AIDS Care.* 2015;27(8):1014–1019.	South Africa, years not specified	Former OVC ages 18–25, both male and female	Standard community child and youth care workers with an addition of food gardens, income generating projects, safe parks, youth life skills development, developing job opportunities, child protection program, education support program, substance abuse prevention	Cross-sectional ex-post evaluation: ex-participants in standard care and in standard care with additional components were surveyed	Psychosocial well-being, HIV risk behavior, unwanted pregnancy, intergenerational sex, partner violence, binge drinking, employment, income, hope for future	» Men reported less binge drinking in the intervention group (12% compared to 31% in the control). » More participants in the expanded program were employed (21% as compared to 12%). » 17pp more in the intervention group had some income (46% compared to 29%). » 12.9% of ex-participants of the expanded program reported some kind of HIV risk behavior as compared to 19.7% in the control group.

may still be less effective than UCTs for HIV reduction if the income effect on HIV prevention is large and CCTs exclude some beneficiaries who could have benefited from UCTs.

The first evidence on the impact of cash transfers on HIV came from Baird et al.,[21] who utilized a cluster-randomized controlled trial (cluster-RCT) to evaluate a cash transfer program targeted to adolescent females and young women in Zomba, Malawi. Targeting 13- to 22-year-old never-married females, the study found that the combined cast transfers arm, (i.e., those in the CCT or the UCT arm) reduced the odds of being HIV-positive at the one-year follow-up by 64% among those in school when the program started, with no impact among out-of-school youth at baseline (note that the out-of-school strata only had the CCT arm). Exploratory secondary analysis suggests that this impact was largely due to increased incomes rather than increases in school enrollment and attainment. The effects dissipated two years after the end of the program. We discuss this project in detail as one of the two case studies discussed in the next section.

In terms of CCTs, two other studies used HIV infection as an endpoint. Pettifor et al.[32] assessed the effect of a CCT on HIV incidence among young women in rural South Africa. Young women ages 13 to 20 randomly assigned to the intervention group received about US$10 and their parent or guardian received about US$20 every month, conditional on the young woman attending 80% of school days per month. Young women were eligible to receive the cash each month in which they met the attendance criteria up to a maximum of three years. The authors found no impact of these relatively large cash transfers on school attendance, dropout rates, and HIV or HSV-2 (herpes simplex virus—type 2) incidence during the program.

Özler[33] discussed this study and noted five key issues that may have handicapped the intervention toward no impact. First, households in the study area were already receiving South Africa's Child Support Grant (CSG), which, on average, provides nearly 20% of monthly household expenditures among is beneficiaries. The CCTs in this intervention doubled this amount. One can imagine that moving from receiving no support to $30 may lead to very different impacts on a number of outcomes than moving from $30 to $60. Second, the eligibility criteria for the program was "girls aged 13–20 years if they were enrolled in school grades 8–11, not married or pregnant, able to read, they and their parent or guardian both had the necessary documentation necessary to open a bank account, and were residing in the study area and intending to remain until trial

completion" (p. e981),[31] which may not include young women most vulnerable to HIV infection. Third, school attendance rates during the three-
year study period were extremely high at 95%, which makes it impossible
to reduce HIV through enrollment gains. Fourth, the trial was individually
randomized, which, while good for power, leaves the study vulnerable to
bias from spillovers (contamination effects) between individuals in the
same school or community. Fifth, inference is also threatened by potential bias from differential loss to follow-up between treatment and control
groups. Hence, the conclusion of no impact should be interpreted with
these limitations in mind.

Caprisa 007,[34] a cluster-RCT in 14 rural schools in South Africa, also
studied the effects of a CCT program on HIV in South Africa. Students
in grades 9 and 10 in all schools received a life skills program called "My
Life! My Future!" Students in the intervention arm also received a cash
incentive of a maximum of US$17.50 quarterly for any combination of
four conditions being met: 80% quarterly participation in the life skills
program, attaining a passing score in a six-month academic test, an annual HIV test, and a one-off report on a community project. The median amount received was US$60 over the course of the intervention.
The authors reported that the intervention reduced HSV-2 incidence by
30%. Unfortunately, the study was not adequately powered to detect HIV
incidence. The authors further noted that only about one third of the
conditions were actually met. (Note that there is currently no published
paper from this trial, and, hence, additional details of the trial and final
findings are pending.)

There is also a small literature on the impact of UCTs on HIV risk;
however, other than Baird et al.,[21] none actually measured a biomarker
endpoint. South Africa's CSG is a means-tested, UCT program (about
US$21 per month as of October 2014) that is paid to the parent or care-
giver of children under the age of 18, targeted to single caregivers making
less than $2,500 per year and married couples making less than approx-
imately $5,000 per year. Using quasi-experimental methods, Heinrich,
Hoddinott, and Samson[35] found that receipt of the CSG is associated with
delayed sexual debut and a reduction of sexual partners—perhaps suggestive of a reduction in transactional sex. Their results also point to the
importance of the CSG continuing through adolescence.

Handa et al.[36] studied the impact of the Government of Kenya's Cash
Transfer for Orphans and Vulnerable Children on sexual debut. The program provided US$20 per month unconditionally to the main caregiver

in the household. Comparing 28 communities randomly assigned (50:50) to treatment and control, they found that the program reduced the odds of sexual debut by 31% among 15- to 25-year-olds. There were no statistically significant effects on secondary outcomes, such as condom use, number of partners, and transactional sex.

Educational Support

Direct educational support through provision of school fees and materials also attempts to eliminate economic barriers to education. Schooling subsidies, in cash or kind, are akin to CCT programs, in that they are only available for those who are enrolled in and/or attend school.

Duflo, Dupas and Kremer[37] conducted a randomized evaluation involving 328 schools (children were, on average, 13.5 at baseline and 20.5 at final follow-up) in western Kenya to compare the effectiveness of two programs conducted stand-alone or jointly. The first provided free uniforms to upper primary school students (two free uniforms over the last three years of primary school), and the second involved an HIV education program where three teachers in each primary school received government-provided training to help them deliver Kenya's national HIV/ AIDS curriculum (which emphasized abstinence). The authors found that the education subsidies alone led to significant reductions in school dropout, pregnancy, and marriage among girls in the near future and school attainment, marriage, and childbearing by age 16. The HIV education program implemented alone did not impact any of these outcomes. However, for girls, the HIV education program led to more early pregnancies within marriage and fewer early pregnancies outside of wedlock. Implementing the two programs jointly caused fertility to fall less than the education subsidy alone, but HSV-2 prevalence was significantly lower. The authors propose a model that is consistent with these findings, in which choices between committed and casual relationships, rather than unprotected sex alone, affect pregnancy and sexually transmitted infections (STIs). The study was not adequately powered to detect difference in HIV incidence. These findings point to the potentially important complementarity between direct educational/economic support and behavior change communication interventions—an area where more research is needed.

Outside of Dupas et al.,[36] studies in the educational support space examining HIV risk factors using with experimental or quasi-experimental identification both focus on orphans and have small sample sizes, making it impossible to detect effects on biomarker endpoints. Cho et al.[39] evaluated a small-scale intervention ($N = 105$), also in western Kenya, that provided adolescent orphans ages 12 to 14 school fees, uniforms, and a "community visitor," who monitored school attendance and helped to re-solve problems that would lead to absence or dropout. Similar to Duflo et al.,[36] the authors found that after one year those in the treatment group were less likely to drop out of school, commence sexual intercourse, or report attitudes supporting early sex. Biomarkers were not assessed as part of this study. However, after two years, Hallfors et al.[38] found null effects. Using a mixed-methods approach, the authors noted that focusing more on adolescents transitioning from primary to secondary school (as opposed to an age-based approach) as well as utilizing a school-based in-tervention instead of individual randomization within a community (with lots of potential for negative spillovers) may lead to better results. They also highlighted the importance of measuring biomarkers.

Hallfors et al.[39] used an RCT in rural eastern Zimbabwe to test whether comprehensive support to keep orphan adolescent girls in school (with a package that is very similar to that in Cho et al.,[40] which included fees, uniforms, and a school-based helper to monitor attendance and resolve problems) could reduce HIV risk factors. All orphan girls in grade 6 in 25 primary schools were invited to participate in the study in fall 2007 ($N = 329$). The intervention reduced school dropout by 82% and mar-riage by 63% after two years and increased gender equitable attitudes. As noted in Hallfors et al.,[37] one reason this program may have had more success than the similar program in western Kenya was the school-based randomization. Hallfors et al.[41] returned three years later to assess longer term impacts—comparing a comprehensive (five-year) intervention group with a delayed (1.5-year) partial intervention group. The comprehensive five-year intervention continued to reduce the likelihood of marriage and improve school retention, but there was no difference between the two groups on HIV or HSV-2 biomarkers.

Savings and Microcredit

Savings and microcredit are provided to young women (often in the same package) to support them to pay for school or to start their own businesses. Some savings accounts are matched to promote savings, some cannot be accessed until certain times, and various models ranging from group saving to matched individual accounts are used. The type of model varies by the target population. For example, younger girls' savings are often individual (rather than group-based), accessible by their family or guardians, and aim to provide financial support to stay in school. Older girls' savings are more likely to be group-based, associated with microcredit, and serve to support vocational endeavors. Hence, these programs may affect income and/or schooling. Unlike transfer and subsidy programs, however, programs that alter livelihood activities can have heterogeneous effects on risky behaviors depending on the context and circumstances. The evidence on the impacts of savings and microcredit for this particular population is mixed and limited, which we summarize in the following discussion.

The savings and microcredit programs targeted at youth for HIV prevention are generally able to improve savings and incomes (if that is their target). A program in Uganda significantly increased savings in the savings and financial education group, with the group with only savings experiencing a slight increase in savings but still more than that experienced by the control group.[42] A cluster-RCT in Uganda on matched savings accounts plus financial education found that 92% of adolescents had savings at study completion as compared to 43% in the control.[43] A pilot microcredit and life skills program in Zimbabwe did significantly improve the proportion of girls having their own income (44%, as compared to 6% at baseline) and the proportion of girls having their own savings (88%, as compared to 0% at baseline).[44]

The tie to HIV risk is more tenuous, both due to the lack of studies and the ways in which HIV-related outcomes are measured. Many studies measured intentions, attitudes, or knowledge related to HIV. Although these measures may be relevant, individuals reporting that they plan to use a condom at their next sexual encounter (or report knowing that they should) is multiple steps away from a significant reduction in the risk of HIV infection. Both an evaluation in Uganda and an evaluation in India (the only evaluation in this group conducted outside of SSA) found improvements in knowledge of HIV with savings interventions that included health information.[41,45] Three other evaluations conducted in Uganda on orphans that involved usual orphan care plus financial education and matched savings accounts found significantly improved attitudes and/or intentions around HIV and HIV behaviors with the addition of financial interventions.[44,46,47]

The results from studies with more concrete HIV-related outcomes were mixed. An evaluation in Kenya on a combined savings, microcredit, and training on reproductive health and business program found that intervention girls were significantly more like to insist on condom use (62%) as compared to those in the comparison group (49%). A unique evaluation that studied the impacts of a microfinance program for women on household and community members did not find an effect on the rate of unprotected sex among the youth living in the households with intervention women.[25] Young women in the intervention group, however, were more likely to have received HIV testing (29%) compared to those in the control condition (18%) and were less likely to have had unprotected sex at last sexual encounter (55%) compared to the control condition (78%). Also, an evaluation in Uganda that included a control condition, a savings-only, and a savings-plus financial education group demonstrated some possible drawbacks of savings-only interventions.[41] Girls in the savings-only group experienced significant increases in verbal harassment and indecent touching as compared to the girls who had both savings and social support, financial education, and health information.[41] This is similar to other studies suggesting that building economic assets without considering other social assets can threaten the safety of young girls in some communities.[48] Three evaluations measured HIV as an outcome. Two evaluations were not powered to detect changes in HIV.[43,47] The other evaluation measured HIV incidence in control and intervention communities, not among intervention participants, and did not find a significant difference between communities.[25]

Taking a closer look at the SHAZ! trial conducted in Zimbabwe,[43,47] there were significant problems with the initial design of the program. It was originally designed as microcredit loans for 16- to 19-year-old out-of-school orphans, with additional business development and life skills training plus mentorship. The feasibility study[47] found that while significantly more adolescents reported to have their own savings and income, there was no significant change in condom use (the study was not powered to detect changes in HIV or HSV-2). They also had trouble repaying loans and supporting their small enterprises, with the most successful individuals with some previous experience, capital, and/or family support.[47] The study team concluded that the original model was not the best livelihood option to reduce risk among females in late adolescence in this context.[47]

Vocational and Entrepreneurial Training

Vocational training aims to provide individuals with specific marketable skills, so that they can support themselves through wage jobs or self-employment. Young people in many developing contexts do not gain the skills needed for many jobs or endeavors in school, and young women are particularly disadvantaged. Similar to vocational training, entrepreneurial training is focused on providing individuals with the skills to start and manage their own businesses. Many of these programs not only provide training, but also provide some links to jobs or credit for further training or to start businesses. Evaluations of these programs that examine HIV-related outcomes often include some life skills or sexual and reproductive health education as well.

Most of the evaluations in this domain did not measure the incidence of HIV or other STIs. The two evaluations that measured HIV incidence are the same noted in the savings and microcredit section, and they were underpowered to measure those outcomes.[43,47] That being said, there are a number of studies on vocational training programs that measured sexual behaviors among young men and women.

A randomized control trial (RCT) in Liberia found that those who had participated in skills training had an 18-point increase in participation in an income-generating activity,[27] while another RCT in Uganda on vocational training found a 35% increase in participation in an income-generating activity.[22] There was also documentation of increased earnings. An apprenticeship program in Uganda found that employment increased from less than half of the participants ever having a job to 86% employed for the previous three months postintervention.[49] The macroeconomic situation can influence these results. In the Liberian program, there was both a job skills track and a business development track. Although there was greater demand for the job skills track upon initiation of the program, eventual employment rates were twice as high in the business development track because there were so few jobs available even with the necessary skills.[27] Other studies reference challenging economic environments as well.

For HIV-related outcomes, many studies found that with increased income and employment came decreased risky sexual behaviors from adolescent girls. Condom use was 50% greater in the intervention group in a cluster-RCT in Uganda after a combined life skills and vocational skills training program.[22] Other studies showed similar increases.[50–52] A few studies also documented a decrease in number of partners or sexual initiation.[43,48–50,53] Only one study measured transactional sex—an RCT in Zimbabwe that involved life skills and vocational training as well as a microgrant—and it documented that participants were less likely to participate in transactional sex.[43] One of the largest RCTs in this domain, among nearly 2,000 girls not enrolled in school in Liberia, found increases in savings and employment after skills training but no significant change in sexual risk behaviors or fertility.[27]

There is not as much evidence on the effect of these types of programs on boys, but the few studies in existence suggest a very different effect on HIV risk resulting from raising incomes of young men. In particular, an evaluation in Kenya on orphans and vulnerable children receiving vocational and health training demonstrated that while girls in the program had half the odds of having their sexual debut, boys in the program had twice the odds. Similarly, girls in the program had one third the odds of unprotected last sex, while boys in the program had three times the odds of unprotected last sex.[50] This mirrors evidence from studies of cash transfers or income shocks, which suggests that increased income among young men can be associated with more risky sexual behavior,[54] or at least not have the protective effect shown in girls.[34] The evidence for this effect on boys receiving vocational programs is still limited, and there are other areas where increased income showed positive effects in HIV-related incomes. For instance, one combined economic and gender empowerment program in South Africa on out-of-school youth showed that men were more likely to have an HIV test after the intervention (increasing from 57.3% to 69.1%).[28] Another combined program in South Africa found that male participants reported less binge drinking (12%) than the control group (31%).[51]

Two Examples: SIHR and ELA

We discuss two cluster-RCTs in more detail: SIHR and ELA.

Schooling, Income, and Health Risk

SIHR,[21] mentioned briefly in the previous section, evaluated the impact of the Zomba Cash Transfer Program in Zomba, Malawi, on HIV and numerous risk factors for HIV. Here, we describe this study in more detail, as it provides important insights into the potential and limitations of cash transfers for HIV prevention.

SIHR tracked the lives of a sample of young women who were enrolled in the study as never-married 13- to 22-year-olds in Zomba, Malawi in 2007. Outside of a small city, also named Zomba, the district is rural, characterized by low educational attainment and few opportunities for formal employment, especially for women. As of 2009, this district was the third poorest in Malawi (in the study sample, real monthly per-capita exchange rate comparable consumption in 2008 was US$20.60). Secondary school completion rates were low. In the SIHR sample, among baseline schoolgirls, half of whom had completed primary school at baseline, only 17.0% had completed secondary school as of 2012.[55] Although most individuals age 15 and older participate in some form of employment, the majority do not receive a formal income. This context is typical for many parts of rural Africa and, hence, is an important environment in which to understand the potential for interventions like cash transfers. HIV rates in Zomba are also high. At baseline, HIV prevalence among 15- to 24-year-old women was 9.1% compared to 2.1% among males of the same age. Moreover, HIV prevalence among women ages 15 to 49 in Zomba was 24.6%, compared to a national average of 13.3%.[56] Given the low education and employment rates, and high HIV prevalence, Zomba provided the perfect setting to test the potential for cash transfers as a HIV prevention tool.

Treatment was randomly assigned, first at the enumeration area (EA) level: 88 to treatment and 88 to control. All baseline dropouts in treatment EAs received CCTs, while a further experiment was performed within the larger cohort of baseline schoolgirls. For them, 46 EAs were assigned to CCTs, 27 were assigned to UCTs, and 15 were assigned to receive no transfers to study spillovers (from baseline dropouts in those EAs). The average total transfer to the household of $10 per month for 10 months a year was nearly 10% of the average household consumption expenditure of $965 in Malawi in 2009.[57] This falls in the range of cash transfers as a share of household consumption (or income) in other countries with similar CCT programs. The transfers were offered to all eligible females in the target demographic and were not targeted by poverty status. Offer letters were distributed in December 2007; payments began in February 2008 and continued through the end of 2009. Four rounds of data took place: Round 1-Baseline (2007), Round 2 (2008), Round 3 (2010), and Round 4 (2012).

Beneficiaries receiving UCTs simply had to show up at a local distribution point each month to pick up their transfers. Monthly school attendance for all beneficiaries in the CCT arm was monitored, and payment for the following month was withheld for any student whose attendance was below 80% of the number of days school was in session. However, participants were never removed from the program for failing to meet the attendance condition, meaning that if they subsequently had satisfactory attendance, their payments would resume.

Along with a multitopic questionnaire administered to both the head of household and the core respondent in the target demographic, which collected detailed information about schooling status, health, dating patterns, sexual behavior, and so on, home-based voluntary counseling and testing for HIV (during Rounds 2–4) were conducted by Malawian nurses and counselors certified in conducting rapid HIV tests through the Ministry of Health HIV Unit HCT Counselor Certification Program.

As reported in Baird et al.,[21] 18 months after its inception, the cash transfer program decreased the prevalence of HIV by 64% and HSV-2 by 76% among baseline schoolgirls. Self-reported levels of frequency of intercourse and age-disparate sex were also lower in the combined inter-vention group at the 12-month follow-up. Individuals in the intervention group were also more likely to be enrolled in school during the 2008 school year than were those in the control areas. For baseline dropouts, al-though school reenrollment was substantially higher and the likelihood of having been married at 12-month follow-up was lower in the intervention group than in the comparison group, the prevalence of HIV or HSV-2 did not differ significantly between the two groups. For self-reported sexual activity at 12-month follow-up, only the self-reported frequency of sexual intercourse was significantly lower in the intervention group.

A first question of interest is, What was the behavior change through which the cash transfer program impacted HIV? Secondary analyses suggested that the program effects were concentrated among a small group of girls, who were sexually active at baseline and continued being active during the program (*always active*).[58] The program impact on HIV in this group was partially due to a reduction in the number of lifetime sexual partners and frequency of unprotected sexual activity but may also owe, in some part, to a significant increase in partner's safety. Among this group, more than one out of five girls in the control group reported having a sexual partner age 25 or older, while the same figure was less than 2% among the same group of girls in the treatment arms.[59] The *always active* young women in the combined treatment arm had younger partners and had partners who were more likely to be tested for HIV. These findings lend support to the idea that girls in the treatment arm were more likely to choose safer (younger) partners and to have sexual intercourse with them less frequently.

A second question of interest is whether these impacts were driven by schooling or income. The story for HIV seems to be very similar to the one that Baird, McIntosh, and Özler[60] outlined for marriage and pregnancy. Baird et al.[58] showed that while both the CCT and UCT led to increased enrollment, the impact in the UCT arm was only 43% as large as the impact in the CCT arm.[59] The CCT arm also improved attendance and test scores—thus indicating that the CCT outperformed the UCT in terms of schooling outcomes per dollar spent. On the other hand, marriage and pregnancy was delayed in the UCT arm, with no impacts in the CCT arm. This result—improved education concentrated in CCT, but delays in marriage and fertility in the UCT—proved a bit of a conundrum because we know from existing evidence from SSA that reducing school dropout should led to declines in teen marriage and pregnancy rates.[36,61–63] The basic explanation is that improvement in the CCT arm was achieved at the cost of denying transfers to noncompliers (girls who, for one reason or another, did not comply with the schooling condition), who are shown to be particularly at risk for early marriage and teenage pregnancy.

The story is similar when it comes to HIV and HSV-2 risk. As described in Özler,[60] schooling is clearly an important correlate of STI status. Among the control group, the probability of being infected with at least one STI (i.e., HIV, HSV-2, or both) was 2.9% for those attending school regularly at the 12-month follow-up, compared with 14.7% among those who were not. However, for UCT beneficiaries, the parallel findings were 2.9% and zero, respectively. These results are suggestive of a strong income effect on HIV risk, as there were no conditions in the UCT arm and minimal schooling effects to influence risky sexual behavior.

As with the previous discussion of the educational support programs, it is also interesting to consider whether the short-term impacts were sustained postintervention. Baird et al.[59] investigated the medium-term impacts of the Zomba cash transfer program two years after the intervention ended on a host of outcomes. Although the overall story is complex, there are no sustained impacts on HIV or HSV-2, with complete catch-up during the two-year postprogram period. This result is again consistent with the short-term evidence that income support, and not educational attainment, drove the short-term results. The positive income shock may have empowered young women to make safer choices while they had a steady income, but, in the absence of the accumulation of some type of capital (human, financial, physical, or social), these effects disappeared with the cessation of that income support.

The SIHR study illustrates the potential and limitations of cash transfers for HIV prevention among adolescents. The results highlight the importance of income above and beyond the schooling impacts but raise many questions about the duration and timing of interventions that can lead to sustained impacts on welfare in general and HIV incidence specifically.

The Empowerment and Livelihood Study

The ELA program in Uganda[22,64] (described in the previous section) was designed to empower adolescent girls through life skills and vocational training. It provides a good example of a rigorous evaluation of the types of vocational programs that attempt to mediate structural factors that influence high HIV rates among adolescent girls.

The ELA program targeted 14- to 20-year-old women in 100 randomly selected communities in Uganda, with 50 communities serving as controls (receiving none of these services). In treatment communities, activities are organized through "adolescent development clubs" led by a female mentor and held after school. Life skills training covered topics including menstruation, pregnancy, STIs, HIV/AIDS, family planning, rape, negotiation and conflict resolution, leadership, and legal rights. Vocational skills training included training in a broad array of skills including hair dressing, tailoring, computing, agriculture, poultry rearing, and small vendor enterprise. Specific vocational training was supplemented with courses in financial literacy, negotiation, and accounting. The clubs also hosted recreational activities including dramas, singing, dancing, and playing games.

Data were collected at baseline, two-year follow-up, and four-year follow-up. At baseline, 5,966 adolescent females were surveyed, of which 4,888 were tracked at two-year follow-up and 3,964 at four-year follow-up. Twenty-one percent of girls in communities where clubs were offered participated in the voluntary program. Of those girls, 84.6% participated in life skills training and 52.6% participated in vocational training.

The evaluation found an increase in the HIV knowledge index in treated communities from baseline to endline. The probability of having a child decreased significantly in treatment communities, which show a 24% decrease in fertility at two-year follow up with sustained impacts at the four-year follow-up. The proportion of sexually active girls who report always using a condom increased from a baseline of 44.6% to a midline of 57.6%—this impact dissipates two years after the program. The proportion of girls who reported having sex unwillingly in the past year decreased from 17.4% to 11.3% in treatment communities at midline and remained at endline.

Economic outcomes also improved throughout the program. The proportion of girls involved in any income-generating activity increased from 10.2% to 17.0% by midline and 15.1% at endline, almost entirely driven by an increase in entrepreneurial activities.

This evaluation shows that a combined intervention providing information and skills can improve health and earnings among adolescent females and young women. It also shows that it is possible to simultaneously increase employment and decrease risky behaviors. Bandiera et al.[22] also argued that HIV educational programs are unlikely to be effective if the economic factors that drive risky behaviors are not addressed in a two-pronged approach. These results also suggest a sustained impact of the combined intervention two years after the completion of program activities.

Although this study demonstrated significant improvements in both economic and health outcomes, it did not measure HIV incidence or prevalence. Although the study did measure HIV knowledge and behaviors, we do not know the direct effect on HIV infection. This program was relatively intensive in terms of staff time and budget, and while found to be cost-effective, scaling to a district or national level would be expensive and pose various other issues.

Although the program was effective in Uganda, a recent evaluation shows that the same program did not replicate this success in Tanzania.[65] The same combined life skills and vocational skills training program was implemented in 100 communities in Tanzania, with 50 communities serving as controls. In 50 of the 100 treatment communities, microfinance was also provided. This study found none of the same improvements in social or economic outcomes that the Ugandan evaluation[22] found. The study authors did find that the addition of microfinance did increase the take-up of services, from 19% in communities with microfinance, 13% for club-only communities, and 7% in the control communities. The authors also documented significant differences in implementation due to more limited funds in Tanzania, a delay in implementation, and lack of supervision of field sites. While this evaluation does not discount the outcomes found in the ELA program in Uganda, it does suggest that there may be some issue with scaling similar programs, that cultural context needs to be addressed, and that changes from the original design can be detrimental to targeted outcomes.

Discussion and Recommendations for Policy and Research

The literature examining the relationship between economic and education intervention interventions and HIV risk for young women in SSA, while growing, is still nascent. Focusing on four main types of structural interventions—cash transfers, educational support, savings and microcredit, and vocational training—we see glimmers of promise, but there are still many more questions than answers. These uncertainties generally arise from a lack of high-quality studies, rather than contradictory evidence. For example, secondary analysis on the evaluations detailed in the ASPIRES systematic review[24] found that across different interventions and subpopulations, measures of HIV were unfortunately underpowered to detect meaningful change.[66] Additional large-scale cluster-RCTs are needed before embarking on concrete discussions of scale and cost-effectiveness. We now summarize some key findings, limitations, and suggestions for next steps across the four intervention types.

Although the importance of income on HIV risk is highlighted by studies of CCT and UCT programs, the analysis of cash transfers does raise questions on the importance of improved educational outcomes for HIV reduction. The observational data clearly show a negative correlation between school enrollment and HIV prevalence. However, marginally increased levels of schooling do not show effects on HIV. Whether this is simply an issue of power (meaning that researchers need treatments powerful enough to cause much larger effects on schooling) or that exogenous changes in schooling—even large changes such as those seen among baseline dropouts in SIHR—do not lead to significant reductions in HIV incidence is a question that remains.

In terms of educational support, its link with HIV and HSV-2 reduction is weak at best, but this may not yet be a reason to abandon it as part of a cost-effective HIV prevention strategy. Given the small number of trials, more work is needed to understand the effects of improved schooling, if any, on HIV and HSV-2. We recommend that future studies use communities as the unit of treatment rather than schools, as HIV incidence among schoolgirls is small and therefore hard to detect. We also recommend that future studies target a random sample of more general populations—either all adolescents or those from poor households. To account for the possibility that the effects may primarily come from improved school attainment later, rather than school enrollment now, studies should be planned for long-term follow-ups, such as those in Duflo, Dupas, and Kremer.[36] Finally, future studies should be powered to detect meaningful effects on HIV. Similar to cash transfers, it is unlikely that educational support will be cost-effective as a stand-alone strategy for decreasing HIV, but considering social benefits of these interventions— both in terms of future outcomes and from current redistribution, it could be part of a broader strategy toward improved health and education.

The evidence on savings and microcredit's effect on HIV behaviors is also mixed, and there is no rigorous evidence pertaining to HIV incidence or prevalence (or other biomarkers). The evidence that does exist suggests that microcredit is most accessible to those girls already less vulnerable and could be most supportive of older, out-of-school young women in less challenging macroeconomic environments. Savings could be an avenue for young girls and their families to support school attendance, and matched savings provide an added bonus (similar to cash transfer models). Given convincing evidence that negative income shocks increase the likelihood of risky transactional sex among women,[19] those designing interventions should consider whether cash transfers, insurance, or savings are the most effective method for among young, vulnerable women.

With vocational training, and not dissimilar from challenges in the CCT and educational support space, one challenge these programs face is targeting. Those most at risk in most communities are the poorest, and the structure of many of these programs makes participation of the most vulnerable females challenging. For example, the RCT in Liberia studying a combined program of vocational and life skills training to almost 2,000 girls found that employment increases were concentrated among the middle wealth quintile.[27] They missed the poorest (and the wealthiest) quintile. Other programs that include a savings element, which is sometimes combined with entrepreneurial training, can edge out girls who have nothing to save (both young girls and the poorest girls). Providing vocational training for formal employment is still dependent on the availability of jobs within the community. Structuring programs to feasibly identify those most vulnerable to adverse outcomes as adults, including HIV infection, may be a desirable design element for such programs.

We conclude with five recommendations for future research and policy:

1. **More well-funded and well-designed large-scale cluster-RCTs:** If we truly want to understand the ability of structural interventions to prevent HIV among young women in SSA, we are going to need well-powered studies of HIV incidence, paying particular attention to study design (e.g., eligibility, targeting, level of intervention, amounts). These will be expensive, require long-term follow-up, and benefit from true multidisciplinary work between economists and experts in HIV.

2. **Simulations and modeling:** Alongside additional large-scale cluster-RCTs, modeling can help further our evidence based on the potential for these types of interventions to impact HIV.[67,68] This can complement experimental work in three important ways: it can (i) help highlight the likelihood of success given the underlying context and proposed study design; (ii) allow for better study design, including realistic power calculations; and (3) allow for learnings beyond the specific scope of the study.

3. **HIV-positive youth/young men:** As currently designed, these interventions ignore youth who are already HIV positive and tend to ignore young men. More thought is needed on whether these types of interventions can also be effective for HIV-positive youth, as well as the importance of complimentary interventions for young men.

4. **Behavioral change communication:** We need more multiarm trials like Dupas et al.[36] that combine structural interventions with more traditional behavioral change communication. We don't know much about the complementarities between the two types of interventions. These combination strategies could illustrate how best to support young women at risk, both through knowledge and through improved resources.

5. **Cost-effectiveness:** It is unlikely that these strategies are going to be cost-effective in terms of HIV incidence as a singular outcome. The benefit–cost ratio of these interventions needs to be thought of in terms of the full set of outcomes that are being altered. Researchers and policymakers need to think about impacts on HIV as part of a broader agenda of improving the health and well-being of young people.

References

1. Williams S. Africa's youth: The African Development Bank and the demographic dividend. *New African.* 2012:30–31.
2. UNAIDS. *HIV Prevention among Adolescent Girls and Young Women.* Geneva: Joint United Nations Programme on HIV/AIDS; 2016.
3. UNICEF, UNAIDS, UNESCO, et al. *Opportunity in Crisis: Preventing HIV from Early Adolescence to Young Adulthood.* Geneva: UNICEF; 2011.
4. Ramjee G, Daniels B. 2013. Women and HIV in sub-Saharan Africa. *AIDS Res Ther.* 2013;10(30).
5. Kharsany ABM, Karim QA. HIV infection and AIDS in sub-Saharan Africa: current status, challenges and opportunities. *Open AIDS.* 2016;10:34–48.
6. Stoebenau K, Heise L, Wamoyi J, Bobrova N. Revisiting the understanding of "transactional sex" in sub-Saharan Africa: a review and synthesis of the literature. *Soc Sci Med.* 2016;168:186–197.
7. Abdul-Quader AS, Collins C. Identification of structural interventions for HIV/AIDS prevention: the concept mapping exercise. *Public Health Rep.* 2011;126(6):777–788.
8. An overview of structural prevention introduction. 2015. Available at: https://aidsfree.usaid.gov/resources/pkb/structural/overview-structural-prevention. Accessed October 30, 2017.
9. World Bank. *World Development Report 2018: Learning to Realize Education's Promise.* Washington, DC: World Bank; 2018.
10. World Bank. *Reaching Girls, Transforming Lives.* Washington, DC: World Bank Education Global Practice; 2016.
11. McCoy S, Kangwende A, Padian NS. Behaviour change interventions to prevent HIV among women living in low and middle income countries. *AIDS Behav.* 2010;14:469–82.
12. Jukes M, Simmons S, Bundy D. Education and vulnerability: the role of schools in protecting young women and girls from HIV in southern Africa. *AIDS.* 2008;22(4):S41–S46.
13. Hargreaves JR, Morison LA, Kim JC, et al. The association between school attendance, HIV infection and sexual behavior among young people in rural South Africa. *J Epidemiol Community Health.* 2008;62(2):113–119.
14. Beegle K, Özler B. Young women, rich(er) men, and the spread of HIV. Paper presented at: International Food Policy Research Institute; April 5, 2007; Washington, DC.
15. Wojcicki JM. "She drank his money": survival sex and the problem of violence in taverns in Gauteng Province, South Africa. *Med Anthropol Q.* 2002;16(3):267–293.
16. Shelton JD, Cassell MM, Adetunji J. Is poverty or wealth at the root of HIV? *Lancet.* 2005;366(9491):1057–1058.

17. Wines, M. Durban Journal; As AIDS continues to ravage, South Africa "recycles" graves. *New York Times*. July 29, 2004.

18. Halperin D, Epstein H. Seizing the opportunity to capitalize on the growing access to HIV treatment to expand HIV prevention. *Lancet*. 2004;364:4–6.

19. Hallman, K. *Socioeconomic Disadvantage and Unsafe Sexual Behaviors of Young Women and Men in South Africa*. Working Paper 190. New York: Population Council; 2004.

20. Robinson J, Yeh E. Transactional sex as a response to risk in western Kenya. *Am Econ J Appl Econ*. 2011;3(1):35–64.

21. De Walque D. *Who Gets AIDS and How? The Determinants of HIV Infection and Sexual Behaviors in Burkina Faso, Cameroon, Ghana, Kenya and Tanzania*. Working Paper 3844. Washington, DC: World Bank; 2006.

22. Baird S, Chirwa E, McIntosh C, Özler B. The short-term impacts of a schooling conditional cash transfer program on the sexual behavior of young women. *Health Econ*. 2010;19:55–68.

23. Bandiera O, Buehren N, Burgess R, et al. *Empowering Adolescent Girls: Evidence from a Randomized Control Trial in Uganda*. Washington, DC: World Bank; 2012.

24. *Definition of Youth*. New York: United Nations Department of Economic and Social Affairs; 2017:1–3. Available at: http://www.un.org/esa/socdev/documents/youth/fact-sheets/youth-definition.pdf. Accessed October 30, 2017.

25. Swann M. Household economic strengthening interventions to address HIV prevention, care, and treatment outcomes: a comprehensive evidence review. Paper presented at: 19th International Conference on HIV/AIDS and STIs; December 2017; Abidjan, Côte d'Ivoire.

26. Pronyk PM, Hargreaves JR, Kim JC, et al. Effect of a structural intervention for the prevention of intimate-partner violence and HIV in rural South Africa: a cluster randomised trial. *Lancet*. 2006;368(9551):1973–1983.

27. Pronyk PM, Kim JC, Abramsky T, et al. A combined microfinance and training intervention can reduce HIV risk behaviour in young female participants. *AIDS*. 2008;22(13):1659–1665.

28. Adoho F, Chakravarty S, Korkoyah DT, Lundberg M, Tasneem A. *The Impact of an Adolescent Girls Employment Program: The EPAG Project in Liberia*. Working Paper 6832. Washington, DC: World Bank Africa Region Poverty Reduction and Economic Management Unit & Human Development Network Social Protection and Labor Unit; 2014.

29. Jewkes R, Gibbs A, Jama-Shai N, et al. Stepping stones and creating futures intervention: shortened interrupted time series evaluation of a behavioural and structural health promotion and violence prevention intervention for young people in informal settlements in Durban, South Africa. *BMC Public Health*. 2014;14:1325.

30. de Walque D, Dow WH, Nathan R, et al. Incentivising safe sex: a randomised trial of conditional cash transfers for HIV and sexually transmitted infection prevention in rural Tanzania. *BMJ Open*. 2012;2(1):e000747.

31. Fiszbein A, Rüdiger Schady N, Ferreira FHG. *Conditional Cash Transfers: Reducing Present and Future Poverty.* Washington, DC: World Bank; 2009.

32. Pettifor A, MacPhail C, Hughes JP, et al. The effect of a conditional cash transfer on HIV incidence in young women in rural South Africa (HPTN 068): a phase 3, randomised controlled trial. *Lancet Global Health.* 2016;4(12) e978–e988.

33. Özler B. The importance of study design (why did a CCT program have no effects on schooling or HIV?). Aprill 24, 2017. Available at: http://blogs.worldbank. org/impactevaluations/importance-study-design-why-did-cct-program-have-no-effects-schooling-or-hiv. Accessed October 30, 2017.

34. Abdool Karim Q, Leask K, Kharsany A, et al. Impact of conditional cash incentives on HSV-2 and HIV prevention in rural South African high school students: results of the CAPRISA 007 cluster randomized controlled trial. Paper presented at: 8th IAS Conference on HIV Pathogenesis, Treatment & Prevention; July 19–22, 2015; Vancouver, Canada. Abstract TUAC0101LB.

35. Heinrich CJ, Hoddinott J, Samson M. Reducing adolescent risky behaviors in a high-risk context: the effects of unconditional cash transfers in South Africa. *Econ Dev Cultural Change.* 2017;65(4).

36. Handa S, Halpern CT, Pettifor A, Thirumurthy H. The government of Kenya's cash transfer program reduces the risk of sexual debut among young people age 15–25. *PLoS One.* 2014;9(1) e85473.

37. Duflo E, Dupas P, Kremer M. Education, HIV, and early fertility: Experimental evidence from Kenya. *Am Econ Rev.* 2015;105(9):2757–2797.

38. Hallfors DD, Cho H, Mbai I, Milimo B, Itindi J. Process and outcome evaluation of a community intervention for orphan adolescents in western Kenya. *J Community Health.* 2012;37(5):1101–1109.

39. Hallfors DD, Cho H, Rusakaniko S, Iritani B, Mapfumo J, Halpern C. Supporting adolescent orphan girls to stay in school as HIV risk prevention: evidence from a randomized controlled trial in Zimbabwe. *Am J Public Health.* 2011;101(6):1082–1088.

40. Cho H, Hallfors DD, Mbai I, et al. Keeping adolescent orphans in school to prevention human immunodeficiency virus infection: evidence from a randomized controlled trial in Kenya. *J Adolesc Health.* 2011;48:523–526.

41. Hallfors DD, Cho H, Rusakaniko S, et al. The impact of school subsidies on HIV-related outcomes among adolescent female orphans. *J Adolesc Health.* 2015;56(1):79–84.

42. Austrian K, Muthengi E. Can Economic assets increase girls' risk of sexual harassment? Evaluation results from a social, health and economic asset-building intervention for vulnerable adolescent girls in Uganda. *Child Youth Serv. Rev.* 2014;42(2):168–175.

43. Jennings L, Ssewamala FM, Nabunya P. Effect of savings-led economic empowerment on HIV preventive practices among orphaned adolescents in rural Uganda: results from the Suubi-Maka randomized experiment. *AIDS Care.* 2015;28(3):273–282.

44. Dunbar MS, Dufour MK, Lambdin B, Mudekunye-Mahaka I, Nhamo D, Padian NS. The SHAZ! Project: results from a pilot randomized trial of a structural intervention to prevent HIV among adolescent women in Zimbabwe. *PLoS One.* 2014;9(11):1.

45. Spielberg F, Crookston BT, Chanani S, Kim J, Kline S, Gray BL. Leveraging microfinance to impact HIV and financial behaviors among adolescents and their mothers in West Bengal: a cluster randomized trial. *Int J Adolesc Med Health.* 2013;25(2):157–166.

46. Ssewamala FM, Alicea S, Bannon WM, Ismayilova L. A novel economic intervention to reduce HIV risk among school-going AIDS orphans in rural Uganda. *J Adolesc Health.* 2008;42:102–104.

47. Ssewamala FM, Han C, Neilands TB, Ismayilova L, Sperber E. Effect of economic assets on sexual risk-taking intentions among orphaned adolescents in Uganda. *Am J Public Health.* 2010;100(3):483–488.

48. Dunbar, MS, Maternowska MC, Kang MJ, et al. Findings from SHAZ!: a feasibility study of a microcredit and life-skills HIV prevention intervention to reduce risk among adolescent female orphans in Zimbabwe. *J Prevent Interven Community.* 2010;38(2):147–161.

49. Rotheram-Borus MJ, Lightfoot M, Kasirye R, Desmond K. Vocational training with HIV prevention for Ugandan youth. *AIDS Behav.* 2012;16(5):1133–1137.

50. Goodman ML, Kaberia R, Morgan RO, Keiser PH. Health and livelihood outcomes associated with participation in a community-based empowerment program for orphan families in semirural Kenya: a cross-sectional study. *Vulnerable Child Youth Stud.* 2014;9(4):365–376.

51. Goodman ML, Selwyn BJ, Morgan RO, et al. Sexual behavior among young carers in the context of a Kenyan empowerment program combining cash-transfer, psychosocial support, and entrepreneurship. *J Sex Res.* 2016;53(3):331–345.

52. Visser M, Zungu N, Ndala-Magoro N. ISIBINDI, creating circles of care for orphans and vulnerable children in South Africa: post-programme outcomes. *AIDS Care.* 2015;27(8):1014–1019.

53. Boungou Bazika, JC. Effectiveness of small scale income generating activities in reducing risk of HIV in youth in the Republic of Congo. *AIDS Care.* 2007;19(Suppl 1):23–24.

54. Kohler HP, Thornton R. Conditional cash transfers and HIV/AIDS prevention: unconditionally promising? *World Bank Econ Rev.* 2012;26(2):165–190.

55. Baird S, McIntosh C, Özler B. *When the Money Runs Out: Do Cash Transfers Have Sustained Effects on Human Capital Accumulation?* Working Paper 7901. Washington, DC: World Bank; 2016.

56. National Statistical Office (Malawi), ORC Macro. *Malawi Demographic and Health Survey 2004.* Calverton, MA: National Statistical Office and ORC Macro; 2005.

57. World Development Indicators. 2010. Available at: https://data.worldbank.org/data-catalog/world-development-indicators. Accessed November 3, 2010.

58. Özler B. Cash transfers: what have we learned so Far? What are the implications for policy? What more do we need to know? 2011. Available at: http://blogs. worldbank.org/impactevaluations/publicsphere/cash-transfers-what-have-we-learned-so-far-what-are-the-implications-for-policy-what-more-do-we-need. Accessed October 30, 2017.

59. Baird S, Özler B. Transactional sex in Malawi. In: Cunningham S, Shah M, eds. *Handbook of the Economics of Prostitution*. Oxford: Oxford University Press; 2016:165–187.

60. Baird S, McIntosh C, Özler B. Cash or condition: evidence from a randomized cash transfer program. *Q J Econ*. 2011;126(4):1709–1753.

61. Özler B. A cash transfer program reduces HIV infection among adolescent girls. Washington, DC: World Bank; 2010. Available at: http://siteresources. worldbank.org/DEC/Resources/HIVExeSummary(Malawi).pdf.

62. Ferré C. *Age at First Child: Does Education Delay Fertility Timing? The Case of Kenya*. Working Paper 4833.Washington, DC: World Bank; 2009.

63. Osili UO, Long BT. Does female schooling reduce fertility? evidence from Nigeria. *J Dev Econ*. 2008;87:57–75.

64. Bandiera O, Buehren N, Burgess R, et al. *Women's Empowerment in Action: Evidence from a Randomized Control Trial in Africa*. Washington, DC: World Bank; 2017.

65. Buehren N, Goldstein M, Gulesci S, Sulaiman M, Yam V. *Evaluation of an Adolescent Development Program for Girls in Tanzania*. Working Paper 7961. Washington, DC: World Bank Africa Region Office of the Chief Economist & Gender Cross Cutting Solution Area; 2017.

66. Ahner-McHaffie T. How household economic strengthening programs are measuring HIV outcomes: A secondary analysis (Master's thesis). Washington, DC: George Washington University; 2017.

67. Abuelezam NN, McCormick AW, Fussell T, et al. Can the heterosexual HIV epidemic be eliminated in South Africa using combination prevention? a modeling analysis. *Am J Epidemiol*. 2016;184(3):239–248.

68. Halloran ME, Auranen K, Baird S, et al. Simulations for designing and interpreting intervention trials in infectious diseases. BioRxiv Paper: 198051.

4

Enhancing Access to Safe and Secure Housing

Julia Dickson-Gomez and Katherine Quinn

Overview

The HIV epidemic increasingly has been found to be influenced by myriad structural, cultural, political, and societal forces, including the shortage of affordable housing in the United States and other high-income countries (HIC) and in low- and middle-income countries (LMIC). This shortage has led to literal homelessness (sleeping on the streets, shelters, or other places not meant for human habitation), inadequate or uninhabitable housing, and high rates of housing mobility/instability among the urban poor. In both HIC and LMIC, the housing crisis is associated with overcrowding and unaffordable housing. The housing crisis in LMIC has led to the proliferation of informal (or slum) settlements. All of these factors (homelessness, unstable housing and frequent evictions/moves, overcrowded, and inadequate shelter) have been associated with higher HIV risk and prevalence rates and poorer outcomes among those living with HIV. Although the association between unstable housing and HIV is well established in the United States and other HIC, the process of understanding these associations (including engagement in HIV care and antiretroviral adherence) in LMIC has just begun.

HIV prevalence rates among samples of homeless populations has been found to be as high as 10%[1] compared to less than one-half of 1% among the general US population.[2] Estimates indicate that the homeless are three to nine times more likely to become infected with HIV than persons who are housed.[3-7] There are numerous pathways linking housing status and HIV risk. For example, growing evidence indicates that housing status, security, and stability are significantly associated with HIV-related risk-taking behaviors,[8] including exchanging sex for money, drugs, or a place to stay.[9,10] In one study, 19% of the homeless and 15% of those unstably housed had recently exchanged sex for money, drugs, or a place to stay.[9] These risks are often magnified for homeless and unstably housed women, who have significantly higher odds of using illicit drugs and having multiple sex partners and are susceptible to doubling up with friends or acquaintances and exchanging sex for shelter or money,[11] which in turn has been shown to increase women's exposure to violence and sexually transmitted infections.[12,13] Homeless people living with HIV (PLH) are more likely to abuse alcohol, use and inject drugs, share needles, exchange sex, and have a greater number of sexual partners.[9,14,15] Homeless and unstably housed youth and young adults are similarly vulnerable to HIV; homeless youth are at an up to 10 times greater risk for contracting HIV than stably housed youth[16] due to substance use, multiple sexual partners, and survival sex to meet basic needs as well as greater numbers of sexual partners than their stably housed counterparts.[17-19] Furthermore, adverse childhood events (ACEs) during periods of homelessness, and following these periods, are pervasive among homeless youth.[20] The vast majority of homeless individuals report experiencing at least one ACE before the age of 18, and over one-half report having experienced four or more ACEs including parental loss, emotional neglect, emotional, physical, and sexual abuse, and substance abuse.[21] Homelessness is also a problem that affects low-income families. From 2007 to 2012, family homelessness in the United States, for example, increased by 13% at the same time that homelessness has been reduced in other populations such as the chronically homeless with disabilities (19%) and veterans (17%).[22,23] An estimated 1.35 million children experience homelessness each year, and families with children constitute approximately 40% of the total homeless population.[24,25] It is likely, given the strong association of ACEs and HIV in later life, that childhood homelessness increases the odds of becoming infected with HIV, especially later homelessness.

In addition to contributing to HIV risk, homelessness and housing instability among PLH are strongly associated with poorer HIV outcomes. Furthermore, approximately one in 12 PLH in the United States has an unmet need for housing assistance,[26] and at least one-half of all PLH report experiencing homelessness or housing instability at some point in their lives.[27] Homelessness and unstable or otherwise inadequate housing is associated with higher rates of HIV risk behaviors, poorer access to healthcare, lower adherence to antiretroviral therapy (ART), and poorer health outcomes.[26] Homeless PLH are more likely to delay entry into HIV care and less likely to have regular HIV care. Further, they are less likely to receive optimal HIV treatment, less likely to adhere to ART than stably housed persons, and at greater risk for poor health outcomes and early death.[8,28–31] Compared to stably housed persons with HIV, PLH who lack stable housing are more likely to engage in sex exchange, have unprotected sex with an unknown status partner, and use and inject drugs.[14] Furthermore, PLH lacking stable housing are more likely to delay HIV care, more likely to have lower CD4 counts and higher viral loads, more likely to have poorer access to regular care, less likely to receive ART, and less likely to adhere to ART.[8,27,29,32] Homeless PLH face considerable barriers not only to accessing care but to maintaining that care to achieve optimal health outcomes. Compared to PLH who are housed, homeless PLH who are engaged in HIV treatment are more likely to stop taking ART.[29] Without stable housing, PLH may be less able to adhere to the demands of complex treatment regimens and are more likely to engage in high-risk sex or drug behaviors.[32]

Homeless and unstably housed PLH face numerous additional health challenges. Routine access to quality medical care and receipt of and adherence to ART are essential in improving HIV outcomes. Homeless PLH are more likely to be uninsured, to have visited an emergency department, and to have been admitted to a hospital compared to their housed counterparts.[29] Additionally, homeless PLH often have other physical comorbidities including hepatitis C and tuberculosis,[8,33] which can further compromise health.

HIV risk and poor HIV health outcomes among homeless and unstably housed individuals are also partially driven by the comorbidities that increase HIV risk and make HIV treatment and ART adherence more difficult. For example, approximately one-third of homeless individuals experience substance use disorders (SUDs),[34] and there is a disproportionately high rate of psychiatric disorders among the homeless.[35,36] Among homeless PLH, those with poorer general mental health and greater levels of depression have lower levels of ART adherence.[37]

In this chapter, we first explore literature that examines in more depth the kinds of precarious housing that leads to greater HIV risk and the limited research on the effects of the urban housing crisis on

HIV in LMIC. We then describe structural interventions that have been attempted to address the association between homelessness/housing instability and HIV risk. These can be sorted into several categories. First are programs intended to provide housing to the homeless, those at risk of homelessness, or PLH including permanent supportive housing (PSH), housing subsidies (such as Housing Choice vouchers), and public housing. Shortcomings of these interventions are that while they have been demonstrated to be successful in reducing HIV risk and health outcomes for PLH, they have generally not improved the neighborhoods in which people live. The neighborhoods surrounding those experiencing housing insecurity, both in HIC and LMIC (as in informal settlements), have been shown to have a significant effect on HIV risk and HIV morbidity and mortality. This chapter thus reviews interventions that focus on improving conditions of neighborhoods and their effects on HIV risk. Finally, overcrowding and the relationships with co-residents are both important in understanding HIV risk and health outcomes for PLH. In LMIC, interventions have focused on improving housing conditions in informal settlements, but the effects of these on HIV risk have not been evaluated. Other interventions have focused on increasing social capital, and increasing access to health-care through peer health educators and location of clinics and harm-reduction prevention services within communities.

In the second half of the chapter, we review recent research addressing gaps in the literature. The first study presented explored the variability in PSH models and, ultimately, the comparative effectiveness of different PSH models on housing stability, HIV, and health outcomes for PLH. We then present data on the HIV risks associated with different kinds of low-income communities (including informal settlements and downtown areas) on HIV and drug risk in El Salvador. This study further examined the reasons for homelessness among some participants.

Multidimensional Definitions of Housing Status and Stability

Although the vast majority of research dichotomizes homeless versus housed, homelessness is only one housing status that can contribute to heightened HIV risk and poor HIV outcomes. Unstable, unafford-able, or otherwise inadequate housing can similarly result in increased HIV risk and poor HIV outcomes, and researchers have increasingly called for an examination of housing as a multidimensional construct,[38] suggesting that dichotomous measures of housing stability obscure important differences.[39,40] Unstable housing can include temporarily living with friends, family, or sexual partners. Low-income residents who rent often suffer from precarious housing as rent often exceeds 50% of their incomes. In these cases, receiving housing subsidies can improve housing stability. A dose-response relationship exists wherein those with more precarious housing situations have greater drug use frequency and more frequently engage in sexual risk behaviors.[41] Individuals who are literally homeless tend to be at greater risk than those who are precariously or marginally housed (e.g., doubled up), both of whom are at greater risk than those who are stably housed.[9,19]

Qualitative research has provided further support to demonstrate the importance of understanding the effects of various types of housing status on HIV risk. Our research[42] looked at how housing status impacted HIV risk and drug use behaviors, comparing those using shelters, doubled up with friends or family, and independently housed. Residents noted that the ubiquitous drug use in shelters, as well as the stress of homelessness, made it difficult for them to refrain from drug activity. Doubling up with family or friends had varied impacts on drug use, depending on the type of relationship the participant had with his or her roommates. Those living with drug-using friends found it difficult to abstain from drug use, whereas living with non-drug-using family members served as a protective factor against drug use. Those who were receiving housing subsidies were less likely to allow their apartments to turn into drug use sites than those who did not receive subsidies.[42]

Housing stability has been defined as individuals' degree of transience, or the number of moves or evictions a person has had within a specified amount of time.[43–46] Residential instability is associated with greater drug and sexual risk behaviors. Frequent changes to one's housing situation may disrupt social networks and neighborhood ties, impede resource acquisition, and inhibit access to clean syringes, subsequently contributing to HIV risk.[43,47] For example, risky injection drug practices increase among injection drug users as housing stability decreases,[19] and individuals who experience changes in housing situation are more likely to have condomless sex or exchange sex for drugs, money, or a place to stay.[9,45] Such relationships are also evident among individuals who simply perceive they are likely to lose their current housing. When drug users believe they are going to be evicted, they often increase drug and sexual risk behaviors in response to the stress of an imminent eviction and, because they stop paying rent, that money is spent on drugs.[48] Little research, however, has examined reasons for moving, which may play an important role in HIV risk. Forcible moves, including evictions, may increase stress, limit opportunities to utilize existing resources or social networks, and increase risk behavior. In contrast, individuals may choose to move to improve their living conditions or distance themselves from harmful or negative social environments, which may ultimately reduce HIV risk behaviors.[43]

The Global Housing Crisis and HIV

Most research on the relationship between housing instability, homelessness, and HIV has been conducted in HIC.[49] This is in spite of the fact that the urban housing crisis is even more acute in LMIC. Many low-income urban residents reside in "informal settlements" or squatter settlements that often consist of makeshift housing from salvaged or inexpensive materials and lack basic infrastructure such as sewage, potable water, garbage collection, and electricity.[50–52] In the developing world, 881 million people are estimated to be living in slums, constituting over 50% of the urban population in sub-Saharan Africa and Latin America,[50,53,54] with some estimating that 70% of urban populations in sub-Saharan Africa live in slums.[55,56] Studies have shown the higher rates of HIV and high rates of hepatitis B and C co-infection in informal settlements compared to other urban areas, including other "formal" low-income urban neighborhoods and rural rates.[57,58] In South Africa, HIV rates in informal settlements are double those in formal areas.[51,59] Residents in urban slums have also been found to have poor adherence to ART and to frequently drop out of care.[56]

Other research has examined housing stability among the urban poor in LMIC and found an association between housing instability and HIV. For example, research with female sex workers in Andhra Pradesh, India, found greater residential instability was associated with increased sexual risk behaviors including condomless sex, recent sexually transmitted infections, and physical and sexual violence.[47]

Several interlocking factors have been hypothesized to contribute to the higher HIV prevalence in informal communities and poorer health outcomes among PLH. First, residents of urban slums are often invisible to government officials who do not want to legally recognize them and provide for their housing needs or find it difficult to perform formal censuses of the highly transient and often mistrustful residents of informal settlements.[60,61] This makes planning for health services for residents of informal settlements difficult, and many settlements do not have any health services, or they have an inadequate number of health services located within their communities.[51] Community violence also contributes to the difficulties of providing healthcare within informal settlements as healthcare workers may be attacked or feel unsafe in informal settlements and residents may be restricted in their movements from one to other parts of the city because of gang control.[62,63] Further, the stigma of being a resident of an informal community and lack of transportation limits access to health services located outside of informal communities for many residents.[64] Lack of basic services and high rates of poverty, including food insecurity, make it more difficult to adhere to ART.[51] Higher rates of HIV and lower access to ART and HIV medical care may increase viral load, making it more likely that residents of informal communities will become infected with HIV.

Missing from much of this literature is the recognition that not all informal or low-income communities in LMICs, or even within particular cities, are the same, and there may be wide and as yet undiscovered disparities in the health among them.[57,61] For example, some informal communities in LMICs have undergone a process of legalization and housing and infrastructure improvement and have their own systems of self-governance.[65] Others within the same city may be in the process of obtaining this but are more recent in origin. In other countries, legalization and improvement of informal communities has been opposed by governments who do not want to give legitimacy to these settlements.[53] Further, most research conducted to date has failed to recognized that some urban residents in LMIC are literally homeless, sleeping on the street as opposed to makeshift shelters. An exception to this is studies of street children have been categorized roughly as "on the street" and "of the street" with children who are "on the street" spending much of their time working on the streets but still having considerable contact with and living with family members. "Of the street" youth, on the other hand, both sleep and work on the street with limited contact with family.[66] All street youth have been found to have elevated HIV risk, with "of the street" children generally at higher risk.[67–74] However, many adults in LMIC also sleep on streets.[75]

Structural Interventions to Address the Link between Housing and HIV

Permanent Supportive Housing

A growing body of research indicates that PSH is an effective structural intervention to improve the physical and mental health of the chronically homeless. A subpopulation of homeless, the chronically homeless, are more likely to have severe mental illness (SMI) and SUDs, conditions that increase their risk for HIV infection, transmission, and poor clinical outcomes for PLH.[37,76,77] A preponderance of research shows that the chronically homeless are able to remain in housing if provided with subsidized supportive housing[78-81] and that persons residing in supportive housing show improved quality of life,[80,82,83] reductions in substance use,[84] and reductions in incarcerations.[85] The research is not as clear, however, in whether placing chronically homeless PLH in supportive housing increases their CD4 count or decreases their viral load. In a randomized controlled trial in which homeless PLH were randomized into receiving immediate, Housing Opportunities for People With AIDS–funded housing or customary care conditions, Wolitski et al.[79] found no significant changes between the experimental condition and customary care control in HIV viral load or CD4 count. However, they found that participants who had been homeless during follow-up had 2.5 times the odds of having a detectable viral load as those who had not experienced homelessness.[79] As approximately one-half the participants in the control condition received housing before the end of the study period, the authors hypothesized the study was underpowered to detect changes in HIV disease progression.[79] Conversely, more recent research found that HIV risk behaviors and sexual activity increased among chronically homeless individuals who were transitioning into permanent supportive housing,[86] suggesting a need for continued research into whether and how housing can mitigate HIV risk.

Supportive housing has become the dominant model in the United States for providing housing and services to the chronically homeless, a population with multiple physical and mental health and social service needs.[87-91] Between 2006 and 2010, the number of available supportive housing units increased from 176,830 to 236,798.[88] Although there is evidence to support the effectiveness of supportive housing on improving housing stability, quality of life, mental health, and health outcomes, to our knowledge, no research to date has compared the effects of different supportive housing models on these outcomes or examined their relative economic efficiency. This is important because "supportive housing" is an umbrella term that covers programs that differ in many important characteristics. PSH programs grew in popularity after the success found in the Pathways to Housing program in New York City, a "Housing First" program that was developed as an alternative to prevailing continuum of care models in which mentally ill or substance-abusing individuals are required to "earn" access to housing by completing treatment programs and achieving sobriety.[83,92] Little research has explored the fidelity with which the original Housing First model has been implemented in practice, although some research suggests that the lack of clear guidelines for replication has led to significant departures from the model.[90,93]

The initial Housing First paradigm included scattered-site housing to provide consumers choice in their housing and to allow them to "mainstream" into community settings, to allow consumer choice in terms of whether or not to engage in supportive services, to provide Assertive Community Treatment (ACT) to engage participants in services, and a harm-reduction philosophy in which consumers were not required to achieve sobriety and were directly, or nearly directly, placed into housing. However, qualitative research of the Federal Collaborative Initiative to Help End Chronic Homelessness found a great diversity of supportive housing programs which diverge in many ways from the original model. These include differences in housing configuration, with many programs using project-based instead of scattered-site housing which may preclude integration into the community and limits consumers' choice of housing. In addition, in some projects the agency rather than consumers holds the lease, again potentially limiting consumer choice. Programs also differed in the extent to which housing management and supportive services were separated.[87] PSH programs also vary in the way that services are delivered and types of services provided.[81,94–96] The initial Housing First models provided ACT which involves intensive, personalized, direct, and highly accessible case management and service delivery for clients.[83] Case management services are provided at different intensities.[97] Finally, programs differ in the other types of supportive services they provide[96] and whether they follow a harm-reduction approach or require abstinence from substance abuse from clients.[96,98] These differences in implementation may affect consumers' health and housing outcomes.[87] Research is needed that compares the effectiveness of different supportive housing models in maintaining stable housing, decreasing HIV risk behaviors, and improving health outcomes including ART adherence, viral load, and CD4 counts for those living with HIV.

The ability to conform to the original components of the Housing First model is not just a matter of these having been imprecisely defined. Many factors of the social context including housing availability, funding constraints, community partners and local politics, and organizational factors including organizational mission, size, resources, and years of staff training may constrain the implementation of supportive housing programs.[87,93] Whether a site is project-based or scattered-site may depend on the availability of rental housing, landlords' willingness to rent to the chronically homeless, or the demands of the particular funding source. In turn, the number of available units and available housing configurations limits consumer choice. Further, Housing First is an ideal often not achieved in practice. Because supportive housing units are limited, there are usually long waiting lists, and applicants may wait months before obtaining housing.[99] Thus many applicants may enter drug treatment or transitional housing before a unit becomes available.[100]

Perhaps the greatest limitation to PSH as a structural intervention is that it has not yet been scaled up nearly enough to meet the need. As mentioned, homeless families have largely been left out of the expansion of PSH. Nationally, less than 15% of all permanent supportive housing units are available for families.[23] Further, eligibility criteria for family supportive housing stipulate that they must have experienced chronic homelessness, defined as having been homeless for a period of 12 months or experiencing four episodes of homelessness in the past three years and having a disabling condition including a serious mental illness, SUD, or HIV/AIDS. This leaves an enormous gap in affordable housing for low-income families. Indeed, recent research suggests that families with school-age children experience more housing instability than other low-income residents from evictions or other involuntary moves.[101–104] Further, the service needs of formerly homeless low-income families are not being met. Subsidized housing comes with no supportive services and the case management and other supportive services in family supportive housing are often designed only for the adult who holds the lease and not their dependent children.[25,105,106] Further, PSH units are still often located in impoverished and distressed neighborhoods. Neighborhood distress had been shown to be a significant factor predicting HIV risk and infection.[107–111] However, these are also limitations of Housing Choice vouchers or other subsidies to help pay for housing.

Housing Subsidies

Since the mid-1970s, the dominant model for US federal housing policy has shifted from unit-based programs to tenant-based vouchers and certificates. This shift occurred in response to the negative views of public housing, the deteriorated condition of many public housing buildings, and as an effort to de-concentrate poverty in inner-city neighborhoods.[112–115] Since the 1990s, many public housing projects have been demolished and replaced by mixed-income housing. Mixed-income housing is a deliberate effort to construct housing for both low- and moderate-income groups.[116] This type of housing is often the result of private non-profit and public partnerships and can therefore receive funding from federal, state, or local sources. However, while the federal government provides rental assistance to approximately 4.6 million low-income renters, more than twice as many who are eligible for the programs based on income (9.7 million) receive no federal housing assistance.[117] Further limiting low-income and homeless persons access to housing subsidies, the federal "One Strike and You're Out" law (P.L. 104-120, Sec.9), passed in 1996, allows federal housing authorities to consider drug and alcohol abuse and convictions by people and their family members when making decisions to evict them from or deny access to federally subsidized housing, although states may ignore this law.

Housing subsidies have generally been found to increase residents' housing stability and improve housing status. Aidala et al.[9] found that homeless or unstably housed HIV-infected individuals whose housing status improved over time were less likely to use hard drugs, use or share needles, exchange sex, or have unprotected sex at last intercourse as compared to those whose housing situation did not change. Research has also demonstrated that formerly homeless individuals who receive housing are more likely to cease or reduce drug and sexual risk behaviors.[28]

One of the limitations of housing subsidies, besides it being woefully underfunded to meet housing needs, is that subsidies and PSH have not consistently shown that recipients can use vouchers to move into better neighborhoods in spite of its potential to allow residents to move to neighborhoods of their choice.[118] As mentioned previously, neighborhood disorder is strongly and consistently related to HIV risk and prevalence.[107,111] Although some studies have found that housing voucher holders are less likely to live in distressed neighborhoods than public housing residents,[114,119,120] other research has found that voucher holders are more likely to reside in distressed neighborhoods than unsubsidized renter households,[113,119] particularly among African American voucher holders.[113] A study of former residents of Atlanta, Georgia, public housing who were relocated after their complex was torn down using housing subsidies showed that most participants experienced improvements in their neighborhood conditions after relocation in economic disadvantage, violent crime, and male to female sex ratios. Further, they found that participants who experienced greater post-relocation neighborhood improvements experienced greater reductions in partner risk and partner concurrency.[121]

Neighborhood Interventions

Surprisingly few interventions have focused on improving neighborhood conditions to improve HIV risk and retention. Many neighborhood-level interventions both in LMIC and HIC have focused on ways of improving access to HIV testing, prevention, and care within communities that are most affected by HIV.[109,122] For example, Nunn and colleagues conducted locally targeted HIV media campaigns, used outreach workers to administer HIV tests door-to-door, and worked with primary health clinics in affected neighborhoods to routinize HIV testing. Interventions in informal settlements in LMIC have used lay health workers to spread HIV prevention messages, promote HIV testing, and encourage PLH to continue treatment.[61,62] These interventions have been found to be effective in improving and sustaining ART adherence, retention in clinical care, and HIV outcomes.[123]

However, evidence suggests that neighborhood disparities in HIV cannot be explained solely in terms of access to HIV prevention and care.[111] A great deal of research has found that among low-income neighborhoods, those with higher levels of informal social control over public spaces, greater community cohesion, and a sense of community efficacy are less likely to experience HIV disparities.[111] Several interventions have used empowerment and community action to increase these factors both in LMIC countries and the inner-city United States. Examples from the United States include interventions to convert vacant lots and abandoned buildings into public areas such as community gardens and youth action groups, among others. These have shown some effects on sense of community cohesion and community efficacy among those who participate in them.[124,125] To our knowledge, no community empowerment intervention has been evaluated for its effects of HIV outcomes. Within LMIC, most researchers and advocates call for working with residents to improve the living conditions and infrastructure of informal communities, including obtaining land rights for residents.[52,53] Because of the failure of many "top-down" housing approaches which when built were largely unaffordable to the lowest income urban residents and because LMIC, which has few resources to provide housing for all its residents, housing projects have largely been rejected.[53] However, the effects of such community improvements on HIV risk and care has not been studied to date.

HIV Prevention Interventions for Homeless Youth

To our knowledge, no research to date has tested interventions to provide housing to homeless youth as a structural intervention to reduce HIV. A few studies have tested HIV prevention interventions for homeless youth; most of these have focused on reducing individual risk behavior and have shown limited impact on reducing high-risk sexual behavior.[126–130] Interventions that combine case management or substance abuse treatment have demonstrated more promising results in decreasing the number of sexual partners and increased condom use.[131,132]

Applied Example: Comparison of Supportive Housing Models for HIV and At-Risk Chronically Homeless

The Center for AIDS Intervention Research, Medical College of Wisconsin, in partnership with the AIDS Foundation of Chicago and the Center for Health and Housing is currently conducting research to compare the effectiveness of different models of PSH in Chicago on the housing stability and health outcomes of formerly chronically homeless people, including HIV-related sexual risk behaviors, substance use, and, for PLH, their engagement in HIV care and medication adherence. The research consisted of two phases. In the first phase, we conducted semi-structured interviews with key personnel in 30 different supportive housing agencies. In total, 65 in-depth interviews were conducted including 32 directors of supportive housing programs and 35 case managers. At least two participants in different roles were interviewed at each agency. In the second phase, we conducted longitudinal surveys with 889 supportive housing residents in a stratified sample to represent different PSH models to determine the effects of different models and their individual components on housing stability, substance use and sexual risk, and health outcomes.

In-depth interview data were analyzed to come up with a typology of different PSH models and key factors that differed in different PSH models. Details about in-depth interviews and the analysis process can be found in previous publications.[133] Results from our in-depth interview indicate that there are six basic types of PSH in the Chicago metropolitan area.[133] As shown in Table 4.1, supportive housing programs can be categorized as either *project based* or *scattered site*. Within these two broad categories, supportive housing can be distinguished by three different social services models, all of which can be provided in project-based or scattered-site units. *Low-intensity case management programs* are those in which face-to-face case management services are provided less than monthly and the case manager to client ratio is greater than 1:20, often times as high as 1:40 or 1:60.

Intensive case management programs provide face-to-face case management more frequently. Client visits occur at least monthly and often as frequently as once a week. The case manager to client ratio has a maximum of 1:20 and most frequently is 1:15 or less. Finally, the *behavioral health model* is characterized by agencies that specialize in providing housing and case management services for the severely mentally or medically ill. These programs offer a range of healthcare, psychosocial, and other services, many of which are provided by agency staff. Behavioral health or medical models can be further characterized by whether they use *clinical case managers, community treatment services (CTS)* or *ACT.* CTS and ACT are team approaches, and thus it is more difficult to specify a case manager to client ratio since a team of staff members often work with individual clients. Typically, the frequency of meetings between clients and members of the CST or ACT teams are once a week or more.

All of the basic housing models can be further divided by whether they provide social or clinical services in addition to case management

Table 4.1 Social Services Model

	Low-Intensity Case Management	Intensive Case Management	Behavioral Health Model
Project-Based Housing Units	#Agencies = 3 #Programs = 14 #Units = 800+	#Agencies = 9 #Programs = 16 #Units = 330+	#Agencies = 4 #Programs = 7 #Units = ?
Scattered-Site Housing Units	#Agencies = 2 #Programs = 2 #Units = 70+	#Agencies = 17 #Programs = 46 #Units = 1,111+	#Agencies = 3 #Programs = 7 #Units = 184+

and whether case management is provided 24 hours a day. Each of the six types described previously can also differ in the extent to which they use a harm-reduction approach. At the time of the study, although all PSH programs offered immediate housing upon referral from the Central Referral List without any preconditions of drug and alcohol abstinence or psychiatric treatment, PSH programs in Chicago do vary in the extent to which they use a harm-reduction approach once participants are housed. We define *harm reduction* as programs that do not require residents to be abstinent from drug or alcohol use or to comply with a psychiatric treatment program in order to maintain their housing.

Different supportive housing configurations are more common for different service delivery models than others (see Table 4.1). For example, in low-intensity case management, project-based housing is by far the most common type with 88% of the units being project-based. Intensive case management programs tend to be associated more frequently with scattered-site housing, with 81% of the scattered-site units using this approach. These trends are often due to logistics, as it may be more time consuming to track participants in scattered-site housing, thus necessitating lower case manager to client ratios. However, it is also due in part to differences in organizational philosophy which may stem from different organizations' histories and missions. Finally, as shown in Table 4.2, there

Table 4.2 **Multinomial Logistic Regression for Scattered-Site Housing Configuration[a]**

Housing Configuration	B	SE	Wald	df	Sig.	Exp(B)	95% Confidence Interval for Exp(B)	
							Lower Bound	Upper Bound
Scattered Site Intercept	2.091	.372	31.581	1	.000			
SMI	.547	.187	8.572	1	.003	1.728	1.198	2.491
Female Gender	−.912	.194	22.067	1	.000	.402	.275	.588
Years Housed	−.549	.083	44.342	1	.000	.577	.491	.679

Note. SE = standard error; df = degrees of freedom; SMI = severe mental illness.
[a] Forward stepwise with two-way interaction effects.

are more supportive housing programs than supportive housing agencies. In other words, many agencies have more than one program, and some of these programs would fit into different cells in the table.

In-depth interviews suggest that there is no reason a priori to believe that any one PSH model is superior to others as there are advantages and disadvantages to each model.[133] Scattered-site housing offers clients more options of where to live than project-based housing. However, the amount of choice that consumers have in scattered-site housing is in practice limited by housing affordability and landlord willingness to rent to supportive housing recipients. In addition, some case managers felt that some residents were isolated in their new communities and took additional measures to try to get residents to know their neighborhoods. A sense of community was easier to create in project-based supportive housing, as residents and staff organized many building activities. However, project-based housing could also create a sense of re-institutionalization, particularly in the few programs that reported heavy "monitoring" of residents' behaviors. Case managers reported that harm reduction can be difficult for some residents in project-based housing as they may find that others' drug use triggers their own relapses. Finally, while project-based housing facilitated easier access to case managers, this could cause overdependence among residents. Scattered-site housing required considerable travel time for many case managers, which limited their access.

Results also indicated few clear advantages to any particular service provider model. The original Pathways to Housing model promoted use of an ACT team. In our study, very few agencies had programs that used ACT or CST teams. These were large organizations that had historically provided community mental health treatment. For smaller organizations with few residents, ACT or CST teams were impractical due to cost and staffing. Many service providers in low-intensity case management programs wished to decrease their case manager to client ratios, citing the increasing needs of the homeless population they were serving. However, higher client to case manager ratios are possible in project-based housing where travel time is not an issue. In addition, some case managers in intensive case management programs reported that residents' needs decrease considerably over time, particularly if they have resided in the program for several years. A more flexible approach to determining the level of case management, based on client need, may be more cost-effective in the long run. The extent to which programs were able to provide additional "wrap-around" services also varied by agencies' size and missions. Although most agencies partnered with other agencies to get needed services for their clients, access was a problem for mental health treatment with long wait times.

Most supportive housing programs in Chicago used a harm-reduction approach to their clients' drug and alcohol use and psychiatric symptoms, only intervening when behaviors were disturbing neighbors or when they were in danger of being evicted. In these cases, case managers would work with housing management and the client to modify the behavior so that residents could keep their housing. In scattered-site housing, residents were often able to stay in the program even if eviction prevention failed as they were moved into new units. A few agencies rejected a harm-reduction approach and took steps to monitor residents' drug use and punished residents who were caught using by restricting visitors or eviction. Some agencies had both harm-reduction and abstinence-based programs. Case managers of abstinence-based programs argued that there was a need for such programs for those who were trying to achieve sobriety. Indeed, some case managers of project-based harm-reduction programs acknowledged that residents' drug/alcohol use could trigger relapses in those who were trying to remain straight/sober. For homeless persons waiting for housing, it may be difficult to reject any housing opportunity, even if they are not ready to be abstinent. Thus as one case manager reported, many will agree to abstinence-based housing just to get off the street and ultimately end up leaving the program.

Baseline Surveys

We have recruited and conducted longitudinal surveys with 889 supportive housing residents from agencies that participated in the in-depth interviews. We conducted a total of four assessments: baseline immediately after enrollment, and 6, 12, and 18 months after the baseline assessment. We used the typology of housing types to conduct a stratified sample of different supportive housing types to the extent possible. This was limited due to the fact that some models (i.e., scattered site, intensive case management) were far more prevalent than others (i.e., scattered site, low-intensity case management).

Surveys assessed (a) primary outcomes, including substance use, injection and sexual risk behaviors, housing satisfaction and stability; health quality of life; and—among PLH—HIV medical care attendance, CD4, viral load, and ART adherence; (b) personal characteristics that could affect these outcomes, such as mental illness diagnoses and symptoms, HIV, and SUD; and (c) recent episodes of incarceration, inpatient treatment for psychiatric or nonpsychiatric disorders, participation in outpatient mental health programs, and participation in inpatient and outpatient substance abuse treatment programs. In addition, we used the MINI Diagnostic Survey to assess current or past mental illness and SUDs. Other measures included housing satisfaction. Type of PSH program and individual program components (e.g., scattered site versus project based) gathered from Phase I are the main predictors in the analysis.

In order to begin to assess whether the CRS list resulted in less optimal placement of residents with more serious mental illness and SUD, we tested for associations between having a SMI diagnosis, SUDs, or dual diagnosis on housing configuration and service provision. Those in fixed-site, low-intensity case management programs were significantly less likely to report having SMI, SUD, or dual diagnoses. Those in fixed-site behavioral health programs were significantly more likely to report SMI, SUD, or dual diagnoses. The odds ratio for being in a scattered site housing type versus project-based housing is greater for those who met the SMI criteria (odds ratio [OR]: 1.73; 95% confidence interval [CI] 1.20–2.49), less for female (OR: 0.40; 95% CI .28–.59) and less for those who had been in housing longer. The OR for being in an intensive case management versus a low intensity case management housing service type, as shown in Table 4.3, was greater for those who have been homeless the longest (OR: 1.27; 95% CI 1.07–1.49); the OR for being in a behavioral health versus a low-intensity case management housing service type was greater for those who met the SMI criteria (OR: 1.43; 95% CI 1.94–5.76), less for female (OR: 1.20; 95% CI .31– .94), and less for those who have been in housing longer (OR: 0.996; 95% CI .58–.91). Two-way interactions between SMI, SUD, or dual and participant demographics were not significant at the .05 level. Thus it appears that those with more SMI or dual diagnoses are receiving more intensive behavioral health services. Longitudinal analyses will help to determine whether this reflects those who are able to maintain stable housing in different PSH types, in other words whether those with SMI, SUD, or dual diagnoses are more likely to drop out of low-intensity case management programs.

Finally, we looked at housing satisfaction scores for participants housed in each of the PSH types shown in Table 4.4. Different items on the housing satisfaction scale were endorsed by residents who are in project-based versus scattered sites. No significant differences were found in housing satisfaction based on service configuration (high intensity, low intensity,

Table 4.3 Multinomial Logistic Regression for Service Model[a]

Service		B	SE	Wald	df	Sig.	Exp(B)	95% Confidence Interval	
								Lower Bound	Upper Bound
Intensive Case Management	Intercept	.010	.467	.000	1	.983			
	SMI	.359	.231	2.405	1	.121	1.432	.910	2.254
	Female Gender	.185	.218	.724	1	.395	1.204	.785	1.845
	Years Homeless	.235	.085	7.738	1	.005	1.265	1.072	1.493
	Years Housed	-.004	.095	.002	1	.966	.996	.827	1.199
Behavioral Health	Intercept	.830	.561	2.189	1	.139			
	SMI	1.207	.278	18.876	1	.000	1.432	1.939	5.760
	Female Gender	-.610	.281	4.710	1	.030	1.204	.313	.943
	Years Homeless	.111	.104	1.125	1	.289	1.265	.910	1.371
	Years Housed	-.325	.116	7.864	1	.005	.996	.576	.907

Note. SE = standard error; df = degrees of freedom; SMI = severe mental illness.

[a] Forward stepwise with two-way interaction effects.

Table 4.4 Housing Satisfaction by Housing Configuration

	Fixed Site	Scattered Site	P value
The place I live in is close to social services I need.	No 79 (15.9%) Yes 419 (84.1%)	No 86 (25.7%) Yes 249 (74.3%)	.000
The place I live in is close to public transportation.	No 61 (12.2%) Yes 441 (87.8%)	No 27 (8.0%) Yes 312 (92%)	.05
I have enough privacy where I live.	No 105 (20.8%) Yes 400 (79.2%)	No 38 (11.2%) Yes 301 (88.8%)	.002
People often intrude upon my space.	No 357 (71.8%) Yes 140 (28.2%)	No 270 (81.1%) Yes 63 (18.9%)	.002
The place I live in is large enough to suit my needs.	No 183 (36.5%) Yes 318 (63.5%)	No 52 (15.3%) Yes 288 (84.7%)	.000
The place I live in is rundown.	No 417 (83.6%) Yes 82 (16.4%)	No 248 (74.5%) Yes 85 (25.5%)	.001

or behavioral health). Participants who lived in project-based housing were more likely to report that the place they live in is close to social services they need ($p = .0001$), were less likely to feel that they had enough privacy in the place that they live in ($p = .002$), and were more likely to feel that people intrude upon the place they live in ($p = .002$). Those in scattered-site housing were more likely to feel that their housing was close to public transportation ($p = .05$), that the place they lived in was large enough to suit their needs ($p < .0001$), and that the place they lived in was rundown ($p = .001$). Longitudinal analyses will help determine which housing satisfaction factors are related to long-term housing stability and improved health outcomes. We expect housing stability to be a mediator between PSH type and health outcomes, and longitudinal analyses will explore the comparative effectiveness of different models of supportive housing on stability and health outcomes of residents with different mental and physical health issues.

Differences in Risk in Different Low-Income Urban Neighborhoods in San Salvador, El Salvador

Beginning in 2005, our team began research to examine the macrosocial context of different low-income communities in the San Salvador metropolitan area and its relationship to the micro-social context of drug use and sexual risk behaviors (R01DA020350). This research is an example of the kind of work needed to understand the risks associated with different types of low-income communities in LMIC urban areas. San Salvador and its outlying areas have undergone an expansion since the 1950s with the beginning of industrialization. This expansion increased dramatically during the 1980s as a result of internal migration during the war, and displacement from other areas of the city after the 1986 earthquake destroyed many of the *mesones* (i.e., low-income housing for those employed in the informal economy).[134] The development of housing for low-income residents in the San Salvador metropolitan area has followed distinct processes resulting in the three types of low-income community that we compared in our research and that are common throughout Latin America.

Marginal communities are informal settlements and were formed on unoccupied vacant land, often municipally owned, on the banks of rivers or near train tracks or bus terminals. Housing was built on these properties without any central planning or zoning. In the first years of formation of a marginal community, housing often consists of makeshift shelters made of scrap iron and other materials, and sanitation services, electricity, and potable water are often missing. Many marginal communities after several years of existence have gone through a process of legalization with the help of nongovernmental organizations (NGOs) such as the Fundación Salvadoreña de Desarollo y Vivienda. Although this process often results in improvements in the infrastructure and loans from international funders to improve housing quality, such communities are still characterized by residential overcrowding, poor overall infrastructure, poor housing quality, and lack of basic services such as running water or sanitation. In addition, improvements in housing, infrastructure, and services are not uniform and vary considerably among marginal communities, depending on a number of historical factors such as their length of existence, level of community organization, and level of NGO or international support, among others. Marginal communities are populated by residents who work in the informal economy, although they also include residents who work in the formal economy in factories or the service sector.[134–136]

The *Asentamientos Urbanos Populares* (AUP), or "popular urban settlements" were formed as part of a government program in the 1970s that continues to the present to provide low-income housing through loans from the Fondo Social para la Vivienda to low-income workers employed in the formal economy.[137] These communities are often located in the larger metropolitan area of San Salvador, in cities such as Soyapango, Ilopango, and Apopa that are close to the food processing and textile factories of the free-trade zone. Although communities characterized as AUP without exception have access to basic services such as sanitation, potable water, and sewage, these communities are poorly planned and are characterized by residential overcrowding and a lack of recreational spaces.

Finally, *older central communities* in San Salvador have different low-income housing patterns. Prior to the 1986 earthquake many migrants to the capital who worked in the informal economy or domestic service resided in *mesones* in neighborhoods in the center of the city.[134] While much of this housing stock was destroyed in the 1986 earthquake, a number of *mesones* still exist in older central communities, along with other housing options, such as *albergues* (shelters) and motels. Both *mesones* and *albergues* consist of private rooms surrounding communal living spaces. *Mesones* are often of very poor quality and made of adobe. Other low-income residents of these neighborhoods may squat in abandoned buildings. Although older established communities often have basic services such as potable water, sanitation, and sewage, these may not be available in some of the low-income housing (*mesones, albergues,* or abandoned buildings).

Results from qualitative interviews with residents, community leaders and crack users in seven low-income communities (three marginal communities, two AUPs, and three older central communities) differed in their structural characteristics which, in turn, influenced the micro-social context in which drugs were used and sold and HIV risk behaviors occurred.[138–140] Communities differed in their organization of drug selling and drug use. Drug organization varied according to how open or closed drug sales were to noncommunity residents; whether drugs were sold on the street, from fixed sites or from *trances* (places where drugs were used and sold and sex exchanges often occurred); and the participation of crack users in drug sales. Drug use sites included private nonshared spaces, semiprivate spaces such as *trances,* and whether crack users used alone or with other drug users. Drug-selling organization and drug use types together formed three patterns.

In Pattern 1 (one marginal community and one AUP), drug sales were closed to those not residing in the community, crack users played little role in drug distribution, and drugs were used in public or private nonshared spaces. This pattern of drug selling and use was in response to increased police surveillance in these communities and helped drug sellers and users to avoid detection. In both cases, police substations had been established and the communities had a greater than average number of police officers. Community members felt that their communities were being used as demonstration projects in the tough on crime policies being promoted at the time.

In Pattern 2 communities (two marginal communities), drugs were sold mainly from *trances*, although drug users often sold drugs to those who did not reside in the community who waited on main streets in cars. In marginal communities, houses are constructed along narrow pedestrian only *pasajes*, making it difficult for those outside the community to enter without being challenged by residents. Drug use was also most common in *trances*. The difficulty of entering the community, except on foot, also discouraged police presence, and police were easily bribed to turn a blind eye.

Finally, Pattern 3 communities included all three older central communities and were characterized by drug sales on the street, in fixed sites, or in *trances*. Drug selling was open to outsiders as the older central communities were often located in market areas with easy access from major bus routes. Sex work was also common in older central communities, both street level and in brothels. Drug use occurred in multiple locations including on the street, in rooming houses, and in brothels, and sex was often exchanged.

Quantitative surveys were conducted with 444 crack users recruited using respondent driven sampling (RDS). Seeds (n = 22) were selected from each of the low-income communities in which we conducted qualitative studies. RDS resulted in the recruitment of participants outside the original communities. Participants were asked in surveys to name their community of residence and the research team categorized communities as marginal, older central, AUP, or other based on ethnographic knowledge of the areas. Surveys asked participants about their drug and sexual risk behaviors, use of drug use sites, and the social dynamics within these sites.[141] Participants were also offered a free, confidential HIV testing.

Quantitative results verified the qualitative findings that different kinds of drug use sites are more common in different community types. The most common drug use site in AUPs was in private residences while residents of older central communities were more likely to use drugs in public locations. *Trances* were used fairly commonly in both marginal and older central communities but not in AUPs. Motels were used in older central communities but were not used in AUPs or marginal communities. See Table 4.5.

Table 4.5 Type of Drug Use Site Most Common within Community Types

	Marginal Community	AUP	Older Central Community	Other	Between community	
	(n = 83)	(n= 90)	(n = 198)	(n = 48)	Chi-square	Signif.
Drug use site within own community, % (n)	72.3 (60)	80.0 (72)	57.1 (112)	60.4 (29)	16.7 (df = 3)	.001
Sites inside neighborhood	(n = 60)	(n = 72)	(n = 112)	(n = 29)	79.4 (df = 12)	.001
Private residence, % (n)	45.0 (27)	61.1 (44)	6.3 (7)	24.1 (7)		
Public	36.7 (22)	33.3 (24)	61.6 (69)	44.8 (13)		
Motel	0.0 (0)	0.0 (0)	11.6 (13)	6.9 (2)		
Trance	13.3 (8)	2.8 (2)	15.2 (17)	17.2 (5)		
Other	5.0 (3)	2.8 (2)	5.4 (6)	6.9 (2)		
Sites outside neighborhood	(n = 22)	(n = 18)	(n = 84)	(n = 19)	27.4 (df = 12)	.007
Private residence, % (n)	9.1 (27)	27.8 (5)	3.6 (3)	21.1 (4)		
Public	68.2 (15)	27.8 (5)	59.5 (50)	36.8 (7)		
Motel	4.5 (1)	5.6 (1)	13.1 (11)	5.3 (1)		
Trance	4.5 (1)	27.8 (5)	21.4 (18)	26.3 (5)		
Other	13.6 (3)	11.1 (2)	2.4 (2)	10.5 (2)		
Drug use inside versus outside own community						
Chi-square (df = 4)	14.9	20.9	2.9	0.91		
Signif.	.003	.001	.59	.94		

Note. AUP = *Asentamientos Urbanos Populares;* df = degree of freedom.

Risk and protective factors varied among crack use sites. Those who used in *trances*, places where drugs are sold and used, and motels were more likely to exchange sex (p = .000). However, only 13.1% of those who used crack in trances reported that condoms were available in these sites as opposed to 81.5% of those who used crack in motels (p = .000). Whether drugs were used or bought within or outside the community of residence also varied by community type (p < .001). Results are presented in Table 4.6.

Our research also explored community assets that could be used to build a community-based HIV prevention intervention.[65] HIV prevention and care services were concentrated in older central communities, although there were none specifically targeted to crack users. In contrast, there were no HIV prevention campaigns within marginal or AUP communities. Those who resided in marginal communities and AUPs reported that they could receive HIV tests at the Ministry of Health clinics but were reluctant to do so because of fears of stigma, long waits, and mistrust of the Ministry of Health. In fact, 60% of the sample had never received an HIV test in spite of the fact that we found an HIV prevalence rate of 5.6% in our sample.[142] All marginal communities, however, had elected boards of directors that they had formed in the process of legalization.

Table 4.6 Risk and Protective Factors Among Crack Users in San Salvador

	Private Residence (%) (n = 48)	Public (%) (n = 188)	Motel (%) (n = 27)	Trance (%) (n = 61)	Other (%) (n = 18)	Chi-square (df = 4)	Signif.
Gatekeeper control	87.5	21.3	96.3	80.3	44.4	134.6	<.001
Crack sold	10.4	36.2	14.8	95.1	16.7	106.7	<.001
Sex in exchange for drugs or money	33.3	68.6	84.6	78.7	27.8	42.3	<.001
Sex not in exchange for drugs or money	33.3	48.4	65.4	50.8	27.8	10.3	.036
Condoms present	37.5	16.0	81.5	13.1	11.1	66.8	<.001

These boards led to a great deal of community organizing and campaigns, such as clean-up campaigns or replacing lightbulbs.[65]

Based on these results, we developed a multilevel HIV prevention intervention to address some of the barriers to HIV prevention services in the communities (5R01DA020350). The intervention included rapid HIV testing in community sites, social network HIV testing in which crack users received incentives for taking an HIV test and for recruiting their social network members to take an HIV test, community awareness campaigns, and small peer network interventions to encourage HIV prevention norms and behavior. The study used an interrupted time-series analysis of HIV tests taken in community sites before and after the implementation of the Social Network HIV Testing Intervention, and before and after the implementation of the small group Peer Network HIV prevention intervention. We also conducted seven cross-sectional surveys to measure the effects of each component on self-reported sexual risk behaviors timed to occur before and after implementation of each component. Results of the Social Network HIV testing component, in which crack users were offered dual incentives to receive an HIV test and refer other crack users to be tested for HIV, showed a four-fold increase in HIV testing among crack users who may not otherwise have requested services, a result that was highly significant.[143] Results of multiple cross-sectional survey saw a significant increase in exposure to HIV prevention components over time including receiving an HIV testing at our community testing sites, receiving an HIV test after being referred by another crack user in their social networks, and attending the peer-facilitated small group intervention.[144] In addition, exposure to Encuentro components was associated with reductions in sexual risk behaviors such as condomless sex with main and casual partners, and reductions in sex exchanges.[144] Finally, the addition of the peer-facilitated small group intervention led to an additional increase of 10% in HIV testing.

Finally, in conducting our research, we observed that many crack-using participants were literally homeless and sleeping on the streets. We conducted additional in-depth interviews with 28 crack users who were living on the street. Many reported that they were staying on the street because family members no longer allowed them to stay in their homes due to their drug use. In general, participants who were literally homeless used a greater frequency and quantity of drugs. Most interestingly, many reported that they had either been "left behind" to be cared for by other family members when one or both parents emigrated to the United States or that they themselves had been deported after living in the United States for most of their lives.[141] The effects of migration on the global housing crisis warrants further study.

Future Directions

In HIC, access to affordable housing has been demonstrated to reduce HIV drug and sexual risk behaviors and improve health outcomes among PLH. However, there are multiple disparities in who gets access to housing subsidies. In particular, while PSH programs have reduced homelessness among veterans and chronically homeless individuals in the United States, families have largely been left behind in these efforts. Homelessness among families with young children has increased in the past 10 years. Research is needed to elucidate the long-term effects of homelessness on children's future health including their risk for HIV. Interventions to provide access to affordable housing to families are urgently needed. Similarly, the effect of providing housing to homeless youth has not yet been evaluated and interventions to reduce HIV risks among homeless youth have been disappointing.

Most research has shown that housing in PSH programs reduces HIV risk and improves health outcomes for PLH. Some of the exceptions to this trend may be due to the large variety of programs that are captured under the "supportive housing" umbrella. More research is needed to describe the variability in PSH programs and to evaluate which PSH program components result in better health outcomes for residents with different mental and physical health needs. Our team is currently conducting such comparative effectiveness research in one city. Such efforts should be duplicated in other cities that are in different stages of implementing supportive housing. Some states and cities have embraced the housing first approach more readily than others, with some states feeling that such programs may encourage drug use and discourage employment. Research in how supportive housing is implemented could elucidate how the social and political context shapes the form that supportive housing models take.

Research is also needed to explore how social dynamics and physical characteristics of housing affect HIV risk and infection and health outcomes for PLH. Housing characteristics that have been understudied to date include overcrowding, affordability, the relationships with the people with whom a person lives including whether roommates use drugs, and the physical condition of housing. While this research is in its infancy, our team and others have found that factors such as the relationship with whom one lives is an important predictor of HIV. Housing transience also warrants further study. Most research has shown a relationship between greater housing transience and HIV risk and infection. However, most research has not distinguished between positive or negative reasons for moving. Eviction, in particular, may have long-term negative consequences on people's financial well-being, mental and physical health.

An urgent need exists for further research in LMIC countries. In particular, more research is needed to understand how housing shortages have led to different solutions among low-income residents. Informal settlements are but one of many areas that impoverished city residents live. Other housing alternatives include overcrowding in formal housing units in downtown neighborhoods that may be sublet as part of the formal economy. Still other inner-city residents may reside in boarding houses or on the streets. The global housing crisis in urban areas is just beginning to receive research attention and much work needs still to be done to understand the effects of these different housing options on health outcomes.

In LMICs, interventions to reduce HIV or other health risks often focus on improving access to health services in informal settlements. Development specialists advocate for housing and neighborhood improvement by working with residents to obtain legal tenure to their land, thereby obtaining housing and infrastructure improvements. To our knowledge, no research has examined whether improvements in housing and infrastructure have led to reductions in HIV risk. Similarly, in HIC like the United States, neighborhood disadvantage has been found consistently to predict higher HIV risk and prevalence and poorer health outcomes for PLH. If neighborhood conditions are one of the most important social determinants of health, then it follows that improving neighborhood conditions would be a logical target for a structural intervention to reduce HIV disparities.

Housing has been demonstrated to be an effective intervention to reduce the risk of HIV infection and improve treatment engagement and adherence for PLH. The effects of providing adequate and affordable housing, however, are much more far-reaching than their effectiveness in reducing HIV prevalence and incidence. Decent housing in safe neighborhoods with access to potable water and adequate sanitation are basic human rights and efforts to improve housing and neighborhoods in HIC and LMIC would have positive effects on a multitude of health problems that disproportionately affect the poor such as substance use disorders, diabetes, mental illness, cardiovascular disease, among others. It is time to refocus public health attention to improving neighborhood and housing conditions.

References

1. Caton CL, El-Bassel N, Gelman A, et al. Rates and correlates of HIV and STI infection among homeless women. *AIDS Behav*. 2013;17(3):856–864.
2. Hall HI, An Q, Tang T, et al. Prevalence of diagnosed and undiagnosed HIV infection—United States, 2008–2012. *MMWR Morb Mortal Wkly Rep*. 2015;64(24):657–662.
3. Elifson KW, Sterk CE, Theall KP. Safe living: the impact of unstable housing conditions on HIV risk reduction among female drug users. *AIDS Behav*. 2007;11(6 Suppl):45–55.
4. Allen DM, Lehman JS, Green TA, Lindegren ML, Onorato IM, Forrester W. HIV infection among homeless adults and runaway youth, United States, 1989–1992. *AIDS*. 1994;8(11):1593–1598.
5. Culhane DP, Gollub E, Kuhn R, Shpaner M. The co-occurrence of AIDS and homelessness: results from the integration of administrative databases for AIDS surveillance and public shelter utilization in Philadelphia. *J Epidemiol Community Health*. 2001;55(7):515–520.
6. Estebanez PE, Russell NK, Aguilar MD, Beland F, Zunzunegui MV. Women, drugs and HIV/AIDS: results of a multicentre European study. *Int J Epidemiol*. 2000;29(4):734–743.
7. Zolopa AR, Hahn JA, Gorter R, et al. HIV and tuberculosis infection in San Francisco's homeless adults: prevalence and risk factors in a representative sample. *JAMA*. 1994;272(6):455–461.
8. Leaver CA, Bargh G, Dunn JR, Hwang SW. The effects of housing status on health-related outcomes in people living with HIV: a systematic review of the literature. *AIDS Behav*. 2007;11(6 Suppl):85–100.
9. Aidala A, Cross JE, Stall R, Harre D, Sumartojo E. Housing status and HIV risk behaviors: implications for prevention and policy. *AIDS Behav*. 2005;9(3).
10. Auerbach JD, Parkhurst JO, Caceres CF. Addressing social drivers of HIV/AIDS for the long-term response: conceptual and methodological considerations. *Global Public Health*. 2011;6(Suppl 3):1–17.
11. Riley ED, Gandhi M, Hare CB, Cohen J, Hwang SW. Poverty, unstable housing, and HIV infection among women living in the United States. *Current HIV/AIDS Rep*. 2007;4:181–186.
12. Tyler KA, Hoyt DR, Whitbeck LB, Cauce AM. The effects of a high-risk environment on the sexual victimization of homeless and runaway youth. *Violence Victims*. 2001;16:441–455.

13. Mallory C, Stern PN. Awakening as a change process among women at risk for HIV who engage in survival sex. *Qual Health Res*. 2000;10:581–594.

14. Kidder DP, Wolitski RJ, Pals SL, Campsmith ML. Housing status and HIV risk behaviors among homeless and housed persons with HIV. *J Acquir Immune Defic Syndr*. 2008;49(4):451–455.

15. Des Jarlais DC, Braine N, Friedmann P. Unstable housing as a factor for increased injection risk behavior at US syringe exchange programs. *AIDS Behav*. 2007;11(6 Suppl):78–84.

16. Young SD, Rice E. Online social networking technologies, HIV knowledge, and sexual risk and testing behaviors among homeless youth. *AIDS Behav*. 2011;15(2):253–260.

17. Kipke MD, Weiss G, Wong CF. Residential status as a risk factor for drug use and HIV risk among young men who have sex with men. *AIDS Behav*. 2007;11(6 Suppl):56–69.

18. Greene JM, Ennett ST, Ringwalt CL. Prevalence and correlates of survival sex among runaway and homeless youth. *Am J Public Health*. 1999;89(9):1406–1409.

19. Coady MH, Latka MH, Thiede H, et al. Housing status and associated differences in HIV risk behaviors among young injection drug users (IDUs). *AIDS Behav*. 2007;11(6):854–863.

20. Coates J, McKenzie-Mohr S. Out of the frying pan, into the fire: Trauma in the lives of homeless youth prior to and during homelessness. *J Sociol Social Welfare*. 2010;37:65.

21. Larkin H, Park J. Adverse childhood experiences (ACEs), service use, and service helpfulness among people experiencing homelessness. *Fam Society J Contemp Social Serv*. 2012;93(2):85–93.

22. Simonsen-Meehan A, Scholl D. Point-in-time counts mask increase in homeless families living in shelter. 2012.

23. U.S. Department of Housing and Urban Development. 2012 AHAR: 2012 PIT estimates of homelessness. 2012.

24. Gewirtz AH, DeGarmo DS, Plowman EJ, August G, Realmuto G. Parenting, parental mental health, and child functioning in families residing in supportive housing. *Am J Orthopsychiatry*. 2009;79(3):336–347.

25. Quinn K, Young S, Thomas D, Baldwin B, Paul M. The role of supportive housing for HIV-positive mothers and their children. *J Social Serv Res*. 2015;41(5):642–658.

26. Aidala AA, Wilson MG, Shubert V, et al. Housing status, medical care, and health outcomes among people living with HIV/AIDS: A systematic review. *Am J Public Health*. 2016;106(1):e1–e23.

27. Aidala A, Lee G, Abramson DM, Messeri P, Siegler A. Housing need, housing assistance, and connection to HIV medical care. *AIDS Behav*. 2007;11(6 Suppl):101–115.

28. Aidala A, Sumartojo E. Why housing? *AIDS Behav*. 2007;11(6 Suppl):1–6.

29. Kidder DP, Wolitski RJ, Campsmith ML, Nakamura GV. Health status, health care use, medication use, and medication adherence among homeless and housed people living with HIV/AIDS. *Am J Public Health.* 2007;97(12):2238–2245.

30. Smith MY, Rapkin BD, Winkel G, Springer C, Chabra R, Feldman IS. Housing status and health care service utilization among low-income persons with HIV/AIDS. *J Gen Intern Med.* 2000;15(10):731–738.

31. Wolitski RJ, Kidder DP, Fenton KA. HIV, homelessness, and public health: critical issues and a call for increased action. *AIDS Behav.* 2007;11(6 Suppl):167–171.

32. Friedman MS, Marshal MP, Stall R, et al. Associations between substance use, sexual risk taking and HIV treatment adherence among homeless people living with HIV. *AIDS Care.* 2009;21(6):692–700.

33. Sadowski LS, Kee RA, VanderWeele TJ, Buchanan D. Effect of a housing and case management program on emergency department visits and hospitalizations among chronically ill homeless adults: a randomized trial. *JAMA.* 2009;301(17):1771–1778.

34. Gillis L, Dickerson G, Hanson J. Recovery and homeless services: new directions for the field. *Open Health Serv Policy J.* 2010;3(1).

35. Folsom D, Jeste DV. Schizophrenia in homeless persons: a systematic review of the literature. *Acta Psychiatr Scand.* 2002;105(6):404–413.

36. Sullivan G, Burnam A, Koegel P, Hollenberg J. Quality of life of homeless persons with mental illness: results from the course-of-homelessness study. *Psychiatr Serv.* 2000;51(9):1135–1141.

37. Royal SW, Kidder DP, Patrabansh S, et al. Factors associated with adherence to highly active antiretroviral therapy in homeless or unstably housed adults living with HIV. *AIDS Care.* 2009;21(4):448–455.

38. Weir BW, Bard RS, O'Brien K, Casciato CJ, Stark MJ. Uncovering patterns of HIV risk through multiple housing measures. *AIDS Behav.* 2007;11(6 Suppl):31–44.

39. Argeriou M, McCarty D, Mulvey K. Dimensions of homelessness. *Public Health Rep.* 1995;110(6):734–741.

40. Marcus A. *Where Have All the Homeless Gone? The Making and Unmaking of a Crisis.* New York: Berghahn Books; 2006.

41. Dickson-Gomez J, McAuliffe T, Quinn K. The effects of housing status, stability and the social contexts of housing on drug and sexual risk behaviors. *AIDS Behav.* 2017;21:1–14.

42. Dickson-Gomez J, Hilario H, Convey M, Corbett AM, Weeks M, Martinez M. The relationship between housing status and HIV risk among active drug users: a qualitative analysis. *Subst Use Misuse.* 2009;44(2):139–162.

43. German D, Davey MA, Latkin CA. Residential transience and HIV risk behaviors among injection drug users. *AIDS Behav.* 2007;11(6 Suppl):21–30.

44. German D, Latkin CA. Social stability and HIV risk behavior: evaluating the role of accumulated vulnerability. *AIDS Behav.* 2012;16:168–178.

45. Davey-Rothwell MA, Latimore A, Hulbert A, Latkin CA. Sexual networks and housing stability. *J Urban Health.* 2011;88(4):759.

46. Rosenthal D, Rotheram-Borus MJ, Batterham P, Mallett S, Rice E, Milburn NG. Housing stability over two years and HIV risk among newly homeless youth. *AIDS Behav.* 2007;11(6):831–841.

47. Reed E, Gupta J, Biradavolu M, Devireddy V, Blankenship KM. The role of housing in determining HIV risk among female sex workers in Andhra Pradesh, India: considering women's life contexts. *Soc Sci Med.* 2011;72(5):710–716.

48. Dickson-Gomez J, Convey M, Hilario H, Corbett AM, Weeks M. Structural and personal factors related to access to housing and housing stability among urban drug users in Hartford, Connecticut. *Contemp Drug Probl.* 2008;35(1):115–152.

49. Tucker JD, Tso LS, Hall B, et al. Enhancing public health HIV interventions: a qualitative meta-synthesis and systematic review of studies to improve linkage to care, adherence, and retention. *EBioMed.* 2017;17:163–171.

50. Brown VJ. Give me shelter: the global housing crisis. *Environ Health Perspect.* 2003;111(2):A92–A99.

51. Vearey J, Palmary I, Thomas L, Nunez L, Drimie S. Urban health in Johannesburg: the importance of place in understanding intra-urban inequalities in a context of migration and HIV. *Health Place.* 2010;16(4):694–702.

52. Smit W, Hancock T, Kumaresen J, Santos-Burgoa C, Meneses RS, Friel S. Toward a research and action agenda on urban planning/design and health equity in cities in low and middle-income countries. *J Urban Health.* 2011;88(5):875.

53. Stewart J, Balchin P. Community self-help and the homeless poor in Latin America. *J Royal Soc Promotion Health.* 2002;122(2):99–107.

54. Mberu BU, Haregu TN, Kyobutungi C, Ezeh AC. Health and health-related indicators in slum, rural, and urban communities: a comparative analysis. *Global Health Action.* 2016;9(1):33163.

55. Riley LW, Ko AI, Unger A, Reis MG. Slum health: diseases of neglected populations. *BMC Int Health Human Rights.* 2007;7(1):2.

56. Unge C, Södergård B, Marrone G, et al. Long-term adherence to antiretroviral treatment and program drop-out in a high-risk urban setting in sub-Saharan Africa: a prospective cohort study. *PLoS One.* 2010;5(10):e13613.

57. Vearey J. Hidden spaces and urban health: exploring the tactics of rural migrants navigating the city of gold. *Urban Forum.* 2010;21(1):37–53.

58. Kerubo G, Khamadi S, Okoth V, et al. Hepatitis B, hepatitis C and HIV-1 coinfection in two informal urban settlements in Nairobi, Kenya. *PLoS One.* 2015;10(6):e0129247.

59. Vearey J, Richter M, Núñez L, Moyo K. South African HIV/AIDS programming overlooks migration, urban livelihoods, and informal workplaces. *Afr J AIDS Res.* 2011;10(Supl1):381–391.

60. Kyobutungi C, Ziraba AK, Ezeh A, Yé Y. The burden of disease profile of residents of Nairobi's slums: results from a demographic surveillance system. *Pop Health Metrics.* 2008;6(1):1.

61. Scorgie F, Vearey J, Oliff M, et al. "Leaving no one behind": Reflections on the design of community-based HIV prevention for migrants in Johannesburg's inner-city hostels and informal settlements. *BMC Public Health.* 2017;17(1):482.

62. de Snyder, V Nelly Salgado, Friel S, et al. Social conditions and urban health inequities: realities, challenges and opportunities to transform the urban landscape through research and action. *J Urban Health.* 2011;88(6):1183–1193.

63. Buck M, Dickson-Gomez J, Bodnar G. Combination HIV prevention strategy implementation in El Salvador: perceived barriers and adaptations reported by outreach peer educators and supervisors. *Global Qualit Nurs Res.* 2017;4:2333393617703198.

64. Rashid SF. Strategies to reduce exclusion among populations living in urban slum settlements in Bangladesh. *J Health Popul Nutr.* 2009;27(4):574–586.

65. Dickson-Gomez J, Corbett AM, Bodnar G, Rodriguez K, Guevara CE. Resources and obstacles to developing and implementing a structural intervention to prevent HIV in San Salvador, El Salvador. *Soc Sci Med.* 2010;70(3):351–359.

66. Woan J, Lin J, Auerswald C. The health status of street children and youth in low-and middle-income countries: a systematic review of the literature. *J Adolesc Health.* 2013;53(3):314–321. e12.

67. Pinto JA, Ruff AJ, Paiva JV, et al. HIV risk behavior and medical status of underprivileged youths in Belo Horizonte, Brazil. *J Adolesc Health.* 1994;15(2):179–185.

68. Lambert M, Torrico F, Billot C, Mazina D, Marleen B, Van der Stuyft P. Street youths are the only high-risk group for HIV in a low-prevalence South American country. *Sex Transm Dis.* 2005;32(4):240–242.

69. Vahdani P, Hosseini-Moghaddam S, Gachkar L, Sharafi K. Prevalence of hepatitis B, hepatitis C, human immunodeficiency virus, and syphilis among street children residing in southern Tehran, Iran. *Arch Iran Med.* 2006;9(2):153–155.

70. Kissin DM, Zapata L, Yorick R, et al. HIV seroprevalence in street youth, St. Petersburg, Russia. *AIDS.* 2007;21(17):2333–2340.

71. Bal B, Mitra R, Mallick AH, Chakraborti S, Sarkar K. Nontobacco substance use, sexual abuse, HIV, and sexually transmitted infection among street children in Kolkata, India. *Subst Use Misuse.* 2010;45(10):1668–1682.

72. Hillis SD, Zapata L, Robbins CL, et al. HIV seroprevalence among orphaned and homeless youth: no place like home. *AIDS.* 2012;26(1):105–110.

73. Cumber SN, Tsoka-Gwegweni JM. Characteristics of street children in Cameroon: a cross-sectional study. *Afr J Primary Health Care Fam Med.* 2016;8(1):1–9.

74. Avila MM, Casanueva E, Piccardo C, et al. HIV-1 and hepatitis B virus infections in adolescents lodged in security institutes of Buenos Aires. *Pediatr AIDS HIV Infect.* 1996;7(5):346–349.

75. Misganaw AC, Worku YA. Assessment of sexual violence among street females in Bahir-Dar town, North West Ethiopia: a mixed method study. *BMC Public Health.* 2013;13(1):825.

76. Poulin SR, Maguire M, Metraux S, Culhane DP. Service use and costs for persons experiencing chronic homelessness in Philadelphia: a population-based study. *Psychiatr Serv.* 2010;61(11):1093–1098.

77. Pecoraro A, Royer-Malvestuto C, Rosenwasser B, et al. Factors contributing to dropping out from and returning to HIV treatment in an inner city primary care HIV clinic in the United States. *AIDS Care.* 2013;25(11):1399–1406.

78. Lipton FR, Siegel C, Hannigan A, Samuels J, Baker S. Tenure in supportive housing for homeless persons with severe mental illness. *Psychiatr Serv.* 2000;51(4):479–486.

79. Wolitski RJ, Kidder DP, Pals SL, et al. Randomized trial of the effects of housing assistance on the health and risk behaviors of homeless and unstably housed people living with HIV. *AIDS Behav.* 2010;14(3):493–503.

80. Hwang SW, Gogosis E, Chambers C, Dunn JR, Hoch JS, Aubry T. Health status, quality of life, residential stability, substance use, and health care utilization among adults applying to a supportive housing program. *J Urban Health.* 2011;88(6):1076–1090.

81. Slesnick N, Erdem G. Efficacy of ecologically-based treatment with substance-abusing homeless mothers: substance use and housing outcomes. *J Subst Abuse Treat.* 2013;45(5):416–425.

82. Gulcur L, Stefancic A, Shinn M, Tsemberis S, Fischer SN. Housing, hospitalization, and cost outcomes for homeless individuals with psychiatric disabilities participating in continuum of care and housing first programmes. *J Comm Appl Soc Psychol.* 2003;13(2):171–186.

83. Tsemberis S, Gulcur L, Nakae M. Housing first, consumer choice, and harm reduction for homeless individuals with a dual diagnosis. *Am J Public Health.* 2004;94(4):651–656.

84. Collins SE, Malone DK, Clifasefi SL, et al. Project-based housing first for chronically homeless individuals with alcohol problems: within-subjects analyses of 2-year alcohol trajectories. *Am J Public Health.* 2012;102(3):511–519.

85. Clifasefi SL, Malone DK, Collins SE. Exposure to project-based housing first is associated with reduced jail time and bookings. *Int J Drug Policy.* 2013;24(4):291–296.

86. Henwood BF, Rhoades H, Hsu H, Couture J, Rice E, Wenzel SL. Changes in social networks and HIV risk behaviors among homeless adults transitioning into permanent supportive housing: A mixed methods pilot study. *J Mixed Methods Res.* 2017;11(1):124–137.

87. Kresky-Wolff M, Larson MJ, O'Brien RW, McGraw SA. Supportive housing approaches in the collaborative initiative to help end chronic homelessness (CICH). *J Behav Health Serv Res.* 2010;37(2):213–225.

88. Kuehn BM. Medical news and perspectives. *JAMA.* 2012.

89. Dunn JR, Van Der Meulen E, O'Campo P, Muntaner C. Improving health equity through theory-informed evaluations: a look at housing first strategies, cross-sectoral health programs, and prostitution policy. *Eval Program Plann.* 2013;36(1):184–190.

90. Watson DP, Wagner DE, Rivers M. Understanding the critical ingredients for facilitating consumer change in housing first programming: a case study approach. *J Behav Health Serv Res.* 2013;40(2):169–179.

91. Levitt A, Jost J, Mergl K, Hannigan A, DeGenova J, Chung S. Impact of chronically street homeless tenants in congregate supportive housing. *Am J Orthopsychiatry.* 2012;82(3):413.

92. Tsemberis SJ, Moran L, Shinn M, Asmussen SM, Shern DL. Consumer preference programs for individuals who are homeless and have psychiatric disabilities: a drop-in center and a supported housing program. *Am J Community Psychol.* 2003;32(3–4):305–317.

93. Tabol C, Drebing C, Rosenheck R. Studies of "supported" and "supportive" housing: a comprehensive review of model descriptions and measurement. *Eval Program Plann.* 2010;33(4):446–456.

94. Henwood BF, Padgett DK, Smith BT, Tiderington E. Substance abuse recovery after experiencing homelessness and mental illness: case studies of change over time. *J Dual Diagn.* 2012;8(3):238–246.

95. Tsai J, Rosenheck RA. Outcomes of a group intensive peer-support model of case management for supported housing. *Psychiatr Serv.* 2012;63(12):1186–1194.

96. Owczarzak J, Dickson-Gomez J, Convey M, Weeks M. What is" support" in supportive housing? Client and service providers' perspectives. *Hum Organ.* 2013;72(3):254–262.

97. Tsai J, Rosenheck RA. Consumer choice over living environment, case management, and mental health treatment in supported housing and its relation to outcomes. *J Health Care Poor Underserved.* 2012;23(4):1671–1677.

98. Dickson-Gomez J, Convey M, Hilario H, Corbett AM, Weeks M. Unofficial policy: access to housing, housing information and social services among homeless drug users in Hartford, Connecticut. *Subst Abuse Treat Prev Policy.* 2007;2:8.

99. Rosenheck RA. Factors related to rapidity of housing placement in housing and urban development—Department of Veterans Affairs Supportive Housing Program of 1990s. *J Rehabil Res Dev.* 2011;48(7):755.

100. O'Connell MJ, Kasprow WJ, Rosenheck RA. The impact of current alcohol and drug use on outcomes among homeless veterans entering supported housing. *Psychol Serv.* 2013;10(2):241.

101. Desmond M. Eviction and the reproduction of urban poverty. *Am J Sociology.* 2012;118(1):88–133.

102. Desmond M, Shollenberger T. Forced displacement from rental housing: prevalence and neighborhood consequences. *Demography.* 2015;52(5):1751–1772.

103. Desmond M. Unaffordable America: poverty, housing and eviction. *Fast Focus.* 2015;22:1–6.

104. Desmond M. *Evicted: Poverty and Profit in the American City.* New York: Crown; 2016.

105. Lee SS, August GJ, Gewirtz AH, Klimes-Dougan B, Bloomquist ML, Realmuto GM. Identifying unmet mental health needs in children of formerly homeless mothers living in a supportive housing community sector of care. *J Abnorm Child Psychol.* 2010;38(3):421–432.

106. Lorelle S, Grothaus T. Homeless children and their families' perspectives of agency services. *Community Ment Health J.* 2015;51(7):800–808.

107. Adimora AA, Schoenbach VJ. Social context, sexual networks, and racial disparities in rates of sexually transmitted infections. *J Infect Dis.* 2005;191(Suppl 1):S115–S122.

108. Friedman SR, Cooper HL, Osborne AH. Structural and social contexts of HIV risk among African Americans. *Am J Public Health.* 2009;99(6):1002–1008.

109. Nunn A, Yolken A, Cutler B, et al. Geography should not be destiny: focusing HIV/AIDS implementation research and programs on microepidemics in US neighborhoods. *Am J Public Health.* 2014;104(5):775–780.

110. Burke-Miller JK, Weber K, Cohn SE, et al. Neighborhood community characteristics associated with HIV disease outcomes in a cohort of urban women living with HIV. *AIDS Care.* 2016;28(10):1274–1279.

111. Brawner BM, Guthrie B, Stevens R, Taylor L, Eberhart M, Schensul JJ. Place still matters: racial/ethnic and geographic disparities in HIV transmission and disease burden. *J Urban Health.* 2017;94(5):716–729.

112. Newman SJ, Reschovsky JD. Neighborhood locations of Section 8 housing certificate users with and without mental illness. *Psychiatr Serv.* 1996;47(4):392–397.

113. Pendall R. Why voucher and certificate users live in distressed neighborhoods. *Hous Policy Debate.* 2000;11(4):881–910.

114. Anderson LM, Charles JS, Fullilove MT, et al. Providing affordable family housing and reducing residential segregation by income: a systematic review. *Am J Prev Med.* 2003;24(3):47–67.

115. Welch D, Kneipp S. Low-income housing policy and socioeconomic inequalities in women's health: the importance of nursing inquiry and intervention. *Policy Politics Nurs Pract.* 2005;6(4):335–342.

116. Brophy PC, Smith RN. Mixed-income housing: factors for success. *Cityscape.* 1997:3–31.

117. Joint Center for Housing Studies of Harvard University. The State of the Nation's Housing: 2001. December 21, 2006 .

118. Keene DE, Geronimus AT. "Weathering" HOPE VI: the importance of evaluating the population health impact of public housing demolition and displacement. *J Urban Health.* 2011;88(3):417–435.

119. Newman SJ, Schnare AB. ". . . And a suitable living environment": the failure of housing programs to deliver on neighborhood quality. *Hous Policy Debate.* 1997;8(4):703–741.

120. Turner MA. Moving out of poverty: expanding mobility and choice through tenant-based housing assistance. *Hous Policy Debate.* 1998;9(2):373–394.

121. Cooper HL, Linton S, Haley DF, et al. Changes in exposure to neighborhood characteristics are associated with sexual network characteristics in a cohort of adults relocating from public housing. *AIDS Behav.* 2015;19(6):1016–1030.

122. Nunn A, Sanders J, Carson L, et al. African American community leaders' policy recommendations for reducing racial disparities in HIV infection, treatment, and care: results from a community-based participatory research project in Philadelphia, Pennsylvania. *Health Promot Pract.* 2015;16(1):91–100.

123. Nachega JB, Adetokunboh O, Uthman OA, et al. Community-based interventions to improve and sustain antiretroviral therapy adherence, retention in HIV care and clinical outcomes in low-and middle-income countries for achieving the UNAIDS 90-90-90 targets. *Curr HIV/AIDS Rep.* 2016;13(5):241–255.

124. Alaimo K, Reischl TM, Allen JO. Community gardening, neighborhood meetings, and social capital. *J Community Psychol.* 2010;38(4):497–514.

125. Aiyer SM, Zimmerman MA, Morrel-Samuels S, Reischl TM. From broken windows to busy streets: a community empowerment perspective. *Health Educ Behav.* 2015;42(2):137–147.

126. Gleghorn AA, Clements KD, Marx R, Vittinghoff E, Lee-Chu P, Katz M. The impact of intensive outreach on HIV prevention activities of homeless, runaway, and street youth in San Francisco: the AIDS Evaluation of Street Outreach Project (AESOP). *AIDS Behav.* 1997;1(4):261–271.

127. Booth RE, Zhang Y, Kwiatkowski CF. The challenge of changing drug and sex risk behaviors of runaway and homeless adolescents. *Child Abuse Negl.* 1999;23(12):1295–1306.

128. DiCenso A, Guyatt G, Willan A, Griffith L. Interventions to reduce unintended pregnancies among adolescents: systematic review of randomised controlled trials. *BMJ.* 2002;324(7351):1426.

129. Rew L, Fouladi RT, Land L, Wong YJ. Outcomes of a brief sexual health intervention for homeless youth. *J Health Psychol.* 2007;12(5):818–832.

130. Milburn NG, Iribarren FJ, Rice E, et al. A family intervention to reduce sexual risk behavior, substance use, and delinquency among newly homeless youth. *J Adolesc Health.* 2012;50(4):358–364.

131. Slesnick N, Kang MJ. The impact of an integrated treatment on HIV risk behavior among homeless youth: a randomized controlled trial. *J Behav Med.* 2008;31(1):45.

132. Carmona J, Slesnick N, Guo X, Letcher A. Reducing high risk behaviors among street living youth: outcomes of an integrated prevention intervention. *Child Youth Serv Rev.* 2014;43:118–123.

133. Dickson-Gomez J, Quinn K, Bendixen A, et al. Identifying variability in permanent supportive housing: a comparative effectiveness approach to measuring health outcomes. *Am J Orthopsychiatry.* 2017;87(4):414.

134. Stein A. The "tugurios" of San Salvador: a place to live, work and struggle. *Environ Urban.* 1989;1(2):6–15.

135. Zchaebitz U. *Proceso de identificación y selección de tugurizadas a rehabilitar: metodo y resultado.* 1999.

136. Ramirez VA. *Monitoreo y evaluación del componente organizacional y liderazgo del proyecto social de la violencia y delincuenci.* San Salvador: Consejo Nacional de la Seguiridad Publica; 2001.

137. Lungo M. *Economía política de la vivienda en El Salvador.* San Salvador. 2001.

138. Dickson-Gomez J. Factores estructurales relacionados a las drogas y violencia en El Salvador. In: *El impacto de las drogas en la violencia: buscando soluciones.* San Salvador: United Nations Development Program; 2004:111–132.

139. Dickson-Gomez J, Bodnar G, Guevara A, Rodriguez K, Gaborit M. Crack use sites and HIV risk in el salvador. *J Drug Iss.* 2007;37(2):445–473.

140. Dickson-Gomez J. Structural factors influencing patterns of drug selling and use in the San Salvador metropolitan area. *Me Anthropol Q.* 2010;24(2):157–181.

141. Dickson-Gomez J, McAuliffe T, Rivas de Mendoza L, Glasman L, Gaborit M. The relationship between community structural characteristics, the context of crack use, and HIV risk behaviors in San Salvador, El Salvador. *Subst Use Misuse.* 2012;47(3):265–277.

142. Dickson-Gomez J, Lechuga J, Glasman L, Pinkerton S, Bodnar G, Klein P. Prevalence and incidence of HIV and sexual risk behaviors in crack users in the San Salvador metropolitan area, El Salvador. *World J AIDS.* 2013;3(04):357.

143. Glasman LR, Dickson-Gomez J, Lechuga J, Tarima S, Bodnar G, de Mendoza LR. Using peer-referral chains with incentives to promote HIV testing and identify undiagnosed HIV infections among crack users in San Salvador. *AIDS Behav.* 2016;20(6):1236–1243.

144. Dickson-Gomez J. *Exposure and effects of a community-based HIV prevention intervention on crack users in San Salvador, El Salvador.* Storrs: InCHIP, University of Connecticut; 2016.

5

Food Insecurity and HIV/AIDS

Angelina A. Aidala, Maiko Yomogida, and Jennifer Leigh

Overview

Food security is understood to be access, at all times, to enough nutritious food needed for an active and healthy life.[1] The lack of food security is not only an issue of individual experience of hunger or malnutrition but an "intermediary social determinant" of health—the outcome of broader social and economic processes, political, legal, and cultural systems—that shapes the immediate conditions of day-to-day life which facilitate or constrain the ability of individuals and communities to meet their basic needs.[2]

Food insecurity has direct and indirect health consequences and is a leading cause of morbidity and mortality worldwide.[1] In response, global health organizations and the US Department of Agriculture have adopted a structural definition of food insecurity directing attention to the economic and social condition of limited or uncertain access to nutritionally adequate and acceptable food.[3,4] Components of food insecurity include insufficient quality, quantity, or diversity of food intake; inability to access foods of sufficient dietary quality; worry or anxiety over food supplies; and inability to acquire food in socially acceptable ways (e.g., relying on charity, begging, stealing etc.). This chapter summarizes available empirical evidence on the multidimensional links between food insecurity and risk for HIV and outcomes of infection and promising approaches to addressing food insecurity at the individual, community, and policy levels.

Prevalence and Predictors

Rates of food insecurity are highest in developing nations with an estimated one-third of the world population struggling with food insecurity and nutritional deficiencies.[5] Although rates of food insecurity are highest in developing nations, rates are also high in developed nations. For example, one in eight (12%) of US households were food insecure at some time during 2016 with rates much higher among low-income households (38%) and among racial/ethnic minorities (19% among Latino and 22% among black households).[6] Population estimates are similar for Canada and the UK.[7,8]

Food insecurity and the HIV epidemic are inextricably linked. Geographies and populations with food and nutrition challenges are those with high rates of HIV infection. Rates of food insecurity are exceptionally high among people living with HIV (PLWH). Although there have been advances in access to prevention, treatment, and care including nutrition support in resource-poor countries, recent studies continue to document prevalence of food insecurity among PLWH between 65% and 90% in settings as diverse as Haiti,[9] Ethiopia,[10] Senegal,[11] Nigeria,[12] Uganda,[13] and South Africa.[14] Rates in high resource countries such as the United States and Canada are estimated to be between 40% to 70% of all HIV-positive adults, with rates being higher for specific subpopulations.[15-23] Predictors of food insecurity among persons living with HIV include gender, age, low income, depression or other mental health needs, problem alcohol or drug use, and unmet needs for housing and other supportive services.[24] Regardless of subpopulation differences, rates of food insecurity among PLWH are 3 to 10 times as high compared to the rates among the surrounding general population.

Bidirectional Pathways Linking Food Insecurity and HIV/AIDS

As many analysts have observed, these associations between food insecurity and HIV and other indicators of structural inequalities are evidence of the syndemic cycle through which food insecurity and HIV both aggravate and perpetuate each other at the individual, household, and population levels.[25-30] Pathways that link food insecurity and risk for HIV, as well as those affecting course and consequence of infection, include nutritional or physiological, mental health, and behavioral pathways.[25,27] For conceptual analysis of bidirectional pathways between food insecurity and HIV see Weiser and colleagues.[25,31]

Food Insecurity Increases Risk for HIV

Research has shown direct and indirect association between food insecurity and sexual and drug use behaviors that increase risk for HIV infection in both resource poor and resource rich settings.[32-41] Economic and social factors are structural drivers of food insecurity as well as drivers of behaviors increasing risk for HIV (see Figure 5.1). However, studies have shown the effect of food insecurity as an independent predictor of sexual risk behaviors including exchange sex, unprotected anal intercourse, and concurrent partnerships, controlling for education and income indicators, especially among women.[42] Qualitative studies confirm the constrained choices of many women, especially if caring for children, who admittedly exchange sex for money or food.[33] Likewise, food insecurity among drug users is associated with drug behaviors (injecting, sharing injection equipment) increasing risk for HIV—behavioral pathways shaped by broader economic and policy contexts of drug use.[43]

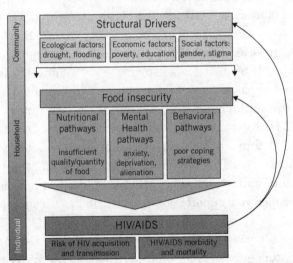

FIGURE 5.1 Conceptual framework for food insecurity and HIV/AIDS linkages
Source: Weiser SD, Young SL, Cohen CR, et al. Conceptual framework for understanding the bidirectional links between food insecurity and HIV/AIDS. *Am J Clin Nutr.* 2011;94(6):1729S–1739S.

In addition to the association of food insecurity and behaviors that put individuals at risk of HIV infection, nutritional or physiological pathways have been identified that further increase susceptibility. For example, micronutrient deficiencies in uninfected, HIV-exposed individuals can impair the integrity of the gut and genital epithelial lining and the differentiation of target cells, as well as cripple other host immune functioning mechanisms, which could, in turn, increase susceptibility to infection.[44,45]

Food Insecurity Is Associated with Poor Outcomes Among People Living with HIV

Among persons diagnosed with HIV, there are nutritional, mental health, and behavioral pathways influencing the bidirectional relationship between food insecurity and HIV morbidity and mortality. Food insecurity and attendant malnutrition have been shown to exacerbate the severity of HIV infection, and HIV infection puts PLWH at a greater risk of experiencing malnutrition.[5,46] When an individual or family member becomes ill with HIV/AIDS and unable to continue the same level of work, loss of income increases the risk of food insecurity, even more so if a productive family member dies.

Food insecurity also affects HIV/AIDS-related physical outcomes through nutritional pathways. Micronutrients such as vitamins A, C, and E, iron, and zinc are all vital for PLWH due to their critical role in immune and other biological functions; however, many PLWH report micronutrient intake levels below recommended levels,[47] findings confirmed by studies using biometric assessments.[21,45,48,49] With increased energy demands and impaired lack of micronutrients to support vital biological processes, malnutrition can increase the risk of opportunistic infections among PLWH. Food insecurity can impact the efficacy of antiretroviral therapy (ART) through biological mechanisms associated with inadequate nutrition, as well as influences on adherence, affecting the health and survival of individuals with HIV even when treatment is available. Lack of sustained viral suppression also contributes to continued forward transmission.[50]

Mental health pathways that link food insecurity and risk for HIV have been well documented in both resource rich and resource poor settings.[51] As is the case for nutritional pathways, poor mental health and food insecurity relationships are bidirectional, and strong correlations between mental illness or symptoms of mental illness and food insecurity have been documented.[52,53] Mental illness (e.g., depression, mood disorders) can limit peoples' ability to earn money for food or to manage daily life to obtain and prepare food—thus increasing risk for food insecurity. A study of pregnant women in North Carolina[54] found that food insecurity was predicted by perceived stress, anxiety trait, depressive symptoms, and external locus of control after controlling for socioeconomic and demographic characteristics. In the Canadian Community Health Survey,[55] mood or anxiety disorder was the strongest predictor of household food insecurity; households with adults with mood or anxiety disorder diagnoses experienced 1.8 times greater odds of household food insecurity.

Food-insecure persons are more likely to have mental illness because of increased stress from not having enough food. This increased stress can lead to depression, chronic anxiety, increased drug and alcohol consumption, and poor overall mental health functioning. A systematic review conducted by Weaver and Hadley in 2009[56] found a strong association between food insecurity and increased mental illness symptoms such as anxiety, stress, and depression from qualitative studies in developing countries. The authors described the qualitative findings by describing "food insecurity as an anxious, stressful, and/or shameful experience." Many of the 11 qualitative studies Weaver and Hadley reviewed focused on women. Food insecurity causes a significant stress for mothers who worry about what children eat. Food insecurity is also a source of shame. People who were forced to pick up food from the trash and parents who cannot afford to buy enough food for children are ashamed of their circumstances. Results from quantitative studies in the same systematic review by Weaver and Hadley suggest a link between food insecurity and symptoms of mental illness, but methodological flaws limit conclusions about direct causation. Among PLWH, Palar et al.[57] investigated the association between food insecurity and subsequent depressive symptoms among PLWH who are homeless or unstably housed in San Francisco. This longitudinal study found that severe food insecurity at a previous time was significantly correlated with increased severity of depressive symptoms after adjusting for confounders.

There are multiple behavioral pathways linking food insecurity to health behaviors affecting management and treatment of HIV as well as behaviors affecting prevention of infection. Health behaviors that may increase risk for poor outcomes among PLWH who are food insecure include sex and drug behaviors but also food-related behaviors such as consumption of cheaper, but nutrition-poor, high-calorie foods.[23,58] Food insecurity and other competing subsistence needs, especially related to housing, are associated with worsened access to and engagement with medical care and treatment regimens—among low-income populations generally, as well as among PLWH.[23,58-61]

Food Insecurity and the HIV Care Continuum

Food security and good nutrition play a significant role in HIV treatment and symptom management. A healthy and regular diet has been shown to reduce negative side effects experienced by PLWH that may further influence nutritional balance, such as nausea and diarrhea.[62] Similarly, food insecurity can play a major role in shaping health outcomes among people living with HIV, specifically in influencing disease progression and treatment efficacy. Recent studies on the health-related effects of food insecurity among PLWH have found that food insecurity can significantly influence both physical and mental health outcomes, as well as access to, and engagement with, medical services and treatment.

Food insecurity has been associated with several HIV-specific and other physical health outcomes. Studies observing the impact of food insecurity on disease progression suggest that food insecurity contributes to worse treatment outcomes, including decreased viral suppression[63] and lower CD4 counts.[64] The overall impact of these HIV-specific outcomes extends to affect overall health and mortality. In a longitudinal study of HIV-positive injection drug users receiving ART, the likelihood of death for those who reported food insecurity at baseline was almost double that of those who did not report food insecurity.[65] This increased mortality among food-unstable individuals was more strongly associated with food insecurity than hunger. The consequences of food insecurity thus not only include those that result from malnutrition but also those that emerge from the psychological instability and unpredictability of living without a dependable food supply. Social factors such as discrimination related to HIV status can influence the ability of food insecure PLWH to access food.[55] In addition, extensive research has shown a relationship between food insecurity and mental health problems, including higher rates of depression,[57] higher severity of depression,[67] and lower quality of life.[68] Indeed, research has found that the impact of unmet subsistence needs can have as great of an effect on mental health outcomes as ART adherence.[69]

Beyond health outcomes, food insecurity plays a major role in engagement with treatment. PLWH who are food insecure are twice as likely to miss scheduled HIV medical appointments.[70] Studies have found that as many as one in four people reported having to choose between accessing food or HIV medication, demonstrating the weighing of health resources necessary for life that occurs among PLWH (such as co-pays or the cost of transportation to obtain medications) who experience food insecurity.[19] Even for those able to access ART, research has shown a negative association between food insecurity and ART adherence, reporting that people who are food insecure demonstrate lower levels of adherence and increased diversion from treatment.[71] The interaction between food insecurity and ART adherence may manifest in complex and dynamic ways. For example, food-insecure patients who were prescribed ART that required food had lower levels of adherence and poorer treatment outcomes.[72]

The effect of food insecurity on ART adherence is even more pronounced in specific subpopulations of PLWH, such as those who are marginally housed or using substances.[73] Among general populations, food insecurity and malnutrition can result in higher rates and longer inpatient stays and more frequent emergency room (ER) visits.[74] The same pattern has been shown among PLWH—food insecurity is associated with increased ER visits and hospital stays, controlling for a range of individual health and service use covariates.[70,75] Food insecurity is not only a biological and psychological problem for PLWH, but it also has significant implications for the healthcare system.

Responding to Food Insecurity and Nutrition Needs

Addressing food and nutrition needs among PLWH or persons at high risk of infection has been recognized since the earliest mobilization of international organizations concerned with social protection and health resources to address the HIV epidemic in developing countries.[1,76] The importance of food and nutrition as a necessary part of treatment for persons with HIV/AIDS was slower to be recognized by major health funding and oversight organizations in the United States and other high-resource nations, but recognition and recommendations have been increasing. The HIV/AIDS Bureau of the US Department of Health and Human Services included a section on the importance of nutrition in supporting the health of PLWH in its 2014 Guide for HIV/AIDS Clinical Care, detailing recommendations for assessing nutritional status and addressing nutrition-related problems. Though it was grouped with other structural determinants of health, nutrition was also recognized as an important structural factor in the 2015 revisions to the National HIV/AIDS Strategy for the United States. The Ryan White Treatment and Modernization Act, discussed in greater detail later in this chapter, recognizes access to nutritious food as a key determinant of health. Further, the Canadian Institutes of Health recognizes food insecurity as an important structural driver of HIV.[77]

However, both the domestic and global response has been primarily direct distribution of food or food subsidies and nutrition education for mitigation of food insecurity and/or nutritional deficiency. The primary types of interventions to address food insecurity have been provision of nutritional supplements or medical tailored food, provision of subsidies to purchase healthy food, and provision of nutritional education and counseling.[78] Recommended, but less common, have been interventions that included *livelihood strengthening*. A review of the United States Agency for International Development's (USAID) Office of Food for Peace food aid program from fiscal year 2003 to fiscal year 2009 evaluated 19 programs providing direct food distribution in 10 countries to PLWH and HIV-affected households for short-term food insecurity mitigation. Inclusion of livelihood strengthening interventions or other provisions focused on achieving long-term solutions to food insecurity were uncommon, and none evaluated outcomes beyond the number of people served.[63] Lessons learned from the earlier phase of direct food provision focused on mitigation include the need to design more comprehensive, cross-sectoral approaches to preventing and resolving food insecurity and malnutrition, including livelihood strengthening and protection.[63] Otherwise, food beneficiaries become dependent on food programs that cannot be sustained indefinitely.

Since 2009, the President's Emergency Plan for AIDS Relief (PEPFAR)/USAID–funded programs have only supported nutritional assessment, counseling, and support (NACS) interventions, intended to encompass the spectrum of activities needed to not only treat food need with nutritional supplementation but also prevent food insecurity by strengthening economic and social protection resources.[76,79,80] Nonetheless, a systematic review of 21 intervention studies in low-resource settings published between 2005 and 2014 found that none of the studies implemented a comprehensive NACS program.[79] As with prior reviews of food and nutrition studies, the evidence was limited for making strong recommendations regarding specific food and nutrition programming to address food insecurity and HIV treatment and health outcomes. The quality of the reviewed studies varied, but equally important the context for programming was very different with regard to baseline food security and nutritional status of household members, stage of HIV infection at diagnosis, resources available at the household, health system, and public services levels, all of which limits cross-study comparisons.[25,37] The authors concluded that based on the limited number of studies of variable rigor and duration, evidence on the impact of food assistance targeted to PLWH and their households show that different forms of food assistance (nutritional supplements, food baskets, vouchers, cash transfers) can have a positive impact on nutritional status and weight, as well as visit and medication adherence; however, impact on disease progression among PLWH and household welfare outcomes needs further study.

Regarding lessons learned from evaluation of interventions to address food and nutrition needs among PLWH in high-resource settings, two recent reviews likewise found little evidence to inform successful models of food and nutrition service provision. McKay et al.[24] identified only five articles, and all were based on studies in the United States or Canada. The main interventions were provision of food through food banks or pantries. None of the interventions addressed broader structural factors to develop resources and resiliency to achieve sustained food security. Although HIV-related outcomes were evaluated, limited sample sizes and cross-sectional designs limited the ability to rigorously evaluate actual impact of the programs. To extend the search for intervention research for review, we conducted a scoping review for any publications through December 2017 and contacted collaborating food and nutrition providers for any unpublished evaluation reports of promising interventions. Five additional studies were identified, discussed next. To add to the currently limited evidence based on food and nutrition intervention studies, we also discuss results from a major observational study investigating need for and response to addressing food and nutrition needs among PLWH in the context of integrated service provision.

Food and Nutrition Services, HIV Medical Care, and Health Outcomes

A research partnership was formed between food and nutrition providers and researchers from the Mailman School of Public Health at Columbia

University. This partnership examined food/nutrition needs and service needs among PLWH to inform program and policy advocacy initiatives. Data were obtained by examining food and nutrition need, service use, and outcomes among a large probability sample (n = 1098) of PLWH in New York City and surrounding suburban counties.[23,58,70,81] Overall rates of food insecurity were high, with over 40% meeting criteria for food insecurity at any interview period during a six-year study period. Over one-half of all study participants received services from a food or nutrition program, most of these (60%) programs were from local community food banks or soup kitchens, with the remainder served by a "medically informed" program indicated by location of services in a medical setting or from a program supported by Ryan White funding, the largest source of government funding in the United States dedicated to the provision of medical and support services for people living with HIV/AIDS.[82] Few programs addressed long-term food and nutrition needs, but analyses shows that 20% to 25% of formerly food-insecure individuals who access services are no longer food insecure by the next interview period (12–18 months later).

To examine outcomes associated with receipt of food and nutrition services, we conducted a series of longitudinal analyses, examining outcomes among PLWH who were food insecure at one interview, received food/nutrition services, and were not insecure by the next interview (referred to here as receiving "effective" food/nutrition services), compared to those who continue to be food insecure.[70]

Food insecurity is associated with worse medical care and health outcomes, and continuing food insecurity is even more strongly associated with poor outcomes (Table 5.1). Previous analyses found that food insecurity was associated with missed medical appointments for HIV, non-adherent ART use or none, ER and hospital inpatient admissions, worse mental and physical health functioning, and unsuppressed viral load.[70] However, formerly food-insecure PLWH who receive food/nutrition services and are no longer food insecure are at much lower risk for these negative outcomes, controlling for a range of client sociodemographic and clinical characteristics and the receipt of supportive services to address co-occurring conditions.[70] For example, odds of missing multiple appointments are one-fourth as high (adjusted odds ratio = 0.26) for formerly food-insecure PLWH who received effective food and nutrition services as for those who continued to be food insecure, and the odds of an ER visit or inpatient stay are about half as high. Receipt of effective food and nutrition services is associated with higher rates of adherent ART use

Table 5.1 Effects of Receiving Effective FNS

	Continued Experience of Food Insecurity or Received Effective FNS					
	Received FNS					
Variable	No	Yes	AOR (95% CI)	β (95% CI)	z	P-value
Healthcare access and use						
Two or more missed appointment, past 6 months	36.0	18.9	0.32 (0.19, 0.55)	—	−4.13	.000
One or more ER visits, past 6 months: %	38.0	25.5	0.56 (0.39, 0.80)	—	−3.15	.002
One or inpatient stays, past 6 months: %	23.0	15.0	0.56 (0.37, 0.87)	—	−2.59	.009
ARV use and adherence						
Adherent ARV use	55.7	67.45	1.82 (1.17, 2.83)	—	2.66	.008
Mental and physical health						
Perceived stress: mean (SD)	6.6 (3.0)	5.3 (2.9)	—	−0.98 (−1.38, −0.57)	−4.73	.000

(continued)

Table 5.1 Continued

	Continued Experience of Food Insecurity or Received Effective FNS					
SF-36 MCS: mean (SD)	41.3 (8.7)	42.9 (8.2)	—	0.69 (−0.48, 1.87)	1.16	.248
SF-36 PCS: mean (SD)	40.9 (11.3)	43.3 (11.7)	—	2.51 (1.22, 3.79)	3.83	.000
Suppressed viral load: %	68.8	76.8	1.30 (0.84, 2.00)		1.16	.244
Viral load >10,000: %	20.8	12.5	0.65 (0.39,1.09)		−1.63	.103
CD4 below 350: %	62.73	56.6	0.67 (0.24, 1.87)	—	−0.76	.450
Sexual behavior						
Number of sex partners past 6 months: mean (SD)	1.4 (4.8)	1.2 (1.9)	—	−0.09 (−0.51, 0.33)	−0.43	.669
Any unprotected sex with negative/unknown status partners, past 6 months: %	14.1	9.09	0.63 (0.36, 1.10)	—	−1.62	.105

Note: FNS = food and nutrition services; AOR = adjusted odds ratio; CI = confidence interval; ER = emergency room; ARV = antiretroviral medication; AOR = adjusted odds ratio; SD = standard deviation; SF-36; MCS = mental component score; PCS = physical component score.

β coefficients are the estimated difference between outcome variable among those food insecure at the previous interview period who received effective FNS (services followed by resolution of food insecurity) and others. P-value is for a test of the effects of FNS, pooling across all follow-up time points while controlling for correlation within person. Analysis based on 453 New York City study participants who were food insecure at one or more interview periods during 2003–2013, 806 observation points. Covariates for this analysis included age, gender, race/ethnicity, poverty level, housing stability, low mental health score (removed for SF-36 MCS outcome), history of problem drug use (cocaine/crack, heroin, or problem drinking), antiretroviral treatment (removed for ARV use outcome), medical case management, social service case management.

and good physical functioning. Viral loads show improvement, but ART medication use is the strongest predictor of suppressed viral load, and increased uptake and adherence to ART was affected by receipt of food and nutrition services.[70,83]

Data are not available that would allow examination of specific service programs. However, results broadly support the recommendation that programs to address food insecurity among PLWH should go beyond providing short-term mitigation of food insufficiency to engage in activities that will improve cross-sector service linkages and the long-term food security and health of PLWH. In the current analyses, programs providing effective food and nutrition services were more often than other food programs classified as "medically informed" (indicating that all would have involved services of a registered dietitian nutritionist to design healthy or medically tailored meals). Food and nutrition providers supported by the US Ryan White program provided the most comprehensive care. They often provided both MNT and food and nutrition services. Medical nutrition therapy covered nutritional diagnostic therapy and counseling services focused on prevention, delay, or management of diseases and conditions and includes an in-depth assessment, periodic reassessment, and intervention provided by a registered dietitian. Food is provided for all or a greater number of meals as needed. Ryan White programs are incentivized to establish service linkages with medical providers and share information with them including tracking nutritional status and HIV clinical indicators. In addition to nutritionists, staffing included case managers or support staff to link clients to safety net providers (e.g., governmental food or income assistance programs). Effective food and nutrition programs likely improve outcomes for PLWH directly by addressing nutritional needs and improving absorption and efficacy of ART as well as indirectly by reducing stress and barriers to care associated with competing subsistence priorities and/or by providing health education and service linkages facilitating access and engagement with medical care.

A Systems Approach to Addressing Food Insecurity and Nutrition Needs

The growing body of evidence linking food insecurity and HIV/AIDS infection and outcomes and the need for cross-sectoral interventions beyond hunger mitigation has led to global policy and program changes. As noted previously, PEPFAR/USAID now supports only programs that adhere to the NACS model, providing a range of activities not only to treat nutritional needs but to enhance food security by strengthening social protection and livelihood resources.[63] In 2011, the UN General Assembly Political Declaration on HIV/AIDS reaffirmed a resolution to integrate food and nutritional support as part of a comprehensive response to the global HIV epidemic.[84] UNAIDS Treatment 2015 provides a framework to scale up and close gaps in the HIV treatment continuum within health and community systems and an expanded understanding of "treatment" to include program activities that address barriers to achieving prevention and treatment goals, including addressing food and nutrition needs.[85]

The emphasis on incorporating food and nutrition interventions with a broader context of structural interventions to achieve HIV prevention and treatment goals is reflected in US domestic policy as well. The Ryan White Treatment and Modernization Act (originally the Comprehensive AIDS Resources Emergency Act), since first enacted in 1990 has recognized the importance of coordinating medical and community-based support services into a system of care and was the first HIV/AIDS program to recognize the vital role of structural interventions to address housing, transportation, and access to nutritious food as key determinants of health.[86] As evidenced by our own previously discussed longitudinal analyses, the Ryan White program has become the gold standard of comprehensive, holistic care for people living with severe and chronic disease. Healthcare reform in the United States required or incentivized by the Patient Protection and Affordable Care Act emphasizes integration of care and new models of care involving health system collaborations with community-level providers of supportive services to improve patient and population health.[87,88]

It is critical to develop and evaluate food and nutrition interventions that go beyond simply remediation of short-term or specialized food and nutrition needs. Although direct provision of nutritious food is likely to be a core service, addressing food insecurity must include addressing contextual or structural factors that limit secure access to nutritious food, including livelihood and/or social protection resources. Figure 5.2 illustrates some considerations for developing food and nutrition interventions using a holistic approach to both address current needs as well as facilitate long-term resolution of food insecurity. Any comprehensive intervention effort would need to attend to cross-sectoral considerations at the community and health systems levels throughout the HIV care continuum.

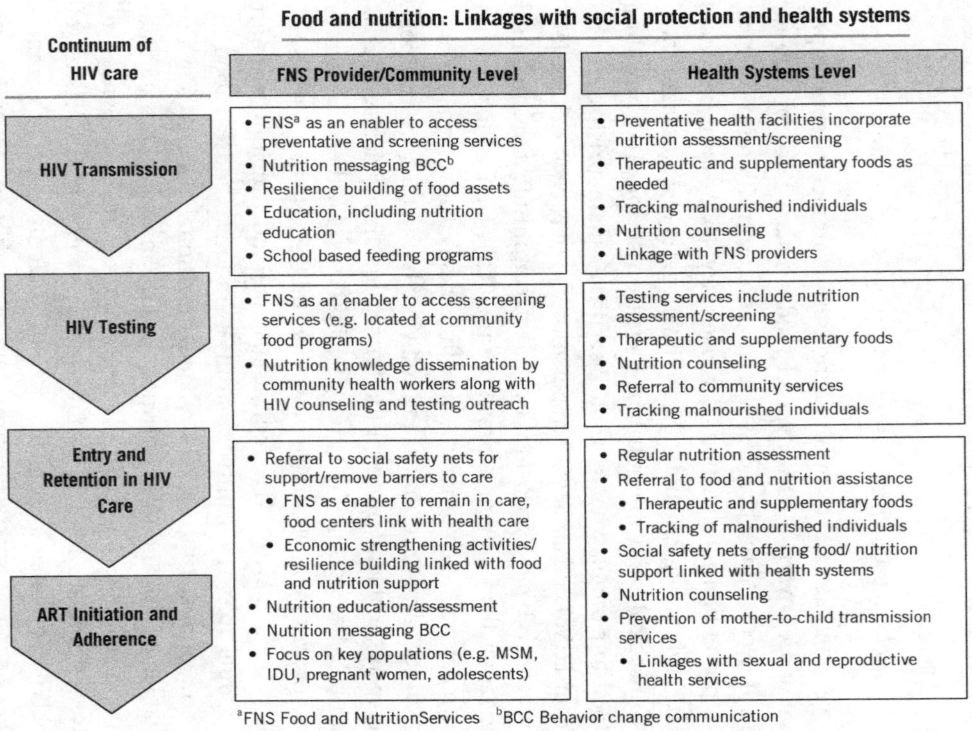

Food and nutrition: Linkages with social protection and health systems

Continuum of HIV care	FNS Provider/Community Level	Health Systems Level
HIV Transmission	• FNS[a] as an enabler to access preventative and screening services • Nutrition messaging BCC[b] • Resilience building of food assets • Education, including nutrition education • School based feeding programs	• Preventative health facilities incorporate nutrition assessment/screening • Therapeutic and supplementary foods as needed • Tracking malnourished individuals • Nutrition counseling • Linkage with FNS providers
HIV Testing	• FNS as an enabler to access screening services (e.g. located at community food programs) • Nutrition knowledge dissemination by community health workers along with HIV counseling and testing outreach	• Testing services include nutrition assessment/screening • Therapeutic and supplementary foods • Nutrition counseling • Referral to community services • Tracking malnourished individuals
Entry and Retention in HIV Care	• Referral to social safety nets for support/remove barriers to care • FNS as enabler to remain in care, food centers link with health care • Economic strengthening activities/resilience building linked with food and nutrition support • Nutrition education/assessment • Nutrition messaging BCC • Focus on key populations (e.g. MSM, IDU, pregnant women, adolescents)	• Regular nutrition assessment • Referral to food and nutrition assistance • Therapeutic and supplementary foods • Tracking of malnourished individuals • Social safety nets offering food/ nutrition support linked with health systems • Nutrition counseling • Prevention of mother-to-child transmission services • Linkages with sexual and reproductive health services
ART Initiation and Adherence		

[a]FNS Food and NutritionServices   [b]BCC Behavior change communication

FIGURE 5.2 Food and nutrition interventions at the food/nutrition service provider, community, and health systems levels throughout the HIV continuum of care.

Adapted with permission from Mehra D, De Pee S, Bloem MW. Nutrition, food security, social protection, and health systems strengthening for ending AIDS. In: Ivers LC, ed. *Food Insecurity and Public Health*. Boca Raton, FL: CRC Press; 2015: 69–89.

This framework, adapted from Mehra et al.,[89] suggests points for interventions at the levels of food and nutrition service provider, the broader community, and health systems throughout the HIV continuum of care. This framework serves as a focal point to discuss current promising models of care that have shown positive outcomes with regard to healthcare and health outcomes, as well as increased food security for PLWH or those at risk of HIV infection.

Types of Food and Nutrition Services

The interventions described in this section are examples of service provision that address variations in type of food assistance appropriate for client health needs. At the broadest level, food and nutrition services can serve as a prevention intervention. Because risky sex or drug behaviors as well as immunological and other physiological changes associated with food insecurity and malnutrition increase risk for HIV, providing healthy food to persons who are food insecure or malnourished can reduce risk for HIV. Food assistance to persons who may be at risk for HIV but not infected is typically provided by general community food and meal programs rather than programs providing medically tailored food or nutrition supplements. Such programs are often widely distributed and have access to vulnerable communities and individuals and thus are in a position to serve as "enablers" of screening for serious dietary deficiencies as well potentially testing for HIV and other illnesses. Further, this access facilitates linkages to other service providers and the healthcare system.

Once diagnosed with HIV, food assistance and nutrition support can play a dual role—as a nutritional intervention to address food insecurity and pre-existing or HIV-related nutritional deficits but also as an enabler to linkage and retention in HIV medical care and adherence to treatment. There are different approaches to provision of medically appropriate food and nutrition services for PLWH, all of which include activities to provide or to link clients to other community services such as safety net providers or livelihood strengthening resources, as well as link with healthcare providers. Types of services include HIV-targeted or HIV-sensitive community food distribution centers or voucher programs for those who are least impaired physically and have resources for food preparation and storage and/or to travel to food distribution sites. *Congregate meal programs* offer nutritional supplements or healthy meals in a group setting. Not only do congregate programs address nutritional needs and increase clients' strength so they can better perform activities of daily living and take and absorb their medications, these programs can also serve to break the isolation of PLWH by providing opportunities to socialize and receive mutual support.[90,91] They can also serve as a site for implementation of additional programming as well as a gateway to additional care services including linking with healthcare systems.

For those whose disease has progressed, or who suffer from disabling comorbidities, home-delivered meals or home-delivered nutritional supplements and food products can be designed to complement their medical treatment. Home-delivered meals or food resources are vital for PLWH who lack the ability to produce or purchase food or meals for themselves or to travel to food distribution centers. Home-delivered food programs ensure that these clients, who are often unable to accomplish the normal activities of daily living, continue to receive the nutrition their condition demands, so that they are able to remain in their home and adhere to their medication regimen. Home-delivered meal providers serve the sickest of the sick, and, without them, many PLWH face increased mortality risk. Home visits can serve multiple additional functions including nutritional education delivered by trained community health workers and monitoring and referral to medical and other services. Home-delivered meal providers are often the first to know if something is wrong with a client given that they visit regularly.

Specific Practice Examples

The awareness of the potential for general food assistance programs to contribute to the fight against HIV has long been recognized by international food relief organizations. For example, the USAID Office of Food for Peace 2006–10 Strategic Plan outlines a number of activities within "food assistance" that go beyond remediation of malnutrition tailored to PLWH or a high risk of infection.[76,92] Supported activities include:

- providing food as an incentive for counseling and testing,
- reducing risky behaviors, using food assistance to incentivize those infected to enter and adhere to medical care and ART treatment,
- supporting community health workers to provide additional care services in addition to food in the home, including home-delivered ART or other medications.

Evaluation results of interventions are methodologically limited but promising (for more information see reviews by Tang et al.[79] and dePee et al.,[5] as well as Van Haeften and colleagues'[76] evaluation of USAID FFA programs).

High-resource countries have had greater awareness of the potential for general hunger relief and programs to serve as strategic intervention sites to address not only food needs but to deliver preventative care and link clients with needed medical care and supportive services. A number of innovative programs have begun in the United States that include partnerships between food banks and healthcare providers to support routine health screenings and needs assessment to food pantry clients and offer those at risk for or living with chronic illness additional services. A promising practice example is the Feeding America Diabetes Initiative.[93] Feeding America is the largest hunger-relief organization in the United States, with 200 food banks and 60,000 food pantries and food programs across the nation. The organization has expanded its mission beyond addressing immediate food needs to also address health more broadly as well as to strengthen pathways out of food insecurity.

As part of the Feeding America initiative, clients coming to food pantries who screen positive for diabetes are offered a "diabetes-friendly" food box containing whole grains, fruits and vegetables, lean meat, and low-fat dairy foods to help them make good choices for their meals. They also access health education classes and diabetes handouts along with nutrition tips and recipes for using the food items in the box. Clients without a regular source of medical care are referred to a local provider who can make sure they get healthcare services, including medication and blood sugar testing supplies, that they need to manage their disease. As part of the project, physicians in the area are trained to talk to their diabetes patients about food access, recognizing that they cannot manage their health if they do not eat the right foods, and they are trained to refer patients to food pantries if they need assistance to afford healthy food.

A pilot test completed at three sites has shown feasibility of screening for diabetes and providing healthy food, healthcare linkages, and other diabetes supports for low-income, food-insecure clients at three food banks. Outcomes included improved diet, improved adherence to treatment regimen, and improved glycemic control. Analysis indicated that the intervention served to reduce cost tradeoffs between purchasing food and paying for medical costs.[94] A clinical research trial is underway to formally test the intervention.

A related approach is "food prescription" programs wherein food-insecure clients receive a prescription from their medical provider that suits their dietary needs. Boston, Massachusetts' Medical Center's Preventive Food Pantry,[95] opened in 2001, brings together primary and specialty medical care with on-site medically tailored food pantry services. Most patients who visit the pantry are at risk for or have chronic diseases. Repeated nutritional and dietary assessments are part of the program. The Food Pantry also offers healthy cooking classes, demonstrating how to cook meals that meet the patients' doctor-recommended nutritional needs.

Other food prescription programs are based on the same model of physician prescription for healthy food but operate outside of the healthcare setting. Clients use prescriptions to receive certain foods at markets (e.g., contracted farmers market and super markets). The Wholesome Wave Produce Prescription program[96] (FVRx) is an example of a food program that has partnered with local medical systems to provide patients with fruit and vegetable "prescriptions." Participating providers enroll patients into the program for four to five months at a time. Doctors and nutritionists provide $1/day per household member in produce prescriptions, which can be redeemed for fresh produce at participating markets and grocery stores.

Another form of assistance programming is known as congregate meal or group feeding programs. These offer a number of advantages for addressing health, mental health, and social support needs beyond addressing food insecurity and nutritional insufficiency. Group settings can facilitate health interventions, especially in low-resource settings where limited expertise may be available for health assessments or educational interventions and facilitating service linkages. Time and resource efficiencies are an advantage of reaching multiple individuals who might benefit from additional care services. Group settings can also provide peer supports that may increase openness to new practices and contribute to positive behavioral change, as well as potentially reducing isolation and stigma associated with HIV status. For example, a group session–based intervention among HIV-infected women in rural India provided nutritional supplements and brought together trained community health workers who provided health education and care and support for accessing existing health services and livelihood resources. The group-setting intervention was associated with improved ART adherence and CD4 counts as well as improved nutritional status.[90]

A promising congregate meal intervention in the United States, Project Open Hand,[97] is informed by the Food is Medicine Coalition,[98] a movement of food and nutrition services providers serving persons with HIV and other chronic illness and advancing public policy that supports access to medically tailored food and nutrition services as a component of medical treatment. The Open Hand, Food = Medicine intervention and evaluation was a collaborative project between Project Open Hand, a meal program in the San Francisco area, and researchers from the University of California San Francisco. Project Open Hand provides three medically tailored meals daily and snacks at 21 dining rooms. The project assists those with AIDS/HIV and other critical illnesses as well as seniors with disabilities. All clients receive nutrition and wellness assessments from registered dietitians who are also available for regular check-ins and advice and assistance with other supportive services such as contracting with a local ride service to ensure clients have transportation to their meal programs. The evaluation of Open Hand's Food = Medicine intervention targeting persons with HIV and/or type 2 diabetes documented positive changes in nutritional and health indicators assessed before and after a six-month period. The intervention provided meals and snacks that compromised 100% of daily caloric requirements and met nutritional guidelines for a healthy diet based on clients' health condition. Amongst study completers, 23 had HIV, 22 had type 2 diabetes mellitus, and 7 had both. Comparing baseline to follow-up, very low food insecurity decreased from 59% to 12%. Statistically significant decreases in symptoms of depression and binge drinking and, among PLWH, adherence to ART increased from 47% to 70%. Benefits of group interaction and support were not measured directly, but, in addition to reduction in symptoms of depression, participants reported reduction in illness-related distress, increased confidence in disease self-management, and, for PLWH, reduction in internalized HIV stigma. Health behaviors improved; in particular tradeoffs were managed more efficiently between spending money on food or healthcare expenses. Use of acute care services (ER visits, hospital inpatient stays) decreased, indicating the potential for significant savings of avoidable healthcare costs.

Yet another type of food assistance approach is home delivery of medically tailored meals and nutrition services. This approach is both a response to a debilitating acute or chronic illness and a preventative measure. Distinct from programs that may deliver food or nutritional supplements to prevent hunger, medically tailored meals are designed to meet specific health goals, identified by a medical provider, of individuals who are unable to provide or prepare appropriate meals for themselves. Programs that provide home-delivered, medically tailored meals address the connection between nutrition and illness most directly. Such services play a crucial role in keeping medically vulnerable people living with HIV (and other chronic illness), alive, healthy, and at home in their communities.

God's Love We Deliver (GLWD) based in New York City has been a leader in HIV nutrition from the earliest days of the epidemic, helping to develop guidelines and best practices for responding to the nutritional needs of PLWH.[99] From its beginning in 1986 delivering restaurant-donated meals by bicycle to homebound PLWH, GLWD now delivers 7,000 meals per day throughout New York City and nearby suburban counties. Meals are individually tailored to meet the nutritional needs of each client and provided free of charge. Medical tailoring begins with medical nutrition therapy (MNT) provided by one of seven licensed registered dietitian nutritionists on staff. MNT covers nutritional diagnostic therapy and counseling services focused on prevention, delay, or management of diseases and conditions and involves an in-depth assessment, periodic reassessment, and intervention as needed. This includes an assessment of nutritional needs, nutritional status, preferences, and food patterns; development of a nutritional treatment plan, including planning for the provision of food and drink appropriate for the individual's physical and medical needs and environmental or cultural conditions; and the provision of nutrition education and counseling for clients and their families. GLWD does not put clients "on specific diets" per se. The goal of the program is for individuals to eat the greatest variety of meals possible and to stay nourished, providing the least restrictive, most varied diet possible within restrictions that may be medically indicated.

GLWD strives to provide food with "love," as their name indicates, which helps address the psychological as well as nutritional needs of their clients. A visit every day from a meal delivery volunteer may be the only social interaction a patient has for the week. In addition to daily meals, GLWD provides special meals for holidays plus a guest meal so that clients can invite a family member or friend to share holiday time with them. Clients receive a personalized birthday cake and greeting cards created by local schoolchildren on their birthday. Breakfast, dinner, and snacks are provided for any children in the household—realizing that when a parent is very ill, the entire family's nutrition needs are compromised and that food-insecure parents will give their meals to the children. Additional meals are also provided to senior caregivers living with GLWD clients.

There are strong links between GLWD and medical care systems. Clients require a medical diagnosis to be eligible for services and nutritionists are in contact with medical providers to discuss medical and nutritional needs. In addition, realizing that many clients may have multiple service needs beyond food issues, GLWD maintains referral relationships with over 50 public agencies and community service providers and works closely with clients to refer them to nearby supportive service providers.

A unique feature of GLWD is the essential role of volunteers. The entire program operates with a small professional staff and the assistance of 10,000 volunteers annually who help with food preparation and delivery. Another distinctive feature of GLWD is its long history of advocacy in support of food and nutrition programs for people living with HIV/AIDS, as well as their history of fighting for understanding and funding support for medically tailored food and nutrition services as a medical intervention for all persons with serious chronic illness. GLWD is the convener of the national Food is Medicine Coalition, bringing together nonprofit, medically-tailored food and nutrition service providers from across North America for the purpose of advancing public policy that supports increasing access to food and nutrition services for persons with HIV or other severe illnesses; promoting research on the efficacy of food and nutrition services on health outcomes and cost of care; and sharing best practices in the provision of medically tailored meals and nutrition education and counseling. The ultimate goal of the Food is Medicine Coalition is to change the structure of resources available to individuals and communities by securing opportunities for reimbursement for food and nutrition services in the public and private healthcare systems, both as these systems exist currently and as they continue to evolve according to healthcare reform efforts.

Efforts continue on many fronts to address social and economic determinants of health that would reduce need for food assistance, as well as expand sources of payment for food and nutrition services when needed. Cross-sector linkages with safety net resources and interventions to strengthen livelihood resources are starting points. Among the program examples described here—Feeding America, Project Open Hand, and GLWD—models of care all include establishing and enhancing cross-sector service linkages with social protection and healthcare providers in the attempt to facilitate system change to improve the conditions of day-to-day life and to reduce food insecurity more broadly defined. However, none directly provide a livelihood-strengthening activity. There are, however, developing program models that address training or other employment or livelihood skills for a longer term solution to food insecurity.

As PLWH are living longer in good health, it is likely that employment skills training as a component of interventions to address food insecurity will become more common. For example, several food and nutrition providers who are partners in the Food is Medicine Coalition support job training programs. Community Services (Massachusetts and Rhode Island) offers to their clients a free 12-week job training program in food service industry. The Open Door has programs in culinary arts and retail for youth between 16 and 21. Harland Alliance (Illinois) provides job trainings through an 11-week Chicago FarmWorks Transitional Jobs program in which participants receive wages working at a farm while completing educational curriculum and receiving job placement support. Both the US and global community of food and nutrition providers increasingly address food insecurity among their clients by providing nutritious food as an immediate solution but also providing service linkages and transferable job skills as a long-term solution.

Promising Multisectoral Interventions in Low-Resource Settings

Recent interventions, one in Malawi and another in Kenya, are good examples of food and nutrition interventions that go beyond short-term mitigation of food insecurity to include both linkages with safety net providers and livelihood strengthening. The Savings, Agriculture, Governance, and Empowerment for Health (SAGE4Health) study[100] evaluated a multilevel intervention in rural Malawi that aimed to improve health and HIV outcomes through a focus on economic and food security. The SAGE4Health intervention was implemented by the CARE International, a nongovernmental organization with the dual goals of improving dietary diversity through trainings in sustainable agriculture and breaking the cycle of poverty through microfinancing programs. The study consisted of four parts: (a) implementing Farmer Field Schools in over 9,000 households, (b) forming 443 Village Savings and Loans Groups, (c) capacity-building trainings and meetings, and (d) training incorporating HIV education and gender empowerment. At the 18-month and 3-year follow-up, intervention recipients demonstrated decreased food insecurity, increased nutritional diversity, and improved economic resilience. In addition, increases in HIV testing and case finding were also observed. The promising results of the SAGE4Health intervention demonstrate the close link between poverty, food security, and poor health outcomes and the need to consider all three of these mediators in intervention design and implementation.

The Shamba Maisha multisectoral intervention conducted in rural Kenya among HIV-infected individuals provides an excellent example of such intervention design and implementation.[27] This study combined agricultural and financial components, driven by demands for more sustainable approaches that address the fundamental causes of food insecurity. The intervention consisted of three components: (a) microfinance loans, (b) provision of pumps that enabled farmers to irrigate crops year-round, and (c) agricultural and financial management training sessions. At a 12-month follow-up, participants in the intervention group demonstrated a statistically significant increase in CD4 + cell counts, as well as significant improvements in food security and frequency of food consumption. Improvements in nutritional, mental health, and behavioral mechanisms contributing to improved outcomes were documented.[27,101] Results of the intervention highlight both the relationship between food security and HIV-related health outcomes as well as the importance of interventions that address immediate needs for food and nutrition but that also target structural drivers of food insecurity.

Cost Considerations

Any attempt to change policy, practice, structures of economic opportunity, and service provision in health and social protection sectors will need to address the issue of cost—both for specific interventions and for scale-up. Unfortunately, information about cost and cost-effectiveness of food and nutrition intervention for persons at-risk for or living with HIV is very limited. There have been efforts using data from studies in Zambia, Uganda, and Mozambique to evaluate costs of including nutritional supplementation as part of clinical care for HIV-positive adults on ART. Estimates range from US$20 to US$60 additional cost per three months based on type of supplement.[102] Considering only mortality benefit, Koethe and colleagues[103] estimate that to attain cost-effectiveness parity with treatment with ART alone, a supplement would need to cost an average of $10.99 per quarter and confer a 20% reduction in both six-month mortality and loss to follow-up. Authors concluded that this threshold would be met for seriously malnourished individuals starting ART (body mass index [BMI] <16.0 kg/m^2) but may not be cost-effective among those in higher BMI strata. However, as they acknowledge, their analysis did not consider cost implications of benefits derived from food assistance for ART adherence. Further, the analysis did not consider additional public-sector health costs associated with food-insecure patients not receiving supplements who are at increased risk of dropping out of care and entering the hospital with advanced disease. Regardless of costs of any specific intervention, the general conclusion of USAID and other international donor programs is that ongoing provision of food assistance to PLWH without addressing broader structural factors that limit self-sufficiency cannot be sustained indefinitely as prevalence increases and HIV-positive individuals live longer lives.[70] Provision of supplementation at a program level will require additional expenditures at a time when many countries are challenged to meet the expanding need for ART services.

Regarding cost threshold and cost effectiveness estimates for food and nutrition services in the United States or Canada, some estimates exist based on comparing cost of services with published information on average costs of healthcare services. For example, the Food is Medicine Coalition collected information on average costs for medically tailored meals among partnering food providers.[98] More than three months of three medically tailored meals per day and supportive services could be provided for the average cost of a single emergency room visit in the United States, which is over $2,000. The cost of three meals a day for an entire year is less than the average cost of an inpatient hospital at $9,700 (all payors).[104,105]

A pilot study of healthcare cost savings associated with the provision of medically tailored meals for adults with HIV and other chronic illnesses was undertaken by MANNA, a food and nutrition provider in Philadelphia, Pennsylvania, in collaboration with researchers from the Center for Collaborative Learning.[106] MANNA serves three medically tailored home delivered meals a day, seven days a week, with no cost to clients. Overtime healthcare costs for 65 MANNA clients were compared with costs for a group of Medicaid recipients matched on gender, age, race, ethnicity, and clinical status.[106] Medical claims data were used to track service utilization and costs. Among the entire group of MANNA clients, average monthly costs dropped from $38,937 to $28,183 when comparing six months prior to six months after receiving services. The average monthly cost for comparison group members' six-month period after baseline was $41,000. Among the HIV-positive subset of MANNA clients (n = 28), mean monthly costs for all health services over the six-month period after starting MANNA food and nutrition services were $16,765 compared to comparison group members living with HIV (n = 300), whose mean medical costs during the same time period were $37,287. Differences were driven by greater numbers and longer length of stay for inpatient care and more discharges to acute care facilities among comparison group members.[99] Despite small sample sizes and other limitations, results of the MANNA intervention study provide encouraging evidence for health and quality of life outcomes for patients, as well as healthcare cost savings, associated with the provision of medically tailored food and nutritional services to patients with HIV and other chronic illness.

Looking Ahead: Next Steps Toward Ending AIDS

The research evidence is clear and consistent: in both resource-limited and high-resource nations, food insecurity increases risk for HIV infection, and HIV infection increases risk for food insecurity. Among persons diagnosed with HIV, food insecurity and unmet nutritional needs are associated with worse medical care, poor functional health, and poor clinical health outcomes. PLWH who are food insecure are less likely to access HIV treatment, remain in care, or remain adherent to their ART regimen. They are less likely to achieve sustained viral suppression, and they are at higher mortality risk. Pathways that link food insecurity and risk for HIV as well as affect course and consequence of infection include direct nutritional or physiological mechanisms and indirect mental health and behavioral pathways.

Addressing food and nutrition needs among PLWH or persons at high risk of infection has been recognized as important since the earliest mobilization of national and international resources to address the HIV epidemic. However, responses in developing and high-resource nations have primarily focused on food distribution or nutritional supplementation for mitigation of nutritional deficiencies—this despite the growing recognition internationally of the social determinants of health and awareness that food insecurity is not only an issue of individual experience of hunger or malnutrition but the outcome of broader social, political, and economic processes which facilitate or constrain the ability of individuals and communities to meet their basic needs. Current major HIV funding and oversight organizations in the United States and globally now emphasize (or require) cross-sectoral interventions at the community and health systems level encompassing activities needed to not only provide nutritional supplementation but also to prevent food insecurity by strengthening social protection and livelihood resources.

Regarding lessons learned from evaluation of interventions to address food and nutrition needs as HIV prevention or treatment interventions, rigorous research has been limited. When evaluated, results of earlier efforts focused on distribution of food or nutritional supplementation found heterogeneous effects on HIV treatment retention, ART adherence, and health outcomes. More recent interventions that encompass a wider spectrum of activities addressing nutritional needs, and also broader determinants of food security by strengthening economic and social protection resources, show substantial promise. Although differences in target populations, implementation contexts, and specific programmatic activities complicate attempts to draw strong recommendations about specific programs, results suggest that cross-sectoral, multilevel interventions are showing positive outcomes for HIV risk and prevention behaviors, engagement in care and ART adherence, HIV health outcomes, reduced potential for forward transmission, and healthcare cost savings.

An important insight is how food programs can serve as "enablers" at each stage of the HIV care continuum. Provision of food and nutrition services helps reduce opportunity costs (time, money, stigma) associated with risk avoidance, accessing testing, engagement with care, and treatment adherence. Regardless of other life challenges, individuals who are food insecure "will come;" they will seek assistance with food and other subsistence needs. This makes food programs ideal points of intervention for delivery of a range of health promotion and disease prevention services—through expansion of services provided by food and nutrition providers themselves or via linkages with healthcare systems. In turn, HIV clinical care settings are strategic sites for a systematic screening and linkage of food insecure PLWH to community providers that address food security and other basic needs, with benefits for adherence and retention in medical care among vulnerable populations. However, for this potential to be realized, system-level changes are needed in program practice to support cross-sectoral collaborations, as well as policy changes, especially with regard to funding to facilitate such collaborations and service integration.

Going forward, it is crucial to develop and evaluate food and nutrition interventions within the broader context of structural interventions that address social determinants of heath. Cross-sectoral interventions at the community and health systems levels that include assessment and monitoring of food and other supportive service needs (e.g., housing), provide health education/ behavioral change communication, and provide or link with other providers to enhance livelihood and/or social protection resources hold the most promise. Indeed, it is difficult to remain hopeful about ending AIDS without understanding and addressing food security as the outcome of broader political, legal, economic, and social systems that shape the immediate conditions of day-to-day life and facilitate or constrain the ability of individuals and communities to meet their basic needs.

References

1. Food and Agriculture Organization of the United Nations, International Fund for Agricultural Development, the United Nations Children's Fund, World Food Programme, World Health Organization (.*The State of Food Security and Nutrition in the World 2017: Building Resilience for Peace and Food Security*. Rome: Food and Agriculture Organization of the United Nations; 2017.

2. Solar O, Irwin A. *A Conceptual Framework for Action on the Social Determinants of Health*. Geneva: World Health Organization; 2010.

3. Bickel G, Nord M, Price C, Hamilton W, Cook J. *Guide to Measuring Household Food Security, Revised 2000*. Alexandria, VA: US Department of Agriculture; 2000.

4. Ziegler J. *Economic, Social and Cultural Rights: The Right to Food*. Report by the Special Rapporteur on the Right to Food. New York: Commission on Human Rights; 2001.

5. de Pee S, Semba RD. Role of nutrition in HIV infection: review of evidence for more effective programming in resource-limited settings. *Food Nutr Bull.* 2010;31(Suppl 4):S313–S344.

6. Coleman-Jensen A, Rabbitt MP, Gregory AC, Singh A. *Household Food Security in the United States in 2015, ERR-215*. Washington, DC: US Department of Agriculture, Economic Research Services; 2016.

7. Sonnino R, Hanmer O. Beyond food provision: understanding community growing in the context of food poverty. *Geoforum.* 2016;74:213–221.

8. Tarasuk V, Cheng J, de Oliveira C, Dachner N, Gundersen C, Kurdyak P. Association between household food insecurity and annual health care costs. *Can M Assoc J.* 2015;187(14):E429–E436.

9. Rebick GW, Franke MF, Teng JE, Gregory Jerome J, Ivers LC. Food insecurity, dietary diversity, and body mass index of HIV-infected individuals on antiretroviral therapy in rural Haiti. *AIDS Behav.* 2016;20(5):1116–1122.

10. Tiyou A, Belachew T, Alemseged F, Biadgilign S. Food insecurity and associated factors among HIV-infected individuals receiving highly active antiretroviral therapy in Jimma zone southwest Ethiopia. *Nutr J.* 2012;11(1):51–19.

11. Benzekri NA, Sambou J, Diaw B, et al. High prevalence of severe food insecurity and malnutrition among HIV-infected adults in Senegal, West Africa. *PLoS One.* 2015;10(11):e0141819.

12. Sholeye OO, Animasahun VJ, Salako AA, Oyewole BK. Household food insecurity among people living with HIV in Sagamu, Nigeria: a preliminary study. *Nutr Health.* 2017;23(2):95–102.

13. Patts GJ, Cheng DM, Emenyonu N, et al. Alcohol use and food insecurity among people living with HIV in Mbarara, Uganda and St. Petersburg, Russia. *AIDS Behav.* 2017;21(3):724–733.

14. Steenkamp L, Goosen A, Venter D, Beeforth M. Food insecurity among students living with HIV: strengthening safety nets at the Nelson Mandela Metropolitan University, South Africa. *SAHARA J.* 2016;13(1):106–112.

15. Normen L, Chan K, Braitstein P, et al. Food insecurity and hunger are prevalent among HIV-positive individuals in British Columbia, Canada. *J Nutr.* 2005;135(4):820–825.

16. Anema A, Wood E, Weiser SD, Qi J, Montaner JS, Kerr T. Hunger and associated harms among injection drug users in an urban Canadian setting. *Subst Abuse Treat Prev Policy.* 2010;5:20.

17. Bowen EA, Bowen SK, Barman-Adhikari A. Prevalence and covariates of food insecurity among residents of single-room occupancy housing in Chicago, IL, USA. *Public Health Nutr.* 2016;19(6):1122–1130.

18. Bekele T, Globerman J, Watson J, et al. Prevalence and predictors of food insecurity among people living with HIV affiliated with AIDS service organizations in Ontario, Canada. *AIDS Care.* 2018;30:663–671.

19. Kalichman SC, Cherry C, Amaral C, et al. Health and treatment implications of food insufficiency among people living with HIV/AIDS, Atlanta, Georgia. *J Urban Health.* 2010;87(4):631–641.

20. Mendoza JA, Paul ME, Schwarzwald H, et al. Food insecurity, CD4 counts, and incomplete viral suppression among HIV+ patients from Texas Children's Hospital: a pilot study. *AIDS Behav.* 2013;17(5):1683–1687.

21. McMahon JH, Wanke CA, Elliott JH, Skinner S, Tang AM. Repeated assessments of food security predict CD4 change in the setting of antiretroviral therapy. *J Acquir Immune Defic Syndr.* 2011;58(1):60–63.

22. Weiser SD, Hatcher AM, Frongillo EA, et al. Food insecurity is associated with greater acute care utilization among HIV-infected homeless and marginally housed individuals in San Francisco. *J Gen Intern Med.* 2012;28(1):91–98.

23. Aidala AA, Yomogida M, Miller-Vazquez R, HIV Food & Nutrition Study Team. *Who Needs Food & Nutrition Services and Where Do They Go for Help?* New York: Mailman School of Public Health, Columbia University; 2012.

24. McKay FH, Lippi K, Dunn M. Investigating responses to food insecurity among HIV positive people in resource rich settings: a systematic review. *J Commun Health.* 2017;42(5):1062–1068.

25. Weiser SD, Young SL, Cohen CR, et al. Conceptual framework for under-standing the bidirectional links between food insecurity and HIV/AIDS. *Am J Clin Nutr.* 2011;94(6):1729S–1739S.

26. Anema A, Vogenthaler N, Frongillo EA, Kadiyala S, Weiser SD. Food insecu-rity and HIV/AIDS: current knowledge, gaps, and research priorities. *Curr HIV/AIDS Rep.* 2009;6(4):224–231.

27. Weiser SD, Bukusi EA, Steinfeld RL, et al. Shamba Maisha: randomized controlled trial of an agricultural and finance intervention to improve HIV health outcomes. *AIDS.* 2015;29(14):1889–1894.

28. Frega R, Duffy F, Rawat R, Grede N. Food insecurity in the context of HIV/AIDS: a framework for a new era of programming. *Food Nutr Bull.* 2010;31(Suppl 4):S292–S312.

29. Kadiyala S, Gillespie S. Rethinking food aid to fight AIDS. *Food Nutr Bull.* 2004;25(3):271–282.

30. Reddi A, Powers MA, Thyssen A. HIV/AIDS and food insecurity: deadly syndemic or an opportunity for healthcare synergism in resource-limited settings of sub-Saharan Africa? *AIDS.* 2012;26(1):115–117.

31. Weiser SD, Palar K, Hatcher AM, Young SL, Frongillo EA. Food insecurity and health: a conceptual framework. In: Ivers LC, ed. *Food Insecurity and Public Health.* Boca Raton, FL: CRC Press; 2015:23–50.

32. Barreto D, Shannon K, Taylor C, et al. Food insecurity increases HIV risk among young sex workers in metro Vancouver, Canada. *AIDS Behav.* 2017;21(3):734–744.

33. Miller CL, Bangsberg DR, Tuller DM, et al. Food insecurity and sexual risk in an HIV endemic community in Uganda. *AIDS Behav.* 2011;15(7):1512–1519.

34. Palar K, Laraia B, Tsai AC, Johnson MO, Weiser SD. Food insecurity is associ-ated with HIV, sexually transmitted infections and drug use among men in the United States. *AIDS.* 2016;30(9):1457–1465.

35. Tsai AC, Hung KJ, Weiser SD. Is food insecurity associated with HIV risk? Cross-sectional evidence from sexually active women in Brazil. *PLoS Med.* 2012;9(4):e1001203.

36. Tsai AC, Weiser SD. Population-based study of food insecurity and HIV trans-mission risk behaviors and symptoms of sexually transmitted infections among linked couples in Nepal. *AIDS Behav.* 2014;18(11):2187–2197.

37. Wang EA, Zhu GA, Evans L, Carroll-Scott A, Desai R, Fiellin LE. A pilot study examining food insecurity and HIV risk behaviors among individuals recently released from prison. *AIDS Educ Prevent.* 2013;25(2):112–123.

38. Barreto D, Shannon K, Taylor D, et al. Food insecurity increases HIV risk among young sex workers in Metro Vancouver. *AIDS Behav.* 2017;21:734–744.

39. Wang EA, Zhu GA, Evans L, Carroll-Scott A, Desai R, Fiellin LE. A pilot study examining food insecurity and HIV risk behaviors among individuals recently released from prison. *AIDS Educ Prevent.* 2013;25:112–124.

40. Tsai AC, Hung JK, Weiser SD. Is food insecurity associated with HIV risk? Cross-sectional evidence from sexually active women in Brazil. *PLoS Med.* 2012:1–10.

41. Tsai AC, Weiser SD. Population-based study of food insecurity and HIV transmission risk behaviors and symptoms of sexually transmitted infections among linked couples in Nepal. *AIDS Behav.* 2014;18:2187–2197.

42. Justman J, Befis M, Hughes J, et al. Sexual behaviors of US women at risk of HIV acquisition: a longitudinal analysis of findings from HPTN 064. *AIDS Behav.* 2015;19:1327–1337.

43. Strike C, Rudzinski K, Patterson J, Millison M. Frequent food insecurity among injection drug users: correlates and *BMC Public Health.* 2012;12:1058–1067.

44. Talluri S, Prabhala ND, Prabhala RH. Influence of nutrition on human immunodeficiency virus infection. In: Watson RR, ed. *Health of HIV Infected People: Food, Nutrition and Lifestyle with Antiretroviral Drugs.* Vol. I. Amsterdam: Academic Press; 2015:117–133.

45. Friis H. *Micronutrients and HIV Infection: a Review of Current Evidence.* Geneva: Department of Nutrition for Health and Development, World Health Organization; 2005.

46. de Pee S, Semba RD. Role of nutrition in HIV infection: review of evidence for more effective programming in resource-limited settings. *Food Nutr Bull.* 2010;31(4):S313–344.

47. Woods MN, Spiegelman D, Knox TA, et a. Nutrient intake and body weight in a large HIV cohort that includes women and minorities. *J Am Diet Assoc.* 2002;102(2):203–211.

48. Campa A, Yang Z, Lai S, et al. HIV-related wasting in HIV-infected drug users in the era of highly active antiretroviral therapy. *Clin Infect Dis.* 2005;41(8):1179–1185.

49. Zachariah R, Fitzgerald M, Massaquoi M, et al. Risk factors for high early mortality in patients on antiretroviral treatment in a rural district of Malawi. *AIDS.* 2006;20(18):2355–2360.

50. Paton NI, Sangeetha S, Earnest A, Bellamy R. The impact of malnutrition on survival and the CD4 count response in HIV-infected patients starting antiretroviral therapy. *HIV Med.* 2006;7(5):323–330.

51. Tsai AC, Bangsberg DR, Frongillo EA, et al. Food insecurity, depression and modifying role of social support among people living with HIV/AIDS in rural Uganda. *Soc Sci Med.* 2012;74(12):2012–2019.

52. Vogenthaler NS, Hadley C, Lewis SJ, Rodriguez AE, Metsch LR, del Rio C. Food insufficiency among HIV-infected crack-cocaine users in Atlanta and Miami. *Public Health Nutr.* 2010;13(9):1478–1484.

53. Vogenthaler NS, Hadley C, Rodriguez AE, Valverde EE, Del Rio C, Metsch LR. Depressive symptoms and food insufficiency among HIV-infected crack users in Atlanta and Miami. *AIDS Behav.* 2010; 15:1520–1526.

54. Laraia BA, Siega-Riz AM, Gundersen C, Dole N. Psychosocial factors and so-cioeconomic indicators are associated with household food insecurity among pregnant women. *J Nutr.* 2006;136(1):177–182.

55. Tarasuk V, Mitchell A, McLaren L, McIntyre L. Chronic physical and mental health conditions among adults may increase vulnerability to household food insecurity. *J Nutr.* 2013;143(11):1785–1793.

56. Weaver LJ, Hadley C. Moving beyond hunger and nutrition: a systematic review of the evidence linking food insecurity and mental health in developing coun-tries. *Ecol Food Nutr.* 2009;48(4):263–284.

57. Palar K, Kushel M, Frongillo EA, et al. Food insecurity is longitudinally asso-ciated with depressive symptoms among homeless and marginally-housed individuals living with HIV. *AIDS Behav.* 2015;19(8):1527–1534.

58. Aidala AA, Yomoigda M, HIV Food & Nutrition Study Team. *HIV/AIDS, Food & Nutrition Service Needs.* New York: Mailman School of Public Health, Columbia University;2011.

59. Weiser SD, Tuller DM, Frongillo EA, Senkungu J, Mukiibi N, Bangsberg DR. Food insecurity as a barrier to sustained antiretroviral therapy adherence in Uganda. *PLoS One.* 2010;5(4):e10340.

60. Riley ED, Moore K, Sorensen JL, Tulsky JP, Bangsberg DR, Neilands TB. Basic subsistence needs and overall health among human immunodefi-ciency virus-infected homeless and unstably housed women. *Am J Epidemiol.* 2011;174(5):515–522.

61. Riley ED, Neilands TB, Moore K, Cohen J, Bangsberg DR, Havlir D. Social, structural and behavioral determinants of overall health status in a cohort of homeless and unstably housed HIV-infected men. *PLoS One.* 2012;7(4):e35207.

62. Macallan DC, Noble C, Baldwin C, et al. Energy expenditure and wasting in human immunodeficiency virus infection. *N Engl J Med.* 1995;333(2):83–88.

63. Feldman MB, Alexy ER, Thomas JA, Gambone GF, Irvine MK. The association between food insufficiency and HIV treatment outcomes in a longitudinal anal-ysis of HIV-infected individuals in New York City. *J Acquir Immune Defic Syndr.* 2015;69(3):329–337.

64. Weiser SD, Frongillo EA, Ragland K, Hogg RS, Riley ED, Bangsberg DR. Food insecurity is associated with incomplete HIV RNA suppression among home-less and marginally housed HIV-infected individuals in San Francisco. *J Gen Intern Med.* 2009;24(1):14–20.

65. Anema A, Chan K, Chen Y, Weiser S, Montaner JS, Hogg RS. Relationship between food insecurity and mortality among HIV-positive injection drug users receiving antiretroviral therapy in British Columbia, Canada. *PLoS One.* 2013;8(5).

66. Miewald C, Ibanez-Carrasco F, Turner S. Negotiating the local food environ-ment: the lived experience of food access for low-income people living with HIV/AIDS. *J Hunger Environ Nutr.* 2010;5(4):510–525.

67. Bansah AK, Holben DH, Basta T. Food insecurity is associated with depression among individuals living with HIV/AIDS in rural Appalachia. *J Appalachian Stud.* 2014;20(2):194–206.

68. Hatsu I, Johnson P, Baum M, Huffman F, Thomlison B, Campa A. Association of Supplemental Nutrition Assistance Program (SNAP) with health related quality of life and disease state of HIV infected patients. *AIDS Behav.* 2014;18(11):2198–2206.

69. Riley ED, Moore K, Sorensen JL, Tulsky JP, Bangsberg DR, Neilands TB. Basic subsistence needs and overall health among human immunodeficiency virus-infected homeless and unstably housed women. *Am J Epidemiol.* 2011;174(5):515–522.

70. Aidala AA, Yomogida M, Vardy Y. *Food and Nutrition Services, HIV Medical Care, and Health Outcomes.* New York: Mailman School of Public Health, Columbia University; 2013.

71. Kalichman SC, Hernandez D, Cherry C, Kalichman MO, Washington C, Grebler T. Food insecurity and other poverty indicators among people living with HIV/AIDS: effects on treatment and health outcomes. *J Commun Health.* 2014;39(6):1133–1139.

72. Chen Y, Kalichman SC. Synergistic effects of food insecurity and drug use on medication adherence among people living with HIV infection. *J Behav Med.* 2015;38(3):397–406.

73. Surratt HL, O'Grady CL, Levi-Minzi MA, Kurtz SP. Medication adherence challenges among HIV positive substance abusers: the role of food and housing insecurity. *AIDS Care.* 2015;27(3):307–314.

74. Malnutrition Quality Improvement Initiative. *Briefing: The Value of Quality Malnutrition Care.* Chicago: Academy of Nutrition and Dietetics; 2017.

75. Palar K, Napoles T, Hufstedler LL, et al. Comprehensive and medically appropriate food support is associated with improved HIV and diabetes health. *J Urban Health.* 2017;94(1):87–99.

76. van Haeften R, Anderson MA, Caudill H, Kilmartin E. *Second Food Aid and Food Security Assessment (FAFSA-2).* Washington, DC: Food and Nutrition Technical Assistance; 2013.

77. Rourke SB, Bacon J, McGee F, Gilbert M. Tackling the social and structural drivers of HIV in Canada. *Can Commun Dis Rep.* 2015;41(12):322–326.

78. Downer SE, Greenwald R, Broad Leib EM, et al. *Food Is Prevention The Case for Integrating Food and Nutrition Interventions into Healthcare.* Cambridge MA: Center for Health Law and Policy Innovation, Harvard Law School; 2015.

79. Tang AM, Quick T, Chung M, Wanke CA. Nutrition assessment, counseling, and support interventions to improve health-related outcomes in people living with HIV/AIDS: a systematic review of the literature. *J Acquir Immune Defic Syndr.* 2015;68(Suppl 3):S340–S349.

80. Langley CL, Lapidos-Salaiz I, Hamm TE, et al. Prioritizing HIV care and support interventions—moving from evidence to policy. *J Acquir Immune Defic Syndr.* 2015;68(Suppl 3):S375–S378.

81. Aidala AA, Yomogida M, Sorgi A, Miller-Vazquez R. Food Insecurity, Medical Care, and Health Outcomes among PLWH in a High Resource Setting: The Importance of Food and Nutrition Services. XIX International AIDS Conference; 2012; Washington DC.

82. US Health Resources and Services Administration. About the Ryan White HIV/AIDS Program. 2016; https://hab.hrsa.gov/about-ryan-white-hivaids-program/about-ryan-white-hivaids-program.

83. Aidala AA, Yomogida M. Medical care and health outcomes associated with food insecurity and receipt of food and nutrition services among persons living with HIV/AIDS. Forthcoming.

84. UN General Assembly. *United to End AIDS: Achieving the Targets of the 2011 Political Declaration Report of the Secretary-General Sixty-fifth Session.* New York: United Nations; 2012.

85. UNAIDS. *HIV/AIDS Treatment 2015.* New York: United Nations; 2012. http://www.unaids.org/en/media/unaids/contentassets/documents/unaidspublication/2013/JC2484_treatment-2015_en.pdf.

86. US Health Resources and Services Administration. A Living History. Washington, DC: Author; 2009. https://hab.hrsa.gov/livinghistory/.

87. Affordable Care Act, Public Law 111-14, §9007(a) 2010 .

88. Peal K, Wassung A, Downer S, et al. *Food is Medicine Advocacy Toolkit: Using Advocacy to Expand Opportunities for Food and Nutrition Services in Public and Private Healthcare Systems.* Cambridge, MA: Center for Health Law & Policy Innovation, Harvard Law School; 2015.

89. Mehra D, De Pee S, Bloem MW. Nutrition, food security, social protection, and health systems strengthening for ending AIDS. In: Ivers LC, ed. *Food Insecurity and Public Health.* Boca Raton, FL: CRC Press; 2015:69–89.

90. Nyamathi A, Sinha S, Ganguly KK, Ramakrishna P, Suresh P, Carpenter CL. Impact of protein supplementation and care and support on body composition and CD4 count among HIV-infected women living in rural India: results from a randomized pilot clinical trial. *AIDS Behav.* 2013;17(6):2011–2021.

91. Geldsetzer P, Francis JM, Ulenga N, et al. The impact of community health worker-led home delivery of antiretroviral therapy on virological suppression: a non-inferiority cluster-randomized health systems trial in Dar es Salaam, Tanzania. *BMC Health Serv Res.* 2017;17(1):160–172.

92. Office of Food for Peace. 2016–2025 Food Assistance and Food Security Strategy. Washington, DC: US Agency for International Development; 2016.

93. Seligman HK, Lyles C, Marshall MB, et al. A pilot food bank intervention featuring diabetes-appropriate food improved glycemic control among clients in three states. *Health Affairs.* 2015;34(11):1956–1963.

94. Community Health Initiatives. Feeding America: On the Front Lines of Health Promotion. Available at; https://hungerandhealth.feedingamerica.org/explore-our-work/community-health-initiatives/ (accessed July 8, 2018).

95. Boston Medical Center. Preventive Food Pantry. 2016. https://www.bmc.org/programs/preventive-food-pantry.

96. Wholesome Wave. Produce Prescription. 2017. https://www.wholesomewave.org/how-we-work/produce-prescriptions

97. Project Open Hand. https://www.openhand.org/.

98. Food is Medicine Coalition. http://www.fimcoalition.org/.

99. God's Love We Deliver. 2018. https://www.glwd.org/.

100. Weinhardt LS, Galvao LW, Yan AF, et al. Mixed-method quasi-experimental study of outcomes of a large-scale multilevel economic and food security intervention on HIV vulnerability in rural Malawi. *AIDS Behav.* 2017;21(3):712–723.

101. Weiser SD, Hatcher AM, Hufstedler LL, et al. Changes in health and antiretroviral adherence among HIV-infected adults in Kenya: qualitative longitudinal findings from a livelihood intervention. *AIDS Behav.* 2017;21(2):415–427.

102. Posse M, Baltussen R. Costs of providing food assistance to HIV/AIDS patients in Sofala province, Mozambique: a retrospective analysis. *Cost Effective Resource Allocation.* 2013;11(1):20–27.

103. Koethe JR, Marseille E, Giganti MJ, Chi BH, Heimburger D, Stringer JS. Estimating the cost-effectiveness of nutrition supplementation for malnourished, HIV-infected adults starting antiretroviral therapy in a resource-constrained setting. *Cost Effective Resource Allocation.* 2014;12(1):10–35.

104. Caldwell N, Srebotnjak T, Wang T, Hsia R. How much will I get charged for this?" Patient charges for top ten diagnoses in the emergency department. *PLoS One.* 2013;8(2):e55491.

105. Pfuntner A, Wier LM, Steiner C. Costs for Hospital Stays in the United States, 2010: Statistical Brief #146. Rockville, MD: Agency for Healthcare Research and Quality; 2013.

106. Gurvey J, Rand, K., Daugherty S, Dinger C, Schmeling J, Laverty N. Examining health care costs among MANNA clients and a comparison group. *J Prim Care Community Health.* 2013;4(4):311–317.

6

Evidence-Based Structural Interventions for HIV Prevention

MICROENTERPRISE AND VULNERABLE
POPULATIONS

Susan Sherman and Kyle Hunter

Introduction

As the HIV/AIDS epidemic enters its fourth decade, there is continued need for evidence-based tools that address the structural factors contributing to HIV risk. Concerted efforts have been made for close to two decades to move beyond individual behavioral and biomedical approaches to preventing HIV transmission and improving health outcomes, particularly in low-resource settings.[1] Yet, an estimated 1.8 million people contracted HIV in 2016, demonstrating a continued need to test and advance novel approaches to prevention.[2]

Microenterprise approaches have been used in the context of both HIV prevention and treatment (e.g., adherence to antiretroviral therapy [ART]) with several highly vulnerable populations including women, female sex workers (FSWs), and low-income HIV-positive individuals. This chapter defines and describes different approaches to microenterprise in the context of HIV prevention. The chapter also includes several case studies with vulnerable populations to evaluate the effectiveness of structural approaches to HIV prevention. The chapter concludes by outlining directions for future policy and research.

Key Concepts

What Is Microenterprise?

Microenterprise—also referred to interchangeably as microfinance and microcredit—is an umbrella term for strategies that increase access to economic resources: banking, small credit lines, savings accounts, business loans, insurance, and livelihood training are all forms of microenterprise. In the context of HIV prevention, microenterprise interventions aim to increase self-efficacy by building personal resources among the poor, in turn combatting one of the most closely linked risk-factors for HIV.[3] Although not a causal factor, the burden of HIV falls primarily on poor people and those lacking access to formal economies; microenterprise aims to provide access to financial tools that are otherwise unavailable and thus reduce behaviors tied to socioeconomic constraints.

Microenterprise interventions can be considered one part of an HIV prevention continuum, a framework that recognizes the multidimensional nature of disease prevention at the population level.[4] In this schema, behavioral, biomedical, and structural approaches to HIV prevention are complementary, rather than competing. Different approaches fall along the cascade of "demand side" (e.g., increasing knowledge of risk), "supply side" (e.g., increasing availability of direct HIV-prevention mechanisms such as condoms), and "adherence" (e.g., structural and behavioral) interventions. This theoretical framework is useful in considering what types of future studies are needed and designs that would complement other HIV prevention efforts with similar populations.

Microcredit, Microfinance, Savings-Led—What Are the Differences?

Existing research has used different models of microenterprise interventions. Although difficult to directly compare across studies, it is important to define the approaches to better understand current and future choices in research. Microcredit is considered a "minimalist" approach to lending in that it usually involves a group-lending process with very small loan amounts, coupled with compulsory savings.[5] These approaches are aimed at people whose economic lives are extremely precarious and for whom taking on significant debt might carry extra risk (e.g., people living with HIV/AIDS). Microfinance on the other hand is considered a "maximalist" approach as it involves slightly larger loans along with additional products or services like micro-insurance or business development training.[5]

The choice of strategy (microcredit versus microfinance) can depend on a host of factors, including organizational objectives, organizational capabilities, client preferences, client needs, local constraints (e.g., technological capabilities for reporting requirements), and—in some countries—regulatory restrictions (e.g., organizational designation of a nongovernmental organization [NGO] means it can only offer a smaller range of services than a microfinance institution [MFI]). An organization may opt to offer only loans if it feels that nonfinancial needs of borrowers (e.g., healthcare) are better addressed by other resources and/or borrowers prefer specific product offerings of another organization (e.g., life insurance). Some lending organizations seek out consumers willing to use their existing products rather than developing new ones, while other organizations lack the capacity to offer more comprehensive microfinance support. Because NGOs are typically non-profit institutions relying on external funding, they may have more resource limitations and offer minimal support, compared with profit-driven MFIs which may have more capacity to offer a multitude of services, whether for a cost to the client or free of charge.[5] Local constraints and regulatory restrictions typically prove to be the greatest factor in deciding whether voluntary or compulsory savings are implemented.[5]

Design of Microenterprise Interventions

Microenterprise in the public health realm explicitly links financial interventions with health/and or education programming. There are three models: *linked*, in which different organizations and different service-delivery staff provide the two services; *parallel*, in which the same organization but different staff provide services; and *combined* programs, in which the same organization and staff provide both elements of the intervention.[6] The cases described in this chapter use different models that may have affected the administration of the programs. For example, the Intervention for Microfinance and Gender Equity (IMAGE) study was designed as a linked program but ended up being run as a parallel.[9]

This chapter features microenterprise approaches to HIV prevention that are designed mainly as *savings-led, vocational training*, and *micro-lending* schemes. Programs may combine elements from multiple domains in their trainings, but in general there is a primary approach driving the program. A savings-led approach emphasizes and incentivizes participants opening savings accounts at local banking institutions. Micro-lending involves providing lines of credit or loans to participants to start small businesses or enroll in job-training programs. Vocational training provides participants with a skills-based training and business development in a specific domain. Cash transfers, in which participants are provided with cash either unconditionally or in exchange for a specific behavior (e.g., school attendance), have limited research evidence in the HIV prevention setting.[7]

Evidence of Program Effectiveness

The existing evidence for the effects of microenterprise interventions on HIV prevention is mixed. Several studies have demonstrated that micro-enterprise has resulted in increased condom use[8] and other reductions in risk behavior, while stopping short of demonstrating a reduction in HIV incidence.[6] What follows are several cases studies from South Africa, Mongolia, the United States, and India, demonstrating the potential for microenterprise interventions among different populations and highlighting gaps in the current literature and areas that need further study.

Microenterprise for Vulnerable Populations at Risk of HIV

Although microenterprise is widely applicable to almost any population, poor women and female sex-workers (FSWs) have been the primary targets of HIV-microenterprise interventions. This is because of their specific vulnerability to HIV acquisition and their pre-existing lack of economic agency in many contexts.

The IMAGE Study

The IMAGE study was a cluster-randomized, prospective intervention in eight pairs of villages located in rural South Africa. The study occurred over the course of two years. The target population was poor women in the Limpopo province. The intervention paired small-group microfinance lending based on the Grameen Bank model with participatory training on understanding HIV infection, gender norms, domestic violence, and sexuality. Outcome measures included intimate partner violence (IPV) in addition to structural-level indicators of women's empowerment.[3]

Overall, the intervention was associated with significant reductions in physical and sexual partner violence among participants but was not associated with reductions in incident HIV. The study also found significant improvements across a broad range of empowerment indicators. There was a demonstrated increase in economic stability and equity and a 55% decrease in IPV over the course of one year, compared to control groups.[9] In a secondary analysis of the intervention, researchers found a greater willingness postintervention to attend HIV counseling and testing, but differences in sexual risk behavior were not found.[3]

The IMAGE study demonstrated that a micro-lending program can increase self-efficacy and women's empowerment and may lead to meaningful reductions in IPV; however, it did not directly demonstrate an effect on HIV incidence or HIV-related sexual risk behaviors. A 2010 analysis of the IMAGE study concluded that the linked/parallel model was suitable for the length of the intervention but that to be sustainable a combined model would be more feasible.[4,6] Overall, the value of IMAGE is that it provided a model on which to base future, large-scale randomized controlled trials by demonstrating the feasibility of combining longitudinal public health interventions with programming that addresses the immediate financial needs of participants.

The Undarga Study

The Undarga intervention was a feasibility study of a group-randomized controlled trial in Ulaanbaatar, Mongolia, conducted from 2011 through 2012. The trial was a structural-level intervention combining savings-led microfinance and HIV prevention trainings targeted to FSWs. Outcome measurements included number of paying sexual partners and number of unprotected sex acts with paying partners. At six-months, those FSWs enrolled in the microfinance-HIV intervention arm reported significant reductions in the number of paying sexual partners and unprotected sex acts compared with those in an HIV prevention intervention alone. The microfinance condition did not have a significant effect on total income of the enrolled FSWs, although it did show reductions in percentage of income from sex-work.

The Undarga program demonstrated that a savings-led microfinance intervention is feasible and effective at altering some sexual risk behaviors. Unfortunately, it did not demonstrate a direct effect on HIV incidence. Many microfinance programs focus on providing small lines of credit and micro-lending, but there is some concern that participants may not understand the implications of taking out loans. Because micro-lending has the potential to become exploitative or increase the marginalization of vulnerable women, a savings-led approach allows participants to build assets without taking on debt.[10,11]

The JEWEL Study

The Jewelry Education for Women Empowering Their Lives (JEWEL) pilot study examined the efficacy of an economic empowerment and HIV prevention intervention targeting FSWs who used drugs in Baltimore, Maryland. It used a vocational-training model combined with financial literacy and marketing skills, encouraging participants to develop individual agency while also providing concrete opportunities to gain income outside the sex trade. The intervention included six 2-hour sessions that taught HIV risk reduction behaviors. It also included training sessions that developed skills in creating and selling jewelry. Behavior change was assessed by a pre- and three-months post-intervention study design. Key outcomes included number of sex partners, drug use, and condom use.

The study found significant reductions in income from sex work, median number of sex-work clients per month, daily drug use, and increased condom use with sex-work clients postintervention.[12] Increased income from jewelry sales was associated with a significant decrease in the number of sex-trade partners at follow-up. Women also reported qualitative increases in self-efficacy, and several women continued making jewelry after the intervention ended, demonstrating its potential for more long-term sustainability.[12] The JEWEL study was the first to establish the feasibility and effects of a microenterprise intervention among FSWs. The success of this study demonstrated the potential benefit of testing and disseminating similar intervention programs.

The Chennai Study

In 2009, a randomized clinical trial among FSWs in Chennai, India, aimed to test the acceptability and efficacy of a microenterprise program on HIV risk behaviors. The Chennai study, like the JEWEL study, aimed to train women in a specific skill rather than involve them in a micro-lending scheme. The intervention taught FSWs to make canvas bags, over 100 hours of training and was coupled with 8 hours of HIV prevention training. At a six-month follow up assessment, women in the intervention arm reported a significantly reduced numbers of sex partners, including paying clients, and they reported significant increases in income.[12] There was no significant change in condom use among participants, although baseline use was already high among FSWs in Chennai, likely due to a previous condom-usage campaign. One other important finding from the Chennai study was that 60% of FSWs had continued involvement in bag making six months after the study ended, suggesting that interventions should consider the potential of their models to be continued even after the formal intervention period ends. Overall, the study demonstrated that microenterprise interventions are successful in both providing FSWs with licit income opportunities and was associated with reductions in HIV risk behaviors.

Microenterprise for People Living with HIV/AIDS

People living with HIV/AIDS (PLWHA) are another population for which microenterprise approaches to support medication adherence and access is under study. PLWHA in low- and middle-income countries face economic obstacles to accessing antiretroviral treatment at both the individual and structural level. Individuals may need to prioritize food, schooling, or other family costs, and on another structural level, they may experience great difficulty accessing healthcare due to distance, lack of services, or inability to travel. Even for those able to access ART, financial losses resulting from HIV are difficult to overcome. These might include job loss, debt from paying for medical care, or food. Food insecurity is another consequence of acute poverty and a driving factor for difficulty in adherence to ARTs as well as increased sexual risk behaviors.[13]

Stigma and discrimination also contribute to PLWHA's increased poverty levels. Unfortunately, microenterprise approaches to reducing stigma are understudied in the literature.[14] Although several microfinance institutions operate in high HIV prevalence areas, most have been cautious to target HIV-infected individuals.

Fortunately, the limited research on microenterprise for PLWHA is promising, despite several concerns with implementation. Concerns about microenterprise initiatives with PLWHA include greater rates of absenteeism, loan default, repayment delinquency, higher drop-out rates, and premature death.[15,16] Many microfinance institutions are reluctant to include PLWHA in their lending schemes due to the possibility of default due to illness or possible death.[17] This leaves an already precarious population even more vulnerable and may exclude those in great financial need.

In one pilot project, conducted in 2007 by the humanitarian organization CARE, a microfinance program targeting PLWHA in Cote d'Ivoire was found to increase income that was then used for HIV-related care. The program was a savings-led, village-level project launched as part of its HIV prevention and mitigation efforts and was evaluated for its effect on the socioeconomic lives of participants and HIV-related stigmatization. In the qualitative analysis, participants reported increased levels of psycho-social support and reduced levels of stigma because of the group aspect of the program. Participants also reported using increased income from the group-savings scheme to pay for ART, which increased adherence and access to an otherwise expensive treatment. Improved health, in turn, then increased the likelihood that community members would loan them money, which then increased their capacity to carry out economic activities, and the use of revenue from intra-governmental agencies to pay for medical expenses improved perceptions of PLWHA as they were viewed as contributors.[17]

A small, two-year study conducted in Cali, Colombia, in 2012–2013 evaluated the effectiveness of a program targeting poor women living with HIV/AIDS using an intervention consisting of separate training modules covering treatment adherence, microenterprise, and access to microfinance (including legal help in setting up small businesses).[6] The study used a pre–post survey research design and found that while treatment adherence increased significantly over the course of the study, only a third of participants (n = 48) started and maintained a small enterprise. The authors proposed that this occurred because microfinance intuitions were reluctant to provide loans to participants with reasonable interest rates.[6] This difficulty offers evidence that though training programs can be effective, stigma and discrimination play a role in access to capital that needs to be taken into consideration.

Most recently, research was conducted on the feasibility of a microfinance program for PLWHA in Uganda. HIV-positive clients of an HIV care organization, Uganda Cares, were enrolled in a group-loan provision program that included ART adherence counseling and business training.

The authors did not track changes in ART-adherence behavior, but they did find that PLWHA benefitted economically from the loan program, suggesting that, when thoughtfully designed, microcredit programs can and should include PLWHA in their programming.[18]

Gaps/Limitations of Current Research and Implications for the Future

Overall, microenterprise interventions have significant potential to play a larger role in HIV prevention efforts particularly for populations living in precarious socioeconomic conditions. In a systematic review of reviews on HIV prevention methods, Krishnaratne and colleagues[19] identified studies of microfinance interventions as having "mixed outcomes," in part due to the lack of multiple, large-scale randomized controlled trials. Other reviews have also demonstrated that microenterprise is a sound approach but currently lacks a large body of evidence.[6]

There are several reasons for the mixed findings regarding microenterprise approaches to HIV prevention. In part, there have simply been too few studies, particularly randomized controlled trials, to draw large conclusions on effectiveness. Several smaller pilot studies have demonstrated significant effects in specific contexts, and there are valuable lessons to be drawn from these efforts. As noted previously, studies have shown promise in reducing proximal risk behaviors rather than incidence of HIV.

Principles for Future Research and Policy

Future research into the effects of microenterprise on HIV incidence should incorporate several principles to build on current knowledge. Based on the studies reviewed here, these principles include (a) scalable programming, (b) sustainable interventions over the long term, (c) savings inclusive or savings led, (d) randomized and/or controlled to the extent ethical and feasible, and (e) targeted to the most at-risk populations.

To demonstrate a viable strategy for high-impact structural change, future interventions must be designed with a larger population in mind. The IMAGE trial demonstrated the potential for large-scale microfinance and health interventions as effective means of influencing behavior. The proliferation of both microfinance and community-level HIV organizations means interventions can be designed to reach significant numbers of people without detracting from the either goal.[20] Similarly, research ought to carefully consider the partnership and delivery models of trainings and finance given local regulations and norms as well as the feasibility of maintaining programs through staffing and material support.

Working with economically vulnerable populations who are also socially marginalized (e.g., sex workers, poor women) requires particular attention to avoid further exploitation, and therefore we recommend future programming take a savings-led or savings-inclusive approach to microenterprise interventions. Though research has demonstrated that even the very poor often have consistently high rates of loan repayment,[20] the preliminary success of savings-led and health interventions with sex workers in Mongolia, as well as with CARE in Cote d'Ivoire, suggest this approach may be a viable way to give access to financial tools without requiring significant risk. Although this review does not discuss country-specific regulatory frameworks around microenterprise and microfinance, they are also important considerations in any policy or programmatic decisions that are made.

Ideally, future research will include randomized controlled trials that specifically examine HIV incidence and risk-related behaviors coupled with microfinance interventions. Though structural-level effects are in some ways more difficult to quantify given the temporality of distal exposures as well as challenges in identifying and measuring the impact of mediating factors, continuing to build evidence for these important tools is critical to HIV eradication efforts.

Finally, from a policy perspective, framing microenterprise approaches to HIV prevention as one part of the "prevention cascade" may help policymakers, grant makers, and other stakeholders (NGOs, banks, microfinance institutions) direct more funding to the field by showing such approaches are complementary to biomedical and individual behavioral approaches to HIV prevention. Moreover, microenterprise approaches can have beneficial "secondary" effects through increasing food security (CARE), reductions in stigma discrimination (IMAGE), reductions in IPV (IMAGE), and self-agency and empowerment (JEWEL) that have been demonstrated in the literature. Significant potential exists for combining public health and development approaches to HIV prevention. Microenterprise represents a practical and evidence-based opportunity for large-scale impact in HIV prevention across populations.

References

1. United Nations Programme on HIV/AIDS. *Report on the Global HIV/AIDS Epidemic.* Geneva: United Nations; 2000.
2. UNAIDS. Global HIV Statistics. Fact sheet, November 2016.
3. Kim JC, Watts CH, Hargreaves JR, et al. Understanding the impact of a microfinance-based intervention on women's empowerment and the reduction of intimate partner violence in South Africa. *Am J Public Health.* 2007;97(10):1794–1802.
4. Hargreaves JR, Delany-Moretlwe S, Hallett TB, et al. The HIV prevention cascade: integrating theories of epidemiological, behavioural, and social science into programme design and monitoring. *Lancet.* 2016;3:e318–e322.
5. Caldas A, Arteaga F, Munoz M, et al. Microfinance: a general overview and implications for impoverished individuals living with HIV/AIDS. *J Health Care Poor Underserved.* 2010;21(3):986–1005.
6. Arrivillaga M, Salcedo JP, Perez M. The IMEA project: an intervention based on microfinance, entrepreneurship, and adherence to treatment for women with HIV/AIDS living in poverty. *AIDS Educ Prevent.* 2014;26(5):398–410.
7. Baird SJ, Garfein RS, McIntosh CT, Ozler B. Effect of a cash transfer programme for schooling on prevalence of HIV and herpes simplex type 2 in Malawi: a cluster randomised trial. *Lancet.* 2012;379(9823):1320–1329.
8. Pronyk PM, Hargreaves JR, Morduch J. Microfinance programs and better health: prospects for sub-Saharan Africa. *JAMA.* 2007;298(16):1925–1927.
9. Pronyk PM, Hargreaves JR, Kim JC, et al. Effect of a structural intervention for the prevention of intimate-partner violence and HIV in rural South Africa: a cluster randomised trial. *Lancet.* 2006;368(9551):1973–1983.
10. Carlson CE, Chen J, Chang M, et al. Reducing intimate and paying partner violence against women who exchange sex in Mongolia: results from a randomized clinical trial. *J Interpers Violence.* 2012;27(10):1911–1931.
11. Dworkin SL, Blankenship K. Microfinance and HIV/AIDS prevention: assessing its promise and limitations. *AIDS Behav.* 2009;13(3):462–469.
12. Sherman SG, German D, Cheng Y, Marks M, Bailey-Kloche M. The evaluation of the JEWEL project: an innovative economic enhancement and HIV prevention intervention study targeting drug using women involved in prostitution. *AIDS Care.* 2006;18(1):1–11.
13. Chop E, Duggaraju A, Malley A, et al. Food insecurity, sexual risk behavior, and adherence to antiretroviral therapy among women living with HIV: a systematic review. *Health Care Women Int.* 2017;38(9):927–944.
14. Viravaidya M, Wolf RC, Guest P. An assessment of the positive partnership project in Thailand: key considerations for scaling-up microcredit loans for HIV-positive and negative pairs in other settings. *Global Public Health.* 2008;3(2):115–136.

15. Datta D, Njuguna J. Microcredit for people affected by HIV and AIDS: insights from Kenya. *SAHARA J.* 2008;5(2):94–102.
16. Barnes C. Microcredit and households coping with HIV/AIDS: a case study from Zimbabwe. *ESR Rev.* 2005;7(1):55.
17. Holmes K, Winskell K, Hennink M, Chidiac S. Microfinance and HIV mitigation among people living with HIV in the era of anti-retroviral therapy: emerging lessons from Côte d'Ivoire. *Global Public Health.* 2011;6(4):447–461.
18. Linnemayr S, Buzaalirwa L, Balya J, Wagner G. A microfinance program targeting people living with HIV in Uganda: client characteristics and program impact. *J Int Assoc Providers AIDS Care.* 2017;16(3):254–260.
19. Krishnaratne S, Hensen B, Cordes J, Enstone J, Hargreaves JR. Interventions to strengthen the HIV prevention cascade: a systematic review of reviews. *Lancet HIV.* 2016;3(7):e307–317.
20. Kim J, Ferrari G, Abramsky T, et al. Assessing the incremental effects of combining economic and health interventions: the IMAGE study in South Africa. *Bull World Health Org.* 2009;87:824–832.

7

Economic Strengthening Approaches with Female Sex Workers

IMPLICATIONS FOR HIV PREVENTION

Andrea Mantsios, Deanna Kerrigan, Jessie Mbwambo,
Samuel Likindikoki, and Catherine Shembilu

Overview

In this chapter we examine different strategies for addressing the economic vulnerability that puts female sex workers (FSW) at increased risk of acquiring HIV. We first discuss the different theoretical approaches to how economic interventions with FSW have been conceptualized and implemented to date. After drawing these distinctions, examples are provided of interventions that have employed different approaches. Focus is placed on those utilizing a community empowerment approach. We argue that it is through this type of approach that FSW can confront their economic vulnerability at the community-level, rather than through programs focused on increasing individual income alone. An applied example is provided by an in-depth look at community savings groups (CSGs) among FSW in Tanzania. We present study findings that suggest the potential these groups have as a structural intervention to improve financial security, reduce HIV risk, and promote community empowerment, thus enabling FSW to confront the economic exclusion they experience as a marginalized community. We conclude the chapter with recommendations for future research and programming.

Contextualizing HIV Risk and Prevention Approaches Among FSW

HIV Vulnerability

FSW bear a disproportionately high burden of disease in the global distribution of HIV. A systematic review and meta-analysis to assess the burden of HIV among FSW in low- and middle-income countries identified a pooled global HIV prevalence of 11.8%.[1] FSW were globally estimated to be 13.5 times more likely to have HIV than other adult women.[1] A recent update to this review including higher income countries found that the sub-Saharan African region continues to have the highest pooled HIV prevalence among FSW at 31.6%, and all countries where FSW had an HIV prevalence of 50% or greater were located in southern Africa.[2]

Multiple and overlapping biomedical, behavioral, and structural factors contribute to heightened risk for HIV among FSW. Behavioral and biomedical factors include multiple and concurrent sexual partners, lack of ability to negotiate consistent condom use (CCU), and untreated sexually transmitted infections (STIs). However, structural factors are increasingly understood as significant factors driving increased risk for HIV acquisition among FSW.[3] Financial security, stigma and discrimination, violence, and legal and policy environments around sex work have all been linked to heightened HIV risk of FSW.[4] These structural factors have been found to be associated with HIV vulnerability through a negative impact on access to HIV prevention services and clinical care for STIs, as well as their role in precluding HIV-protective behaviors such as CCU with clients and other sexual partners.[3]

Structural Interventions

Early HIV interventions among FSW focused on individual behavior change involving peer education, condom promotion, and provision of sexual health services.[5,6] However, as it became widely recognized that interventions addressing structural vulnerabilities were crucial to the success of HIV prevention efforts,[7-9] interventions to address underlying drivers of HIV transmission among FSW took root.[10] Structural interventions with FSW aimed at altering social, economic, political, and environmental factors have focused on reducing stigma and discrimination, gender inequality, and economic vulnerability. Strategies include decriminalizing sex work, promoting access to safer sex work venues, and eliminating violence perpetrated against FSW by clients and police. A recent review paper highlighted multipronged structural interventions as being critical to HIV prevention and treatment efforts with FSW globally.[3]

Community Empowerment Approaches

Structural interventions which are community led and focus on empowering and mobilizing the FSW community are now recognized as having a vital role in addressing HIV among FSW.[11] With a focus on the broader context of social and structural barriers, a community empowerment framework is one in which the community takes collective ownership of strategies to address structural barriers to their health and human rights.[12] A systematic review and meta-analysis of the effectiveness of community empowerment approaches among FSW found that these programs were associated with a 32% reduction in HIV infection, significantly decreased odds of STIs, and an approximately three-fold increase in the odds of consistent condom use between sex workers and their clients across geographic settings.[4] Typically, such approaches begin by promoting cohesion within the FSW community through peer-led activities and then mobilize the collective power of FSW to improve access to social and material resources.[13] The ultimate goal is to empower the sex worker community, in partnership with other actors and groups, to gain access to resources and address the social and structural barriers that contribute to their HIV risk and vulnerability.[12]

Financial Security and HIV Risk

Across geographic settings, FSW are a population often living in poverty and thus balancing competing financial priorities such as food, housing, children's expenses, and medical costs.[14–17] Economic realities for FSW can include low education and lack of skills for formal employment, scarcity of jobs, and low pay.[18,19] There is an established literature indicating the importance of financial insecurity as a driver of HIV risk behaviors such as unprotected sex among FSW.[20–27] For a sex worker facing financial insecurity, factors such as higher pay for sex without a condom may impede her ability to negotiate and demand condom use to protect herself from HIV. Studies in diverse settings indicate that financial insecurity places sex workers in a position of limited power to negotiate condom use and to refuse unsafe sex with clients.[28–32] The impact of using condoms on FSW earnings has been quantified in multiple and diverse settings indicating marked price differences between sex with and without a condom.[33-36] Higher premiums for unprotected sex are particularly compelling when additional pay can help cover basic needs such as food, housing, or health-care for one's family. This underscores the role of financial incentives in decision-making around condom use for economically vulnerable FSW.

In this chapter, we describe different strategies for addressing the eco-nomic vulnerability that puts FSW at increased risk for HIV. We start by pro-viding a framework for understanding the different theoretical approaches to how economic interventions with FSW have been conceptualized and implemented to date. After drawing these distinctions, we provide examples of interventions that have employed different approaches and hone our focus on those utilizing a community empowerment approach. We argue that it is through this type of approach that FSW can confront their economic vulnerability at the community-level, rather than through programs focused on increasing individual income alone. We then provide an in-depth look at organically formed CSGs among FSW in Tanzania. We share findings from our research on these group that suggests their poten-tial as a structural intervention to improve financial security, reduce HIV risk, and promote community empowerment among FSW, enabling them to confront the economic exclusion they experience as a marginalized community. The chapter concludes with recommendations for future re-search and programming and a call to determine how the field of public health will move forward with economic interventions for HIV prevention among FSW.

Economic Strengthening Approaches with FSW

Given the literature indicating the link between financial insecurity and HIV risk behaviors among FSW, economic interventions promoting fi-nancial security among FSW have gained considerable traction.[37] These interventions address the economic conditions of sex workers' lives that contribute to HIV risk and acknowledge the role of economic vulnerability in the lives of FSW including, but not limited to, its impact on sexual decision-making, and they aim to promote financial security as a means to reducing vulnerability to unprotected sex and other HIV risk behaviors. The literature on economic interventions for FSW is limited.[38] Sex worker advocacy groups like the Global Network of Sex Work Projects (NSWP) have called for greater research and program planning focus on addressing the economic realities faced by FSW.[39] NSWP recently published a report documenting economic empowerment programs for FSW in 16 programs in 11 countries around the world.[40] A review of the limited body of peer-reviewed scholarly literature on economic strengthening interventions for FSW has previously been conducted.[38] Instead of cataloging all of them here, we will first highlight the distinct differences in how economic interventions with FSW differ in theoretical approach and design. We then provide examples of programmatic strategies illustrating these varied approaches.

Contrasting Approaches: "Rescue and Rehabilitate" Versus "Sex Work Is Work"

Strategies for increasing financial security of FSW can include microfinance, vocational training and income-generating activities, cooperative banking, and savings and money management. Which of these strategies is the focal point reflects a fundamentally different understanding of and approach to economic empowerment of FSW. Namely, focusing on securing alternative income can be conflated with efforts to rescue or rehabilitate women from sex work, while focusing on the role of savings and money management can promote financial security without intervening on a woman's decision to engage in sex work. Having women leave sex work or engage in rehabilitative economic activity is not necessary to improve the economic conditions of their lives. Focusing on increasing financial security with the income they have from sex work is rooted in a rights-based approach in which sex work is recognized as work. FSW are recognized as workers with the same labor rights and need for financial management mechanisms as other groups working in informal and constrained labor markets.

Individual-Level Versus Community-Level Economic Empowerment

In addition to these distinctly different approaches to economic interventions with FSW, there are also two conceptually different ways economic empowerment programs are designed and implemented. We have organized this section to reflect this fundamental difference. First, we describe interventions that address economic vulnerability of individual sex workers, such as vocational training programs. Next, we describe those that address economic vulnerability of sex worker communities, such as cooperative banks. The available literature on economic interventions with FSW is presented in this way to draw the distinction between the two approaches and provide a foundation for the case study presented later in the chapter. We argue that the case study supports the importance of the latter of these approaches by providing evidence from CSGs among FSW in Tanzania that community-led structural economic interventions may be able to intervene on the overall economic exclusion of FSW as a highly marginalized community.

Addressing Economic Vulnerability of Individual FSW

There are a handful of examples in the literature of programs that sought to address economic vulnerability of FSW by providing skills training or small business development to individual sex workers. These types of programs focused on alleviating the economic vulnerability experienced by women engaging in sex work by increasing their individual financial security. In some cases, their conceptualization may have been based on the rationale that diversifying FSW income increases bargaining power; in other cases, they may have focused on securing alternative income as a means for exiting sex work. All of them used economic strengthening activities paired with an HIV prevention intervention to try to reduce economic vulnerability of individual FSW to HIV.

The Strengthening STD/HIV Control Project in Kenya assessed individual-level effects of adding microcredit finance and business skills training to an HIV prevention intervention for FSW.[41] Program components included microcredit for small business development, business development training, and the promotion of savings practices. Findings based on pre- and postassessment among FSW participating in the pilot (N = 227) revealed that two-thirds of participants had operational businesses by the end of the project. Close to one-half of the women reported having stopped sex work. Further, the weekly mean number of regular sex partners decreased significantly over the follow-up period, and self-reported condom use with all regular partners increased from baseline to survey end.[41]

As another example, The Pi Project provided HIV education and a microenterprise program for tailored canvas bags made by FSW (N = 100) in Chennai, India.[42] The study involved randomizing women to an intervention or a control arm, where they received either microenterprise training and HIV education or HIV education alone, and examining the association of the intervention with sexual risk behaviors. By the end of the program, 75% of participants in the intervention had made at least one canvas bag for sale, and six months after the study ended, 60% were still involved in producing bags. Intervention participants reported a significantly lower number of sex partners and number of paying clients per month at the six-month follow-up compared to control participants. They also reported significant increases in individual income at follow-up. Unfortunately, significant changes in condom use were not reported.[42]

In Mongolia, a randomized clinical trial was conducted among FSW (N = 107) to assess the impact of a program known as Undarga. This was an intervention that combined savings-focused microfinance with an HIV prevention component. The program provided matched savings for FSW, where matched funds could be used for business development or vocational education, as well as training in financial literacy, business development, and mentorship. At the six-month follow-up, women receiving the HIV risk reduction and savings components reported significantly fewer clients and were more likely to report consistent condom use with clients compared to those receiving the HIV prevention component alone.[43] Those receiving both components also had significantly increased odds of reporting no income from sex work, a lower percentage of income from sex work, and increased odds that sex work was not their main source of income.[44]

Collectively, the programs in this section provide examples of approaches focused on increasing the financial security of individual FSW through supplementary or alternative income, through business development and job training and through access to savings. Obtaining supplementary income can be important for FSW when it means they are more able to be selective about the clients they take, including being able to refuse those who do not want to use condoms or are aggressive.[40] Programs focused on securing alternative income as a means for transitioning out of sex work are only appropriate in the case that a woman wants to exit sex work but are not recognizing that this may not be the preference of some FSW. Ability to assess the sustainability and real-world feasibility of these programs is limited by the fact that they were studies involving compensation for study participation and were pilots with relatively small sample sizes.

Addressing Economic Vulnerability of FSW at the Community Level

In contrast to the programs described in the previous section, the programs in this section aim to address the community-level drivers or socio-political drivers of the economic marginalization that FSW experience. These programs provide examples of a model in which economic interventions are situated within community empowerment-based approaches. They illustrate how this approach allows for economic strengthening efforts to occur within the context of socially cohesive FSW communities taking collective action to confront other structural barriers to their health and rights.

Durbar is a well-known multicomponent STI/HIV intervention with sex workers in Kolkata, India. This program was among the first community empowerment-based programs to model an approach to addressing economic vulnerabilities of FSW at the community level.[45,46] The overarching components of the program are an STI/HIV intervention, a sex worker community organization, and a sex worker-led cooperative bank.[45] The cooperative bank, the USHA Multi-purpose Cooperative Society, began providing access to safe and secure savings for FSW by utilizing sex worker "field tellers" who went from house-to-house in their community encouraging their peers to start a savings plan and made regular follow-up visits to collect deposits and report account balances to these women.[45] In their efforts to establish USHA as a registered savings and lending cooperative, FSW faced significant resistance from government officials as they refused to permit a sex worker group to form a cooperative on the grounds of a "morality" clause. The women began a lobbying and advocacy campaign to garner support for their cooperative and succeeded in getting the controversial clause abolished and becoming the first formally recognized cooperative of sex workers in India. In the process, sex work became formally acknowledged by the state as an occupation; the sex worker community gained voice and presence in the political, social, and business sectors; and social norms and perceptions of sex work were changed.[47] Durbar successfully redefined the status of the sex worker community "from socially and economically excluded to an empowered workforce."[46]

The program was shown to reduce the economic vulnerability that affects FSW condom-negotiating capacities with clients by increasing savings among the women.[45,48] In addition to reporting increases in consistent condom use and reductions in HIV prevalence among brothel-based FSW,[49-51] evaluations of Durbar reveal increased collective agency and improved economic status among program participants.[45,52] The USHA cooperative, as a component of the larger Durbar intervention, models how economic empowerment within a community empowerment framework can occur. As exemplified here, it is within the context of forming social cohesion among FSW communities and mobilizing for change that FSW can address economic barriers as part of empowerment strategies that overcome obstacles to social recognition, participation and inclusion, and access to resources.

Another leading multicomponent intervention program with FSW in India is known as Pragati. Applied in Bangalore, this example illustrates the synergy of combining a cooperative bank structure with community mobilization and peer-based HIV prevention activities. The program focused on social and economic empowerment through building capacities of FSW and strengthening individual and collective action. Strategies included capacity development, representation and democratization, fostering leadership, creative advocacy, and alliance-building with stakeholders.[53] A microfinance system was established to provide a savings and credit mechanism for the FSW community. Results from a study of FSW participating in the program showed a significant decrease in STI incidence over a three-year follow-up period. Moreover, the results supported that condom use at last paid sex increased from 77.6% in year 1 to 85.5% in year 3 and to 100% during the fourth year of follow-up.[54] A total of 3,053 FSW had joined as shareholders of the cooperative bank during a three-year period. More than one-half of them (52%) opened savings accounts.[53] A separate study was conducted to understand the impact of collectivization and savings group participation on HIV risk reduction among FSW across three districts in Karnataka and included Bangalore.[55] Study results show that group members in Bangalore were three times more likely to have used condoms with their last client, and both membership in a group and access to a savings and credit cooperative were demonstrated to influence safer sex practices.

Both of these examples of community-led interventions helped change community perceptions and reduce stigma, leading to political and legal change that helped FSW organize and claim their rights.[56] For both programs, it is important to note that mobilizing sex workers was the first step in the process of generating change in the community, and the introduction of an economic empowerment component followed based on responses from the FSW community.

Summary of the Evidence

We are at an important juncture in the field of public health with regard to the use of economic interventions designed for FSW. There have been a handful of economic interventions targeting individual-level financial security which have been assessed in pilot studies and raise a number of questions about impact, scalability, and sustainability. Meanwhile, a body of literature supports community-led responses to the HIV epidemic among FSW, and the examples of community-led economic empowerment efforts in the literature provide evidence of their effectiveness. As we consider the appropriateness of different intervention models to address the deeply rooted social, economic, and political vulnerabilities of FSW, we argue that the need for community-led approaches is clear. The case study in this chapter offers an in-depth look at organically formed CSGs among FSW in Tanzania, examining their potential as an economic empowerment strategy to enable sex workers to address structural sources of HIV vulnerability and ultimately to help them achieve socioeconomic inclusion.

CSGs Among FSW in Tanzania: A Case Study

Context and Sample

Tanzania has a national HIV prevalence of 5.1%; however, the Iringa region in the southwest highlands has a notably higher prevalence of 9.1%.[57] Iringa is characterized by high levels of trade, transport, and migration of seasonal workers, dynamics that create and sustain demand for sex work.[58] Sex work in Iringa occurs mostly in venues such as bars, guesthouses, and truck stops along the major transport and trucking route that traverses the region, the Tanzania-Zambia highway. HIV prevalence among FSW in Iringa is estimated to be 32.9%.[59]

CSGs are an important aspect of multicomponent HIV intervention models in Tanzania. One research study on CSGs was nested within a parent study, known as Project Shikamana (Swahili for "stick together"). This is an ongoing Phase II trial of a community empowerment-based combination HIV prevention study conducted among Tanzanian women at heightened risk in Iringa.[60] The study enrolled venue-based FSW who were consented, tested for HIV, and completed an interviewer-administered baseline survey. Eligibility criteria included being 18 years or older, having exchanged sex for money in the last 30 days, and working at a sex work venue in one of the two study communities. The study communities were matched on demographics and HIV prevalence among the general population. The communities were randomized to either a community-led combination package model including biomedical, behavioral, and structural intervention elements or a standard of care control arm. The FSW community was placed in a leadership role to help tailor, implement, and evaluate the intervention. The sample (N = 496) recruited from the two communities included both HIV-uninfected (n = 293) and HIV-infected (n = 203) women. FSW were recruited from venues using time-location sampling to approximate a representative sample. The study received human subjects research approval from the institutional review boards of Johns Hopkins Bloomberg School of Public Health and the National Institute for Medical Research of Tanzania.

Theoretical Foundations

We situated our research on CSGs among FSW in this cohort within the theoretical orientation of social and economic exclusion[61] to conceptualize the processes by which FSW, as a historically marginalized population, experience structural constraints to their health and rights. Social and economic exclusion entails a lack of opportunities, blocked access to resources and services, and marginalization from decision-making in society and can be understood as a group-level form of discrimination.[62,63] FSW face multiple and multifaceted forms of stigma and discrimination as women, as sex workers, in some cases as poor members of society, and in other cases as persons at risk for, or living with, HIV. Their marginalized status coupled with low education and literacy levels present significant barriers to their ability to access traditional financial institutions, economic activities, and the labor market.[64] For FSW, the interaction of social and economic exclusion limits their access to resources necessary to protect their health. Specifically, in the case of HIV, economic exclusion plays into financial insecurity and economic vulnerability to infection. From this orientation, community empowerment, and economic empowerment within that process, introduce promising strategies for overcoming the complex interaction between social and economic exclusion faced by FSW.

Furthermore, our understanding of sex workers' economic vulnerability to HIV and the potential for empowered FSW communities to address it is situated within the theoretical framing of structure and agency. Sociologist Anthony Giddens proposed a duality in which an individual's agency is influenced by social structure and societal structures are, in turn, simultaneously maintained and adapted through the exercise of individual agency. Through this lens, we recognize the role of contextual factors of sex workers' lives and the critical role social structure plays in determining their health choices but at the same time the collective ability of sex workers to come together to reshape structural constraints.[65] It is through a community empowerment process that FSW can gain both individual and collective agency to effectively address power imbalances and the structural sources of their HIV vulnerability.

Michezo: CSGs Among FSW in Tanzania

Prior formative work conducted by our study team in Iringa identified organically formed CSGs (locally called *michezo* [singular: *mchezo*]) among FSW. *Michezo* are widespread among non-FSW in Tanzania as well and used for general financial security and social support. Similar to group lending strategies and informal local savings cooperatives seen throughout Tanzania and in other parts of the world, members of *michezo* in Iringa regularly contribute a set amount, receive the lump sum of the members' contributions in a rotating payout, and have access to loans for emergency funds. At the start of the group's cycle, members choose a number that dictates when in the cycle they will receive the payout. Each member contributes the group's prespecified amount of money on a regular basis and the payout of the lump sum is given to the member whose turn it is to receive the payout. The length of the cycle is determined by how many members are in the group. The amount of the regular contribution can either be determined by the collector or decided upon by the group.

In order to assess the potential these groups have for improving financial security and better positioning FSW to refuse unsafe sex and negotiate condom use, we used quantitative and qualitative methods. We sought to quantitatively assess the association between participating in a CSG and sexual risk behaviors. We then qualitatively explored the experiences of FSW who participate in these groups to understand the meaning and importance of the groups in their lives and in relation to their work.

Using cross-sectional data from the Project Shikamana baseline survey of venue-based FSW (N = 496), we examined the association between CSG participation and CCU. The primary outcome measure of consistent condom use in the last 30 days was assessed by asking about condom use with new clients, regular clients, and steady non-paying partners, respectively. Participants were asked if they had always, almost always, sometimes, almost never, or never used a condom during vaginal sex in the last 30 days with each partner type. This variable was dichotomized into consistent (always) and nonconsistent (less than always) condom use for each partner type. CSG participation was the primary independent variable of interest and was assessed by a survey question asking participants if they currently participated in a savings group. Our main hypothesis was that participating in a savings group would have a protective effect on HIV risk behaviors.

The cohort had a median age of 25 years (range: 18–55) and the median number of children among the participants was 2 (range: 0–10). The majority of participants were unmarried (82%) and had primary-level schooling or no schooling (71%). A total of 203 women (41%) were HIV-infected, only 31% (62/203) of whom were previously aware of their status. Their median number of years in sex work was five and median number of clients per week was two. Among women reporting sex with new clients in the past 30 days, 40% reported consistent condom use; among those reporting sex with regular clients, 34% reported consistent use; and among those reporting sex with steady, non-paying partners, 21% reported consistent use. Median monthly income was 120,000 Tsh (~ US$55). The majority of participants (71%) had one or more financial dependents. Only 8% of participants had a bank account. Over one-third of the sample (35%) participated in a CSG.

Assessing the Role of CSG Participation in Sexual Risk Behaviors

Logistic regression examined the associations between financial indicators including CSG participation and CCU. When controlling for other characteristics, CSG participation was significantly associated with nearly two times greater odds of consistent condom use with new clients in the past 30 days (adjusted odds ratio = 1.77, 95% confidence interval [CI] 1.10–2.86). Establishing an association between group participation and higher CCU with new clients suggests the potential of CSGs to intervene on economic vulnerability as a structural barrier impeding condom use among FSW. Participating in a CSG was not significantly associated with consistent condom use with regular clients or with steady, non-paying partners in multivariate models. This is consistent with prior research showing that condom use decreases with increasing relationship intimacy.[66–69] In particular, this finding echoes a prior study among FSW in India in which participating in CSGs affected condom use with sex work clients but had not been sufficient to allow FSW to overcome barriers to protected sex with their personal sex partners.[55] Nonetheless, the strength of the relationship we detected between CSG participation and consistent condom use with new clients is important. New clients are often "gateway clients," meaning that a new client can become a future regular client or steady partner.[68] Hence, establishing a norm of CCU with new clients may allow for greater levels of condom use with these other partner types over time, if such transitions occur.

Exploratory mediation analysis indicated that the relationship between CSG participation and CCU was partially mediated by financial security, as measured by total monthly income. The strength of the direct relationship between CSG participation and consistent condom use with new clients was reduced after controlling for monthly income in the model, and the standardized regression coefficients of both the direct effect (β_c=0.18, 95% CI 0.06–0.30) and the indirect effect (β_b = 0.05, 95% CI 0.02–0.10) were statistically significant with approximately 23% of the total effect of CSG participation on consistent condom use being mediated by financial security. Thus there remained a substantial direct effect on condom use with new clients after accounting for the mediation effect of financial security. Identifying a residual positive effect of CSG participation, a benefit beyond financial security alone, that contributes to reduced risk behaviors among FSW was an important finding warranting further study.

As a result of these survey findings, we wanted to gain an understanding of what more was contributing to the effect of savings group participation on condom use in addition to financial security. Thus we sought to learn more from women about what participating in a CSG meant to them in terms of their lives and work. To explore these themes, we conducted qualitative research with a subset of women from the Shikamana cohort who participate in *michezo*.

Exploring the Meaning and Importance of CSGs in FSWs' Lives

We conducted 27 in-depth interviews (IDIs) with 15 FSW, 4 focus group discussions (FGDs) with 35 FSW, and 10 key informant interviews (KII) with group collectors, those tasked with collecting and holding the group money, in the Iringa region. We purposively sampled for women participating in savings groups and sought a diverse sample with regards to age and HIV status. Women who reported CSG participation in a previous study conducted by our team were first recruited into this study to participate in IDIs. Next, using snowball sampling, study participants were asked to recommend other FSW who participated in CSGs for IDIs and FGDs.

Further, 10 women who serve as group collectors were recruited to participate in KIIs by asking study participants to refer their group collectors.

IDI and FGD participants ranged from 20 to 45 years old, with a mean age of 29 years. Among the sample, 80% (40/50) of the women were single. Nearly all (90%) of participants had children and over half (56%) had two or more. Education levels were low, with 38% (19/50) having some secondary school, 60% (30/50) having primary-level education, and one individual having no schooling. Of the 15 FSW who participated in IDIs, 11 of them were HIV-infected. HIV status of FGD participants was not collected to maintain confidentiality of those not wanting to disclose their status to the group. The 10 group collectors who participated in KIIs ranged in age from 22 to 32 years old, with a mean age of 28 years. Eight of the collectors had primary level education and two had some secondary schooling.

Some of the key themes that emerged from this qualitative work included (a) the groups were community established and led, (b) they provided members with both financial and social support, (c) group participation was linked to changes in their HIV risk behaviors with clients, (d) the groups provided members with a sense of solidarity and collectivism, and (e) the groups were anxious to move toward social and economic inclusion. Further description of these themes is provided next.

Community Established and Led

Participants described CSGs forming organically among FSW, often among women who work in the same venue or live near one another, and explained that the groups operate covertly due to fear of stigma from the non-FSW community. Participants spoke specifically about the unique challenges they face as sex workers and the benefit of coming together as a community to support their future livelihoods. One participant who started a group with her colleagues explained:

I called them [her fellow FSW] and we sat at the table. I told them these jobs have an end. Where we are going to get men, there is AIDS, it may reach a point when you lose all the power to work. It may reach a point when you will be worn out, even the men won't desire to sleep with you. In that sense, if we participate in an mchezo you can get money. You may get money and do something meaningful; you may even buy a plot and build a small house of one room. Why don't we participate in an mchezo? They all saw this was a good idea.

—IDI participant, age 30

Women described involvement in group decision-making and adapting the groups to the changing needs of members. One participant recounted when her group decided to increase regular contributions to meet their increasing needs saying:

> *I was part of that decision. Our collector involved all of us in it. We discussed it and decided to increase the amount from 1,000 to 2,000 because life has changed and now people have a lot more needs*
>
> —IDI participant, age 34

Financial and Social Support

Participants saw *michezo* as vital to being able to financially support themselves and their families. The group payouts were considered a necessary supplement to sex work income that allowed them to be able to afford their basic needs. Speaking about the role of *michezo* in the lives of sex workers, one woman said:

> *The advantage of an* mchezo *is that you can improve your financial stability very fast compared to when you save money yourself. I cannot live without an* mchezo; *any sex worker cannot live without an* mchezo . . . *An* mchezo *can help you afford to do a lot of things, big things. When you look at sex workers who are not in an* mchezo, *it's very difficult for them to improve their living standard; they will never improve.*
>
> —IDI participant, age 30

Participating in *michezo* was also described as providing an insurance mechanism in times of need, which left women feeling less vulnerable to financial crises. An important feature of the groups was the ability of members to switch places in the rotation with another member when experiencing particular financial strain. In addition to the value of receiving monetary support, many participants described this aspect of the groups as providing a sense of social support they felt from other members assisting them with their problems. As one woman described:

> *That's how we help each other, not because it's your turn then and you want to just take the money without caring about your friends and their problems. We listen to each other, and we listen to our friends' problems, how big their problems are and how we can help them.*
>
> —IDI participant, age 30

Savings group meetings were sometimes described as opportunities for information sharing, exchanging advice, and addressing group dynamics and community issues. One collector reported that sexual health advice was shared between members during meetings, including encouraging condom use with clients and HIV testing. One group member spoke about the challenge of sex work clients seeking lower prices at different venues in the area and reported that it was during savings group meetings that members would discuss and set the prices they thought should be used by FSW across local venues.

Group Participation and HIV Risk

Participants reported feeling that they had little or no power to negotiate the terms of sex with clients when they knew they did not have enough money to meet their basic needs. However, they unanimously reported that participating in *michezo* created a safety net they utilized when they had immediate financial need, thus safeguarding them against high-risk sex with clients. Many women articulated that knowing they had money from *michezo* allowed them to feel in control of being able to have safer sex with clients. They described a sense of agency to participate in decision-making in their interactions with clients which allowed them to choose when, with whom, and for how much they would provide their services. One focus group participant articulated the sentiment expressed in the group discussion saying:

> *The* mchezo *has helped me a lot. For example, you might get a client, and he will refuse using a condom. But I can decide to refuse because I know even though he doesn't pay me, I have money at home from the* mchezo. *It's different from when you're not in an* mchezo, *you might just go without a condom because you want money. But now I make my own decisions.*
>
> —FGD participant

Complementing our quantitative work, these qualitative findings provided an understanding of some of the ways in which savings group participation contributes to reduced HIV risk behaviors among FSW. As described here, participating in *michezo* can promote individual agency among members to practice HIV-protective behaviors and empowered decision-making, enabling them to more effectively navigate condom negotiation and safer sex with clients.

Solidarity and Collectivism

Many participants described the groups as a network of people who care for one another in times of need. One participant described it as fundamental to how problems are handled in the community saying, "It means when you get a problem, the group is obligated to help you because you are one of them . . . we live by cooperating with each other" (IDI participant, age 35). Participants made it clear that camaraderie within the sex worker community over their shared experiences fueled a sense of solidarity and support within the savings groups. One collector spoke about the need for such groups in order for FSW to be able to help each other through the challenges faced in their work:

> In our group, we sat and thought, because we all do our activities differently. And it happens someone may go to her activities and face problems. You find she comes back with no money at all. There is this and that problem, so we help her . . . we help each other. As a group member who has a problem, we need to do something to help her. We know the whereabouts of one another. So if I go any place and I am harmed, then I just get in touch with my fellows. One will come or maybe send a motorcycle. It's like a certain type of union. We decided to form our own mchezo because of this business that we are doing.
>
> —Group collector, age 30

This quote exemplifies the social cohesion and collective agency the groups appear to foster among FSW. However, while group dynamics were mostly described as fostering solidarity and support, exclusivity within the FSW community was also described. Overall low income and high mobility of FSW in Iringa was described as posing an inherent challenge to FSW savings groups and fueled exclusion of certain women from the groups. Stigma toward FSW who were considered transient and therefore untrustworthy as group members suggested discriminatory practices in group membership.

Moving Toward Social and Economic Inclusion

As participants described exclusion from formal banking due to insufficient income, they explained that savings groups provided them a mechanism within the community that allowed them to safely save money. Group members and collectors alike expressed that their vision for the future was to move their groups into a more formal capacity. They specifically spoke about their desire to gain recognition, register their savings groups with the government, and achieve social inclusion in the broader non-FSW community. One participant said, "My vision, what I see, is being recognized by the community and the media. . . . We are not known anywhere; everything we are doing has to be done secretly" (IDI participant, age 30). While many women thought that registering their groups with the government would improve group functioning by introducing more formal accountability, others were optimistic that this would help them be recognized and respected by society. One focus group participant spoke of wanting to "do something in society so I can be seen as if I am somebody." Another woman said:

> *Sex work is work like any other work. It's just that we are not recognized . . . For example, here in* [town name omitted for anonymity], *we're not recognized at all; I think nobody knows that I am a sex worker. I don't even think people know that we are running an mchezo and we are really helping each other.*
>
> —IDI participant, age 30

Many women spoke with optimism about the future of their groups. Participants reflected on how much their groups had already grown in size and contribution amount. They had clear ambitions for continuing to strengthen and grow the groups and conveyed that registering with the government and becoming formally recognized was a natural next step for them.

The desire expressed by many participants to have their groups registered and their profession recognized underscores their commitment to achieving social and economic inclusion. FSW organizing through the community empowerment process to advocate for and protect their interests in a public way promotes a more open recognition of sex work as a profession.[70] It is through bringing their collective solidarity into the public arena that FSW can begin to access the resources from which they are excluded.[71,72]

Summary of Case Study Findings

Overall, our study findings suggest the promising role of CSGs as a sustainable, community-established and community-led effort to improve financial security and reduce economic vulnerability of FSW to sexual risk with clients. Furthermore, the groups appear to serve as a mechanism through which FSW form social cohesion and can take collective action. The collective agency the FSW in Iringa described forming in *michezo* allowed them to counter their social and economic exclusion vis-à-vis group status.

Returning to the duality of structure Giddens proposed, namely that an individual's agency is influenced by social structure and social structures are maintained through the exercise of individual agency, FSW in Iringa are reshaping social structures by exercising agency in creating informal financial institutions. In turn, by reshaping structure, their opportunities and agency to think and act autonomously are transformed. Through these groups, formed with the intention of confronting economic exclusion, HIV risk-reduction can be achieved. The groups hold potential as an economic empowerment strategy to enable sex workers to intervene on the structural factors contributing to their HIV risk and vulnerability and ultimately to gain access to resources and equity.

The qualitative research described in this case study served as formative work for an economic component of the community-empowerment intervention implemented as part of Project Shikamana, the parent study. Based on these findings, financial security workshops tailored to the needs identified by the FSW community were held at the project's peer-run drop-in center. The workshops included sessions on financial literacy and money management skills, discussions around forming and managing successful *michezo*, and brainstorming ideas for group business projects. There was great interest in forming a Project Shikamana *mchezo* which has since developed into a more complex financial management mechanism within the FSW community participating in these activities. It began with the basic model of weekly contributions and a rotating payout of the lump sum among the group. However, it has evolved to include loans that group members can use to support their own activities and a growing catering business that the women are developing together. The group has opened a bank account and the next step for the catering business has been identified as getting a tax identification numbers so they can write receipts and renting a space to set up a cafeteria where they can serve the food they make. All of this activity has grown out of an *mchezo* formed in the context of a community-empowerment intervention.

Looking Ahead: Next Steps for Economic Strengthening Interventions Among FSW

As presented in this chapter, there are two main models for economic strengthening approaches with FSW utilized to date. These approaches have fundamental differences in whether the focuses is on intervening at the individual level or as part of a community-level effort to alter socio-political and economic barriers. Economic interventions focused on individual-level impact have an important role in promoting individual agency of FSW for empowered decision-making around their work, finances, and savings. However, narrowly focusing on improving individual income alone threatens the success and sustainability of these approaches and the scope of what they can do. It is critical to recognize that in the context of the socio-structural barriers that constrain women's ability to make strategic life choices, structural inequalities cannot be addressed by individuals alone.[72]

While being cognizant of the importance of promoting economic empowerment of individual FSW, focus must be placed on community-empowerment–based approaches given their implications for bringing about social and structural change for the broader FSW community. In line with many of the points outlined in this chapter, a useful model for conceptualizing future work on economic interventions with FSW is provided by Stanton and Ghose's model for multilevel community led approaches to economic interventions.[73] The model identifies three critical tenets on which such programs should be built: meaningful sex worker ownership over the intervention; a multilevel approach addressing sex workers' individual, social, and political sources of risk; and a goal of empowering sex workers as workers, rather than treating them as victims.[73]

The savings groups that are the subject of the case study presented in this chapter were organically formed rather than intentionally implemented, which makes a unique contribution to this field of research. This approach thus utilizes patterns of financial management naturally occurring among FSW in the community. These types of savings groups are an accepted element of Tanzanian society and are commonplace in other sub-Saharan African countries and around the world. Thus they offer a valuable platform for engagement in HIV prevention. This has implications for the conceptualization of HIV prevention programming for FSW. In forming CSGs, FSW in Iringa are working to build financial security and create economic stability for themselves and, in their effort to do so, they have exercised agency to reshape the structures that constrain them. Their increased individual and collective agency around sexual decision-making is a result and additional benefit of that process. The savings groups explored here underscore the need for the process of embracing protective behaviors to be stimulated and supported by communities and driven by their intentions to have their identified needs met. Public health must support structural change to have the fundamental needs of marginalized groups met in order for the adoption of protective behaviors to follow.

The structural-level intervention of CSGs presents an important role for HIV prevention research and programming. HIV researchers should assume the role of determining the effectiveness and strengths of community initiatives and work to disseminate those strategies to others, sharing best practices across networks of sex worker communities and encouraging the exchange of ideas and lessons learned. Community empowerment approaches place value on FSW involvement in research and capacity building within the community to serve various roles within the research process.[74] As illustrated by this study, research should begin by examining what the community sees as the primary problem and study what strategies they have developed for themselves. Researchers can begin by looking at what people are doing and be guided by them and include members of FSW communities in setting the research goals and conducting the research itself. Areas for future research include examining other ways participating in savings groups may lead to improved quality of life and well-being of FSW, including overall health outcomes as well as HIV treatment and care outcomes for FSW living with HIV. Further research on savings groups across diverse settings is also needed to enhance understanding of how savings groups can best be implemented and potentially taken to scale in the unique contexts of different countries around the world.

From a programmatic perspective, our findings highlight the importance of HIV prevention efforts promoting and supporting CSGs as a strategy for community mobilization of FSW to advocate for their health and human rights and tackle the structural barriers they face to adopting HIV protective behaviors. Funding to support capacity building at various levels of group operations would help strengthen the groups and could widen their reach allowing more groups and more FSW in the community to benefit from participation. Increased financial and political support is needed from donors, governments, partner organizations, and other allies if FSW communities are to advance in their efforts to effectively and sustainably overcome barriers to their social and economic inclusion. Because addressing social and economic exclusion requires changing the attitudes of those responsible for policy and in control of resources, programmatic focus should be placed on efforts to assist and support FSW communities in engaging with policymakers and political processes. Supporting FSW in building alliances with other organizations provides a bottom-up way of strengthening the capacity of FSW to advocate for themselves and ensure their needs and priorities are met.[75] NGOs, community-based organizations, and research partners serving as a liaison in such a capacity can help destigmatize sex work, change attitudes among government agencies and police, and may help reduce violence and mistreatment from clients, police, and the broader community.

Key Considerations for Economic Strengthening Activities with FSW Moving Forward

Based on the body of evidence and applied case study presented in this chapter, we offer a series of core tenets for the planning of future programs and research.

- **Adopt a rights-based approach**—Understanding sex work as work and recognizing the health and human rights of sex workers is essential.
- **Involve FSW throughout the process**—When sex workers are involved in the entire process, a program ensures that the real needs of the community are being identified and the strategies to address them are appropriate.
- **Prioritize community empowerment**—Focusing on community empowerment ensures that in addition to reducing economic vulnerability of individual sex workers, programs help FSW confront the economic exclusion they face as a marginalized community.
- **Build on naturally occurring patterns of financial management**—Existing financial mechanisms in the community are already designed to meet the financial needs of FSW; building on them to promote embracing protective behaviors tied to their economic security follows naturally.

- **Incorporate an advocacy component**—Programs aimed at economic empowerment of sex workers must also incorporate an advocacy component to address the stigma, discrimination, and legal and political obstacles to FSW ultimately gaining access to resources and equity.

References

1. Baral S, Beyrer C, Muessig K, et al. Burden of HIV among female sex workers in low-income and middle-income countries: a systematic review and meta-analysis. *Lancet Infect Dis.* 2012;12(7):538–549.
2. Beyrer C, Crago AL, Bekker LG, et al. An action agenda for HIV and sex workers. *Lancet.* 2015;385(9964):287–301.
3. Shannon K, Strathdee SA, Goldenberg SM, et al. Global epidemiology of HIV among female sex workers: influence of structural determinants. *Lancet.* 2015; 385(9962):55–71.
4. Kerrigan D, Kennedy CE, Morgan-Thomas R, et al. A community empowerment approach to the HIV response among sex workers: effectiveness, challenges, and considerations for implementation and scale-up. *Lancet.* 2015;385(9963):172–185.
5. Shahmanesh M, Patel V, Mabey D, Cowan F. Effectiveness of interventions for the prevention of HIV and other sexually transmitted infections in female sex workers in resource poor setting: a systematic review. *Trop Med Int Health.* 2008;13(5):659–679.
6. Foss AM, Hossain M, Vickerman PT, Watts CH. A systematic review of published evidence on intervention impact on condom use in sub-Saharan Africa and Asia. *Sex Transm Infect.* 2007;83(7):510–516.
7. Parker RG, Easton D, Klein CH. Structural barriers and facilitators in HIV prevention: a review of international research. *AIDS.* 2000;14:S22–S32.
8. Blankenship KM, Bray SJ, Merson MH. Structural interventions in public health. *AIDS.* 2000;14(Suppl 1):S11–S21.
9. Gupta GR, Parkhurst JO, Ogden JA, Aggleton P, Mahal A. Structural approaches to HIV prevention. *Lancet.* 2008;372(9640):764–775.
10. Shannon K, Goldenberg SM, Deering KN, Strathdee SA. HIV infection among female sex workers in concentrated and high prevalence epidemics: why a structural determinants framework is needed. *Curr Opin HIV AIDS.* 2014;9(2):174–182.
11. World Health Organization Department of HIV/AIDS. Prevention and treatment of HIV and other sexually transmitted infections for sex workers in low- and middle-income countries: recommendations for a public health approach. Geneva: World Health Organization; 2012 .

12. World Health Organization, United Nations Fund for Population Activities, Population Fund, United Nations Programme on HIV/AIDS, Global Network of Sex Work Projects, World Bank. Implementing comprehensive HIV/STI programmes with sex workers: practical approaches from collaborative interventions. Geneva: World Health Organization; 2013.

13. Kerrigan DL, Fonner VA, Stromdahl S, Kennedy CE. Community Empowerment Among Female Sex Workers is an Effective HIV Prevention Intervention: A Systematic Review of the Peer-Reviewed Evidence from Low- and Middle-Income Countries. *AIDS and Behavior.* 2013;17(6):1926–1940.

14. Tsai LC, Witte SS, Aira T, Riedel M, Hwang HG, Ssewamala F. "There is no other option; we have to feed our families . . . who else would do it?": The financial lives of women engaging in sex work in Ulaanbaatar, Mongolia. *Global J Health Sci.* 2013;5(5):41–50.

15. Gurnani V, Beattie TS, Bhattacharjee P, et al. An integrated structural intervention to reduce vulnerability to HIV and sexually transmitted infections among female sex workers in Karnataka state, south India. *BMC Public Health* 2011;11:755.

16. Bikaako-Kajura W. *AIDS and Transport: The Experience of Ugandan Road and Rail Transport Workers and Their Unions.* London: International Transport Workers' Federation; 2000.

17. Oyefara JL. Food insecurity, HIV/AIDS pandemic and sexual behaviour of female commercial sex workers in Lagos metropolis, Nigeria. *SAHARA J.* 2007;4(2):626–635.

18. Scorgie F, Chersich MF, Ntaganira I, Gerbase A, Lule F, Lo YR. Sociodemographic characteristics and behavioral risk factors of female sex workers in sub-Saharan Africa: a systematic review. *AIDS Behav.* 2012;16(4):920–933.

19. The Synergy Project, University of Washington Center for Health Education and Research. *Room for Change: Preventing HIV Transmission in Brothels.* Washington, DC: US Agency for International Development; 2000.

20. Fitzgerald-Husek A, Martiniuk AL, Hinchcliff R, Aochamus CE, Lee RB. "I do what I have to do to survive": an investigation into the perceptions, experiences and economic considerations of women engaged in sex work in northern Namibia. *BMC Women's Health.* 2011;11:35.

21. Reed E, Gupta J, Biradavolu M, Devireddy V, Blankenship KM. The context of economic insecurity and its relation to violence and risk factors for HIV among female sex workers in Andhra Pradesh, India. *Public Health Reports.* 2010;125(Suppl 4):81–89.

22. Ngo AD, McCurdy SA, Ross MW, Markham C, Ratliff EA, Pham HT. The lives of female sex workers in Vietnam: findings from a qualitative study. *Culture Health Sexuality.* 2007;9(6):555–570.

23. Saggurti N, Jain AK, Sebastian MP, et al. Indicators of mobility, socio-economic vulnerabilities and HIV risk behaviours among mobile female sex workers in India. *AIDS Behav* 2012;16(4):952–959.

24. Phrasisombath K, Faxelid E, Sychareun V, Thomsen S. Risks, benefits and survival strategies—views from female sex workers in Savannakhet, Laos. *BMC Public Health.* 2012;12:1004.

25. Agha S, Chulu Nchima M. Life-circumstances, working conditions and HIV risk among street and nightclub-based sex workers in Lusaka, Zambia. *Culture Health Sexuality.* 2004;6(4):283–299.

26. Onyeneho NG. HIV/AIDS risk factors and economic empowerment needs of female sex workers in Enugu Urban, Nigeria. *Tanzania J Health Res.* 2009;11(3):126–135.

27. USAID Project Search. HIV among female sex workers and men who have sex with men in Swaziland. Washington, DC: US Agency for International Development; 2013.

28. Wojcicki JM, Malala J. Condom use, power and HIV/AIDS risk: sex-workers bargain for survival in Hillbrow/Joubert Park/Berea, Johannesburg. *Social Sci Med.* 2001;53(1):99–121.

29. Urada LA, Morisky DE, Pimentel-Simbulan N, Silverman JG, Strathdee SA. Condom negotiations among female sex workers in the Philippines: environmental influences. *PLoS One.* 2012;7(3):e33282.

30. Adu-Oppong A, Grimes RM, Ross MW, Risser J, Kessie G. Social and behavioral determinants of consistent condom use among female commercial sex workers in Ghana. *AIDS Educ Prevent.* 2007;19(2):160–172.

31. Umar US, Adekunle AO, Bakare RA. Pattern of condom use among commercial sex workers in Ibadan, Nigeria. *Afr J Med Sci.* 2001;30(4):285–290.

32. Bharat S, Mahapatra B, Roy S, Saggurti N. Are female sex workers able to negotiate condom use with male clients? The case of mobile FSWs in four high HIV prevalence states of India. *PLoS One.* 2013;8(6):e68043.

33. Rao V, Gupta I, Lokshin M, Jana S. Sex workers and the cost of safe sex: the compensating differential for condom use among Calcutta prostitutes. *J Dev Econ.* 2003;71(2):585–603.

34. Elmes J, Nhongo K, Ward H, et al. The price of sex: condom use and the determinants of the price of sex among female sex workers in eastern Zimbabwe. *J Infect Dis.* 2014;210(Suppl 2):S569–S578.

35. Gertler P, Shah M, Bertozzi S. Sex sells, but risky sex sell for more. 2003. Unpublished manuscript. Available at http://graphics8.nytimes.com/images/blogs/freakonomics/pdf/GertlerAIDS.pdf

36. Ntumbanzondo M, Dubrow R, Niccolai LM, Mwandagalirwa K, Merson MH. Unprotected intercourse for extra money among commercial sex workers in Kinshasa, Democratic Republic of Congo. *AIDS Care.* 2006;18(7):777–785.

37. Blankenship KM, Friedman SR, Dworkin S, Mantell JE. Structural interventions: concepts, challenges and opportunities for research. *J URH.* 2006;83(1):59–72.

38. Moret W. Economic strengthening for female sex workers: a review of the literature. FHI 360; May 2014.

39. Network of Sex Worker Projects. Sex work and money. *Res Sex Work*. 2006;9.

40. Global Network of Sex Work Projects. *Stepping Up, Stepping Out Project: Economic Empowerment of Sex Workers*. Edinburgh, UK: Author; 2015.

41. Odek WO, Busza J, Morris CN, Cleland J, Ngugi EN, Ferguson AG. Effects of micro-enterprise services on HIV risk behaviour among female sex workers in Kenya's urban slums. *AIDS Behav*. 2009;13(3):449–461.

42. Sherman SG, Srikrishnan AK, Rivett KA, Liu SH, Solomon S, Celentano DD. Acceptability of a microenterprise intervention among female sex workers in Chennai, India. *AIDS Behav*. 2010;14(3):649–657.

43. Witte SS, Aira T, Tsai LC, et al. Efficacy of a savings-led microfinance intervention to reduce sexual risk for HIV among women engaged in sex work: a randomized clinical trial. *Am J Public Health*. 2015;105(3):e95–e102.

44. Tsai L, Witte S, Aira T, Riedel M, Offringa R, Chang M. Efficacy of a microsavings intervention in increasing income and reducing economic dependence upon sex work among women in Mongolia. *Int Social Work*. 2018;61:6–22.

45. Swendeman D, Basu I, Das S, Jana S, Rotheram-Borus MJ. Empowering sex workers in India to reduce vulnerability to HIV and sexually transmitted diseases. *Soc Sci Med*. 2009;69(8):1157–1166.

46. Jana S, Basu I, Rotheram-Borus MJ, Newman PA. The Sonagachi Project: a sustainable community intervention program. *AIDS Educ Prevent*. 2004;16(5):405–414.

47. Durbar. Durbar Mahila Samanwaya Committee. http://durbar.org. Accessed October 1, 2016.

48. Fehrenbacher AE, Chowdhury D, Ghose T, Swendeman D. Consistent condom use by female sex workers in Kolkata, India: testing theories of economic insecurity, behavior change, life course vulnerability and empowerment. *AIDS Behav*. 2016;20(10):2332–2345.

49. Basu I, Jana S, Rotheram-Borus MJ, et al. HIV prevention among sex workers in India. *J Acquir Immune Defic Syndr*. 2004;36(3):845–852.

50. Jana S, Chakraborty AK, Das A, Khodakevich L, Chakraborty MS, Pal NK. Community based survey of STD/HIV infection among commercial sex-workers in Calcutta (India). Part II: sexual behaviour, knowledge and attitude towards STD. *J Communic Dis*. 1994;26(3):168–171.

51. Cohen J. HIV/AIDS in India: Sonagachi sex workers stymie HIV. *Science*. 2004;304(5670):506.

52. Ghose T, Swendeman D, George S, Chowdhury D. Mobilizing collective identity to reduce HIV risk among sex workers in Sonagachi, India: the boundaries, consciousness, negotiation framework. *Soc Sci Med*. 2008;67(2):311–320.

53. Euser SM, Souverein D, Rama Narayana Gowda P, et al. Pragati: an empowerment programme for female sex workers in Bangalore, India. *Global Health Action*. 2012;5:1–11.

54. Souverein D, Euser SM, Ramaiah R, et al. Reduction in STIs in an empower-ment intervention programme for female sex workers in Bangalore, India: the Pragati programme. *Global Health Action.* 2013;6:22943.

55. Pillai P, Bhattacharjee P, Ramesh BM. Impact of two vulnerability reduction strategies—collectivisation and participation in savings activities—on HIV risk reduction among female sex workers. Bangladore: Karnataka Heath Promotion Trust; 2012.

56. Patel SK, Prabhakar P, Jain AK, Saggurti N, Adhikary R. Relationship between community collectivization and financial vulnerability of female sex workers in southern India. *PLoS One.* 2016;11(5):e0156060.

57. Tanzania Commission for AIDS, Zanzibar AIDS Commission, National Bureau of Statistics, Office of Chief Government Statistician, ICF International. *Tanzania HIV/AIDS and Malaria Indicator Survey 2011–12.* Dar es Salaam: Authors; 2013.

58. Beckham S, Kennedy C, Brahmbhatt H, et al. *Strategic Assessment to Define a Comprehensive Response to HIV in Iringa, Tanzania.* Research Brief: Female Sex Workers. Washington, DC: US Agency for International Development; 2013.

59. Tanzania National AIDS Control Program, PSI Tanzania. *HIV Biological and Behavioral Surveys: Tanzania 2013. Female Sex Workers in Seven Regions:* Dar es Salaam, Iringa, Mbeya, Mwanza, Tabora, Shinyanga and Mara; 2013.

60. Kerrigan D, Mbwambo J, Likindikoki S, et al. Project Shikamana: baseline findings from a community empowerment-based combination HIV preven-tion trial among female sex workers in Iringa, Tanzania. *J Acquir Immune Defic Syndr.* 2017;74(Suppl 1): S60–S68.

61. Sen A. *Social Exclusion: Concept, Application, and Scrutiny.* Manila: Asian Development Bank; 2000.

62. Mathieson J, Popay J, Enoch E, et al. Social Exclusion: Meaning, Measurement and Experience and Links to Health Inequalities A review of Literature. Lancaster, UK: Lancaster University; 2008.

63. Dertwinkel T. Economic Exclusion of Ethnic Minorities: On the Importance of Concept Specification. ECMI Issue Brief 19. Flensburg, Germany: European Centre for Minority Issues; November 2008.

64. Dworkin S, Blankenship K. Microfinance and HIV/AIDS prevention: assessing its promise and limitations. *AIDS Behav* 2009;13(3):462–469.

65. Seidel G. The competing discourses of HIV/AIDS in sub-Saharan Africa: discourses of rights and empowerment vs discourses of control and ex-clusion. *Soc Sci Med.* 1993;36(3):175–194.

66. Murray L, Moreno L, Rosario S, Ellen J, Sweat M, Kerrigan D. The role of re-lationship intimacy in consistent condom use among female sex workers and their regular paying partners in the Dominican Republic. *AIDS Behav.* 2007;11(3):463–470.

67. Andrews CH, Faxelid E, Sychaerun V, Phrasisombath K. Determinants of con-sistent condom use among female sex workers in Savannakhet, Lao PDR. *BMC Womens Health.* 2015;15:63.

68. Robertson AM, Syvertsen JL, Amaro H, et al. Can't buy my love: a typology of female sex workers' commercial relationships in the Mexico-U.S. border region. *J Sex Res.* 2014;51(6):711–720.

69. Le MN, D'Onofrio CN, Rogers JD. HIV risk behaviors among three classes of female sex workers in Vietnam. *J Sex Res.* 2010;47(1):38–48.

70. Campbell C. Selling sex in the time of AIDS: the psycho-social context of condom use by sex workers on a Southern African mine. *Soc Sci Med.* 2000;50(4):479–494.

71. Blanchard AK, Mohan HL, Shahmanesh M, et al. Community mobilization, empowerment and HIV prevention among female sex workers in south India. *BMC Public Health.* 2013;13:234.

72. Kabeer N. Resources, agency, achievements: reflections on the measurement of women's empowerment. In: Institute of Social Studies, ed. *Development and Change.* Oxford: Blackwell; 1999:435–464.

73. Stanton MC, Ghose T. Community-led economic initiatives with sex workers: establishing a conceptual framework for a multidimensional structural intervention. *Sex Res Soc Policy.* 2017;14:254–256.

74. World Health Organization, United Nations Fund for Population Activities, Global Network of Sex Work Projects, World Bank. *Implementing Comprehensive HIV/STI Programmes with Sex Workers: Practical Approaches from Collaborative Interventions.* Geneva: World Health Organization; 2013.

75. Kabeer N. *Social Exclusion: Concepts, Findings and Implications for the MDGs.* London: Department for International Development; 2005.

8

Integrating Treatment for Opioid Use Disorders and HIV Services into Primary Care

SOLUTIONS FOR THE 21ST CENTURY

Nabila El-Bassel, Phillip L. Marotta, Louisa Gilbert, Elwin Wu, Sandra Springer, Dawn A. Goddard-Eckrich, and Timothy Hunt

Overview

From 1999 to 2015, the number of opioid overdose deaths in the United States more than quadrupled, claiming more than 180,000 lives.[1] In 2014, a total of 10.3 million individuals misused prescription opioids for nontherapeutic purposes.[2] Presently, more than 1.9 million people have a past-year opioid use disorder (OUD) of which 591,000 involved heroin.[3] The growth of OUD and misuse of prescription opioid medications led to a precipitous increase in injection drug use, thereby creating an explosive context for the spread of HIV.[4] Injection of opioids leads to acquisition and transmission of HIV and related comorbidities such as hepatitis C (HCV) and hepatis B (HBV) and serves as a barrier to accessing and staying in HIV care.[5,6] The 2015 outbreak of HIV associated with injection of prescription opioids (Oxymorphone) in Austin, Indiana, was an unfortunate example of the disastrous consequences of untreated opioid addiction in which 140 cases of HIV emerged in a town with a population of 4,000 over a period of just 1.5 years.[7,8]

Medication-assisted treatments (MAT) are evidence-based strategies for treating OUD that also reduce HIV transmission risk behaviors, improve

HIV treatment outcomes (lower viral load, increased CD4 count, increased retention in care), and lower risk of HCV transmission.[9–17] Despite substantial progress, people with OUD face considerable social and structural barriers to linkage to MAT and behavioral treatments for OUD, as well as barriers to linkage, testing, and treatment for HIV.[18–20] Structural barriers to linkage, testing, and treatment for HIV greatly inhibit the optimization of OUD and HIV services for people who use drugs and inhibits progression through the HIV continuum of care to viral suppression.[21] Receiving HIV and substance use care in two separate locations increases institutional and structural barriers to engagement and retention in services for OUD and the prevention and management of HIV infection.

The public health crisis of OUD and HIV infection in the United States demands solutions that incorporate factors beyond the individual to increase coverage and surmount social and structural barriers to accessing and engaging in drug abuse treatment and HIV care.[22] Given the intertwined nature of substance use and HIV infection, primary care settings are an ideal environment to optimize treatments that addresses use of opioids and other substances and HIV and other medical needs presented by people with OUD. In recent years, buprenorphine-naloxone and extended-release naltrexone became available for use in primary care settings, creating a number of potentially effective MATs for patients with OUD that could be integrated with HIV care in primary care settings.[23,24] Providing care that integrates treatments for OUD (MAT and behavioral) with HIV services into primary care settings enables coordination of otherwise fragmented services.[22,25–28] Receiving a package of evidence-based substance use treatment services for OUD that cater to a patient's needs could improve retention and engagement of people who use heroin or other opioids in HIV primary care settings.[28–30]

In this chapter, we first present the scope of the HIV and drug use epidemics in the United States, then introduce and define drug treatment as HIV prevention. Second, we identify a number of evidence-based pharmacological and behavioral interventions that have been used in integrated approaches of HIV and treatments for opioids in primary care. Third, we introduce, define, and provide models of integrating treatments for OUD with services for the prevention and management of HIV infection in primary care with case studies to illustrate the benefits and advantages of integration of services. Finally, we review multiple structural barriers to integration of substance use treatment into primary care and offer structural strategies to overcoming and implementing integrated OUD-HIV services in primary care settings.

Injection Drug Use and the HIV Epidemic for People with OUD

Sharing needles and contaminated injection equipment are a major mode of HIV transmission worldwide. Approximately 12.7 million people inject drugs globally, of which 13.1% live with HIV.[6] Data from national population-based surveys in the United States show that people who inject drugs (PWID) comprise 2.6% of the population (confidence interval: 1.8%–3.3%) equating to approximately 6,612,488 PWID (range: 4,583,188–8,641,788).[31] Empirical studies suggest that PWID, particularly younger populations, have worse HIV outcomes along the HIV care continuum compared to other populations with HIV.[32,33] PWID are less likely to be linked and retained in care, receive antiretroviral therapy, and achieve HIV viral load suppression, which further increases risk of HIV/HCV transmission. PWID with HIV often initiate antiretroviral therapy (ART) late, many years after they have been diagnosed and after they have experienced an AIDS-defining illness which limits the effectiveness of ART in suppressing HIV infection.[34] Nearly 30% of PWID with HIV in the United States are not linked to HIV care within a month of diagnosis.[32] Less than one-half of men (40.1%) and women (48.6%) who inject drugs and have HIV in the United States have received a prescription for ART.[32] Poor retention in services for the prevention and management of HIV leads to poor HIV treatment outcomes, namely, less viral suppression and lower CD4 counts.[35–37] Less than one-third of men (32.2%) and about 36.5% of women who inject drugs are virally suppressed.[32] In addition to treatments for OUD and HIV, people with OUD often require diagnosis and treatment for coinfections of HCV and HBV.[38] Multiple viral infections complicate care in people living with HIV and lead to poor HIV outcomes such as low adherence to ART, low viral load suppression, and other serious health outcomes such as cardiovascular disease, neurocognitive impairment, and insulin resistance, all of which also affect HIV treatment and adherence to ART.[39,40]

HIV Prevention and Treatment Services in Primary Care Settings

Primary care clinics are in an ideal position to improve rates of testing, initiate HIV care, increase retention, and treat comorbid infections for people with OUD.[41–44] Formerly relegated to specialist settings, primary care clinics are now viable settings to deliver services for the prevention and management of HIV infection.[45] The primary care setting offers opportunities to identify a greater number of people in the general population with OUD and HIV, discuss HIV prevention and infection with patients, and identify at-risk patients who would benefit from more enhanced treatments.[44,45] The Centers for Disease Control and Prevention recommended evidence-based strategies for those who use drugs for the prevention and management of HIV in primary care settings include (a) prevention and treatment of substance use and mental disorders; (b) outreach programs; (c) risk assessment for use of substances; (d) risk assessment for infectious diseases; (e) screening, diagnosis, and counseling for infectious diseases; (f) vaccination; (g) prevention of mother-child transmission; (h) interventions for reducing risk behaviors (risk reduction programs and messages, treatment of substance use and mental disorders to prevent infectious diseases, access to sterile injection and drug preparation equipment, interventions to increase condom efficiency); (i) partner services and contact follow-up; (j) referrals and linkage to care; and (k) medical treatment for infectious diseases.[45]

Comprehensive assessment includes screening for HIV, HCV, and other sexually transmitted infections (STIs); laboratory panels required for primary care medical practice; medical history; psychological status; social circumstances; and family history.[45] At the time of writing this chapter there were no studies examining the delivery of pre-exposure prophylaxis (PrEP) within a package of integrated OUD-HIV services. Studies among PWID show that PrEP reduces HIV infection and transmission, and PrEP adherence ratings are high.[46–49] PrEP is currently available in primary care settings in the United States for HIV prevention with this population.[50,51]

For patients diagnosed with HIV, guidelines from the International Antiviral Society USA Panel inform clinical decision-making about which HIV treatment services are most suited to the multiple needs presented by the patient population.[52] US guidelines recommend screening for STI/viral hepatitis at least once a year to identify cases of infection in PWID and other at-risk populations.[45] Biannual or quarterly clinic visits are recommended for clinical examination and lab testing as needed.[45] Recommendations for HIV-negative PWID in general medicine primary care include annual testing for HIV/STI and viral hepatitis.[45] People with OUD who are HIV-positive often face complications that require ongoing medical monitoring and treatment in primary care.[21] Nonetheless, a number of studies suggest that providing drug treatment and services in primary care settings is feasible and cost-effective, reduces HIV infection, and improves HIV treatment outcomes in the United States and other countries.[53,54]

Drug Treatment as Prevention: Evidence-Based MATs for HIV Prevention

The integration of drug treatment into primary care settings for people with OUD could enhance the prevention of HIV and improve HIV treatment outcomes.[55–61] Addiction specialists are healthcare providers with requisite training and credentials to prescribe and manage MAT and play a critical role in redressing the HIV epidemic among people with OUD.[74] The capacity of treatments for OUD to reduce HIV risk and transmission is known as "drug treatment as HIV prevention."[62,63] Based on a consensus from scientific evidence, MAT is critical to reducing HIV transmission and acquisition and achieving the goal of ending the HIV pandemic by 2030.[64,65] A systematic review among 12 studies and unpublished data examining the effects of MAT on HIV transmission among PWID show MAT was associated with a 54% reduction in risk of HIV infection among PWID.[66] Presently, four MATs are available to reduce opioid use, and they are in the form of *full and partial mu-receptor agonists*: (a) methadone (full), (b) buprenorphine or buprenorphine/naloxone (partial); and *opioid antagonists*: (c) oral naltrexone (NTX) and extended-release naltrexone (XR-NTX), as shown in Table 8.1.[67]

MAT for OUD

The most widely available treatment for opioid addiction is methadone, a full mu-receptor agonist, taken once per day orally.[68] Methadone fully activates opioid receptors throughout the body to ameliorate painful symptoms of withdrawal and unpleasant cravings. Substantial empirical evidence suggests methadone maintenance is effective for stopping or reducing heroin use, decreasing incidence of HIV, suppressing viral load, increasing medication adherence to ART, and increasing retention in

Table 8.1 Medication-Assisted Therapies for the Treatment of OUDs

Medication	MOA	Dosage	OUD	HIV	Primary Care	Advantages
Methadone	Full mu-receptor agonist	Oral daily	↓Heroin, ↓Illicit prescription opioid use ↓Overdose	↑retention in HIV care, viral suppression, medication adherence, ↓HIV, HCV infection, transmission risk behaviors	Not approved	Opiate effects blocks cravings and withdrawal symptoms
Buprenorphin-Naltrexone	Partial mu-receptor agonist	Transmucosal daily	↓Heroin ↓Illicit prescription opioid use ↓Overdose	↑ medication adherence, retention, screenings for HIV, HCV, HBV ↓HIV, HCV infection, transmission risk behaviors	Approved with certification waiver from DEA <276 patients	Opiate effects blocks cravings, naltrexone effects prevent euphoria when injected
Naltrexone	Opioid antagonist	Oral (NXT), daily	No change in heroin, prescription medication, or other opioid use	none	Any primary care provider	No diversion risk, naltrexone effects block euphoria when relapse occurs
		Injection (XR-NXT) monthly	↑time abstinent from opioids	↑viral suppression ↓transmission risk behaviors		

Note. MOA = method of administration; OUD = opioid use disorder; DEA = Drug Enforcement Agency; HVC = hepatitis C virus; HBV = hepatitis B virus; XR-NXT = extended release naltrexone.

treatment.[10,70-73] Despite the merits of methadone as an effective intervention for OUD and HIV prevention, legal barriers prevent the integration of methadone into primary care settings.

Buprenorphine as a partial *mu-receptor opioid agonist* presents some unique advantages compared to other pharmacological medications for OUD. It is prescribed by certified physicians, which eliminates the need to visit specialized treatment clinics and thus widens availability to a larger population.[74] Providers who have delivered buprenorphine to 100 patients for a period of more than a year may apply to lift limits to 275 patients.[24] Studies from the past 35 years emphasize the benefits of buprenorphine in reducing use of illicit opiates and overdose.[66,75,76] Buprenorphine is shown to improve HIV quality of care indicators including medication adherence, retention in care, four infectious disease indicators (HIV, HCV, HBV, syphilis), and screenings for medical conditions in the general population.[61,77] The opioid effects are weaker with buprenorphine than methadone, thus presenting a lower potential for misuse and overdose compared to methadone.[74] If injected, the naloxone component potentiates withdrawal symptoms but, if taken orally, the opiate effects of the buprenorphine prevent withdrawal and cravings.[67] At the time of writing this chapter the Food and Drug Administration (FDA) had approved Bunavail® (buprenorphine + naloxone) as a buccal film, Suboxone® as a film, Zubsolv® as sublingual tablets, and buprenorphine containing transmucosal products for dependency on opioids.[78] Prior empirical literature underscores buprenorphine's promise in primary care settings.[79-84] Fiellin and colleagues[83] examined long-term outcomes with office-based primary care buprenorphine/naloxone treatment in 53 opioid-dependent patients. Two-year retention was 38% during which 91% showed no evidence of opioid use.[83]

Naltrexone is an FDA-approved *opiate antagonist* for treatment of opioid and alcohol use disorders that prevents the euphoric effects of opiates. The daily oral formulation ReVia® or Depade® was approved in 1984 for treatment of OUD, and the injectable once monthly formulation XR-NTX (Vivitrol®) was FDA-approved in 2010 for OUD in the United States.[78] Oral naltrexone is not effective in treatment of OUD due to nonadherence. The extended-release form of Naltrexone consisting of a monthly injection is shown to be a safe and effective method of reducing opioid use.[86-92] In a randomized double-blind placebo-controlled trial of XR-NTX among Russian opioid-dependent persons, XR-NTX increased time of abstinence and reduced HIV risks compared with the placebo group.[88] Studies of

XR-NTX among persons living with HIV found improvements in HIV viral suppression in persons with OUD being released from prison or jail.[93] As an opiate antagonist, naltrexone prevents feelings of euphoria associated with the drug, and there is no diversion risk or potential for abuse.[94] Any medical provider can issue a prescription for naltrexone to treat OUD in medical settings.[67] An important concern of XR-NTX is the requirement to abstain from opioid use prior to initiating treatment.[94] The drop in tolerance resulting from complete abstinence from opioids could result in overdose in the event of relapse for people with OUD receiving XR-NTX.[94]

Screening Brief Intervention and Referral to Treatment for People with OUD

The Screening Brief Intervention and Referral to Treatment (SBIRT) model for substance use provides a tool to link patients to different types of behavioral treatments based on clinical needs and preferences in primary care settings.[95–102] Behavioral interventions for OUD and other substance use disorders are delivered in a number of settings and can range in intensity of treatment from brief intervention (one session) and treatments (two to five sessions) to specialized and intensive treatment programs (more than five sessions).[103] Physicians, physician's assistants, nurses, social workers, and other medical staff screen patients for OUD and other substance use problems to identify those who would benefit from brief interventions or behavioral treatments.[103–105] Evidence-based screening instruments apply thresholds to identify risky drug or alcohol use and are recommended by the National Institute of Drug Abuse.[106] Screening instruments have emerged to address risk factors for OUD in primary care settings including the Clinical Opiate Withdrawal Scale, the McCaffrey Initial Pain Assessment Tool, and the Pain Assessment and Documentation Tool.[106]

Depending on severity of substance use, patients are provided either single (BI) or multiple brief interventions (BT) typically lasting about 5 to 10 minutes or longer in the SBIRT model.[100,101,107] BI and BT help individuals reduce drug use behaviors by increasing insight and awareness into negative consequences of drug use and increasing readiness for change.[108] Gyczynski and colleagues[109] examined SBIRT screening data of over 55,000 patients in New Mexico in which 1,208 received either BI or BT treatment. Participants in the BT group underwent a sharper decline in substance and alcohol use compared to BI. Randomized controlled trials by Saitz et al.[102] and Roy-Byrne et al.[110] could not confirm efficacy of a single-session intervention over treatment as usual (TAU) in primary care settings. Roy-Byrne and colleagues[110] examined data from more than 10,000 patients who were screened in a government subsidized primary care setting. Out of the screened patients, 868 were randomized to either receive a brief single-session intervention or an enhanced TAU group. The single-session intervention did not change drug use of patients compared to the enhanced TAU group. Following behavioral treatment, patients identified as needing additional care are provided access to evidence-based treatments for substance abuse that require more specialized settings including detoxification, stabilization, inpatient, residential, and other types of treatment.[96,101,105]

Models for the Delivery of Integrated OUD-HIV Services in Primary Care to Improve Access to Treatment for OUD and HIV Services

Despite mounting empirical literature showing that MAT reduces HIV transmission and infection and improves HIV treatment outcomes, coverage of MAT for people with OUD remains low or entirely unavailable in many areas.[111] In order to maximize coverage, MAT must be widely delivered through interventions that increase access beyond specialized substance abuse treatment centers for OUD.[14] Delivering MAT in primary care settings enables providers to monitor treatment for medical complications that may accompany OUD (HIV, HCV, HBV, and tuberculosis), which has been found to improve both HIV and OUD treatment outcomes.[28,112,113] Integrated service delivery of treatment for OUD and HIV involves selecting the most suitable combinations of evidence-based strategies for the prevention, treatment and management of HIV and OUD in primary care.[17]

Integration is a combination of service functions designed to improve the delivery of HIV services as well as HIV prevention and treatment outcomes, substance abuse treatment, and other medical and psychological outcomes provided in a single location.[30] Haldane et al.[30] identified a typology of integration to inform service delivery models: (a) *clinical integration* in which primary care providers combine all services in direct practice to patients (i.e., HIV testing and prescribing buprenorphine); (b) *service integration* involving multidisciplinary teams of practitioners from diverse professional backgrounds who provide services to address substance abuse and HIV care needs (i.e., the primary clinic employs addiction physicians to dispense buprenorphine); and (c) *systems integration*, which encompasses collaboration across sectors (i.e., primary care and HIV care) and professional organizations (MAT and HIV care) to improve the delivery of HIV care and substance abuse services.[30] Drawing on prior literature, we offer three models to integrate MAT into HIV primary care for PWID: (a) clinical integration model with primary care providers, (b) service integration model with primary care providers and addiction specialists, and (c) clinical-service integration hybrid model).[30,112]

Clinical Integration Model with Primary Care Providers

In the *clinical integration model with primary care providers* (see Figure 8.1), primary care clinicians provide initiation and maintenance of MAT and services for the prevention and management of HIV.[30,112] Intake and initial sessions include risk assessment for use of substances, risk assessment for infectious diseases, and screening and diagnosis for infectious diseases. After intake and patient assessment, primary care providers deliver risk reduction interventions administer vaccinations for HBV (if needed); prevent mother-to-child transmission; and provide medical treatment of infectious diseases, treatment for mental health disorders and substance abuse, and partner notification services. Primary care providers discuss medication treatment options with HIV positive patients to decide a course of treatment for substance abuse that best fits the clinical needs of their HIV care. The provider follows recommendations for the management of HIV in primary care settings including HAART medication and medication adherence to maximize chances of viral suppression. A case manager and counselor (social worker, substance abuse counselor, or other mental health professional) coordinate services that accompany MAT, such as behavioral interventions including motivational enhancement and cognitive interventions. Case management services including referrals for housing, intimate partner violence, food security, employment, and other psychosocial services that are essential and often included in primary care case management services.

In the clinical integration model with primary care providers, patients are eligible to receive services from HIV care providers that include prescriptions for PrEP and ordering necessary medical tests combined with the delivery of MAT and access to condoms.[51] Primary care clinics that do not offer harm reduction services should issue referrals to syringe

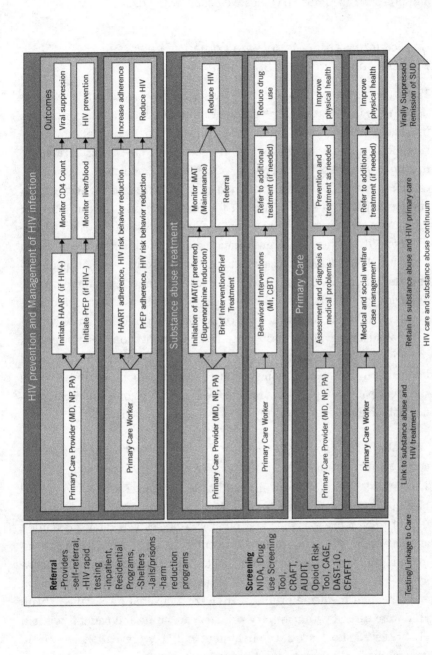

FIGURE 8.1 Clinical integration model with HIV primary care providers

exchange programs where patients can access sterile injection materials and prescribe PrEP for HIV-negative people with OUD.

Service Integration Model with Primary Care Providers and Addiction Specialists

The *service integration model with primary care providers and addiction specialists* (Figure 8.2) involves the coordination of a multidisciplinary team to provide integrated services to people who use drugs. HIV practitioners provide intake, preliminary assessments, and triage to specialized substance abuse treatment providers.[30,112] Following screening, the addiction specialist or counselor collects more information to identify suitable MAT interventions and develops a course of treatment for OUD. The primary care provider initiates and monitors HIV treatment medications without providing treatment for OUD. There is communication among members of the multidisciplinary HIV-addiction specialist clinical team about treatment planning and optimizing care. The addiction specialist provides buprenorphine induction, initiation, and maintenance. Addiction counselors and case managers with human services and counseling backgrounds can deliver behavioral substance abuse treatment including motivational enhancement, cognitive behavioral therapy, relapse planning, and other evidence-based interventions.[114] The addiction specialist model may be most useful with a sufficient patient population of people who use drugs or a smaller population with a greater severity drug use or polydrug use behaviors.[30]

Facilitated Access to Substance Abuse Treatment with Prevention and Treatment for HIV (FAST-PATH)

The FAST-PATH model was funded by the Substance Abuse and Mental Health Services Administration (SAMSHA) to examine service integration of treatments for OUD and other substances with HIV prevention and treatment in an urban medical center through primary care, pharmacological substance abuse treatment, and referral for additional services.[26,28] Two multidisciplinary medical teams, an HIV primary care team and a general medicine primary care team, delivered care. Patients with HIV were treated within an HIV primary care clinic and patients without HIV received substance abuse treatment and HIV prevention services in general medical primary care. Services included primary care, MAT, substance abuse counseling in groups and individually, overdose prevention, HIV sexual risk reduction counseling, and referral to more intensive drug

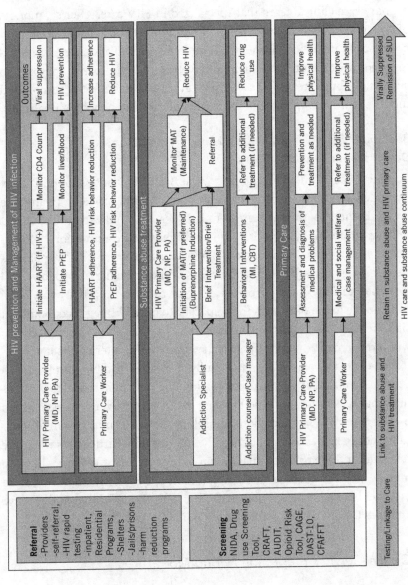

FIGURE 8.2 Service integration model with primary care providers and addiction specialists

treatment services as needed. The addiction counselor or case manager provided group and individual counseling as well as intensive "wrap-around" case management services including housing, childcare, food security, and other services. HIV-positive PWID received treatment by a primary care clinical team that specialized in HIV care. After six months of treatment in the FAST PATH model more than half of patients on buprenorphine no longer met the criteria for OUD. Patients preferred integrated care as more convenient and valued the team-based approach to substance abuse treatment and HIV care.[26] Patients felt the team-based model of care was valuable to the quality of care and benefit of treatment.

Buprenorphine HIV Evaluation and Support (BHIVES) Demonstration Project

Conducted between 2004 and 2009, the BHIVES Demonstration Project examined service integration of buprenorphine and naloxone treatments for OUD and HIV primary care at 10 US sites. Currently, six studies report findings from BHIVES.[25,114–118] The study provided training for HIV primary care providers including an HIV doctor and either a nurse, pharmacist, or drug counselor to provide behavioral counseling and follow-up.[114] Retention and substance use outcomes for patients in primary care were comparable to the outcomes from specialty clinics.[118] Integrated treatment sites included community health centers and HIV/AIDS specialized clinics with providers who were physicians specializing in internal medicine, infectious disease, psychiatry, and family medicine. A buprenorphine/naloxone case manager was incorporated into the treatment model to improve medication adherence. Patients were required to attend weekly group meetings provided by addiction counselors related to buprenorphine medication adherence as a component of the intervention. Participants who were retained for three or more quarters on buprenorphine were more likely to initiate ART and become virally suppressed.[115] Qualitative interviews from 33 patients emphasized high satisfaction with the treatment and positive attitudes toward receiving integrated OUD-HIV care.[116]

Clinical-Service Integration Hybrid Model

The *clinical-service integration hybrid model* involves use of addiction specialists to fulfill a specific task of treatment for OUD and other substances within an otherwise fully integrated primary care provider model (Figure 8.3).[30,112] In the hybrid model, the addiction specialist

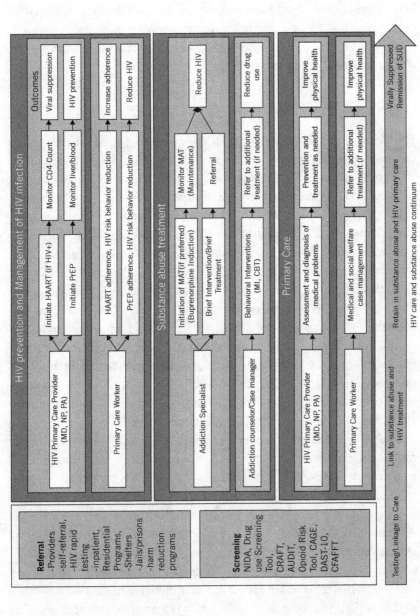

FIGURE 8.3 Clinical-service integration hybrid model

provides on-site buprenorphine initiation that stabilizes patients and transfers the remainder of care to the primary care provider, after the patient has significantly reduced illicit opiate use. One formulation of the hybrid model consists of an addiction specialist who delivers services related to stabilization of substance abuse, buprenorphine induction, and initiation. The primary care provider delivers services related to maintenance while the patient is in recovery from drug use.

Looking Ahead: Next Steps Toward Ending AIDS

The delivery of integrated OUD-HIV services in primary care settings presents opportunities to make progress toward ending AIDS and the HIV epidemic in the United States and globally. The intertwined nature of drug use and HIV require interventions that coordinate multiple evidence-based strategies to meet the clinical needs that patients present in primary care. Overcoming structural barriers to implementing integrated OUD-HIV services are critical to increasing coverage to meet the demands for treatment due to the expanding opioid epidemic in the United States.[119,120]

In this section we review social and structural barriers to implementing integrated OUD-HIV services in primary care. Social interventions mediate the social arrangement and conditions to increase access to health-promoting resources and reduce risks within various social contexts.[121–123] In order to promote integration of drug abuse and HIV treatment in primary care, structural interventions need to target social norms, organizational practices and policies, laws, institutional regulations, and economic and financial conditions.[124–130] Combination prevention recognizes that individual and structural approaches alone are insufficient and call for multilevel interventions that address the intersection of multiple social and structural factors.[120,131,132] We identify multilevel barriers and present solutions at the patient, provider, service delivery, and structural levels (Figure 8.4).

Patient-level barriers include ongoing drug use, comorbid psychiatric conditions, homelessness, food insecurity, chaotic life conditions, employment, and childcare.[124,129,133–135] Nearly one-quarter of patients receiving Ryan White funded HIV/AIDS treatment are homeless, and 81.0% earn less than the federal poverty line.[136] Homelessness and income instability create social conditions that inhibit retention and engagement in care.[137,138] Studies find that unstable housing is associated with higher viral load and lower CD4 count compared to people living with HIV who

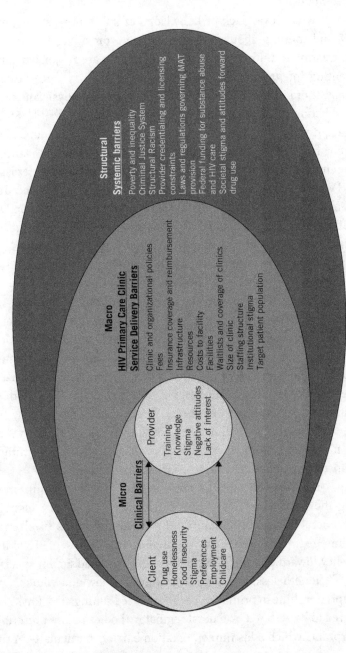

Micro
Clinical Barriers

Client
Drug use
Homelessness
Food insecurity
Stigma
Preferences
Employment
Childcare

Provider
Training
Knowledge
Stigma
Negative attitudes
Lack of interest

Macro
HIV Primary Care Clinic
Service Delivery Barriers

Clinic and organizational policies
Fees
Insurance coverage and reimbursement
Infrastructure
Resources
Costs to facility
Facilities
Waitlists and coverage of clinics
Size of clinic
Staffing structure
Institutional stigma
Target patient population

Structural
Systemic barriers

Poverty and inequality
Criminal Justice System
Structural Racism
Provider credentialing and licensing
constraints
Laws and regulations governing MAT
provision
Federal funding for substance abuse
and HIV care
Societal stigma and attitudes forward
drug use

FIGURE 8.4 Multilevel barriers to integrating treatment for opioid use disorders into HIV care

have secure housing.[137,138] These factors compound the stigma inflicted by negative social norms toward substance use disorders and HIV status in the United States.

At the provider level, lack of knowledge of substance use treatment and HIV and training about treating OUD and providing HIV prevention and treatment among primary care providers are major barriers to implementing integrated OUD-HIV services in primary care settings.[42] Historically, there is a lack of training for primary care physicians on the role of addiction in primary care and HIV treatment.[50,98,101,103] Studies show that physicians in primary care may view substance dependence as different from other diseases by taking a draconian moral stance on nonadherence to treatment that does not factor in the many complex issues facing HIV-positive people who use drugs.[139] Collaboration have occurred between federal agencies including SAMSHA, National Institute on Drug Abuse, and academic professional organizations including the American Psychiatric Association and the American Association for Primary Care to require accredited universities to expand training in substance abuse treatment at the medical school level. Professional training in medical school curricula devotes a relatively small portion of training to working with people who use drugs; thus primary care physicians are often not well prepared to address addiction.[140] After medical school training in the form of continuing professional education must include providing treatments for OUD and other substances in primary care, the impact of drug use on HIV disease progression, and the benefits of treatment for OUD and HIV care continuum outcomes. To surmount the barriers presented by poor training, additional interventions are necessary at the provider level that include in-service training to change knowledge, self-efficacy attitudes, and negative perceptions of treating substance use disorders.

Changes must be made to the credentialing and legal requirements regarding the provision of MAT in primary care. US legal constraints have, in general, discouraged community-based physicians involvement in providing treatments for OUD.[141] Buprenorphine represented a shift in health policy toward providing buprenorphine in nonaddiction specialist settings.[24,74] Nonetheless, there are strict rules on how and who can prescribe buprenorphine in primary care office–based settings.[24,141] Physicians are required to be certified by federal regulatory bodies before prescribing buprenorphine, which adds implementation barriers particularly in rural locations.[24] State and federal regulations particularly around credentialing and provision of MAT create administrative and legal barriers to accessing integrated OUD-HIV services in primary care. Changes to credentialing and legal requirements around providing MAT in HIV primary care could significantly remove barriers to the implementation of integrated substance abuse treatment in HIV primary care. The geographical shortage of physicians with training to treat OUD and addiction counselors create a scarcity of services that leave people who use drugs without care.[142]

Integration of treatments for OUD and services for the prevention and management of HIV into primary care also depends on the staffing structure and size of the clinic. The agency must have the resources to meet demands presented by patients with OUDs with a range of severity.[143] Partnerships between governmental and nongovernmental organizations could ameliorate staffing challenges presenting barriers to integrated OUD-HIV services in primary care. Partnerships could include combinations between state-funded public health employees with university-employed practitioners and researchers. Promoting communication between staff members from addiction and HIV care backgrounds at group clinical supervision meetings could create flows of information and support to prevent staff burnout and improve patient care.

Costs to primary care clinics are another potential structural barrier that may interfere with delivering integrated OUD-HIV services in primary care. Research examining the costs of integrated care suggest an increase in clinic costs to meet the demands of staff training, adding physical resources, lab testing, and other services.[119] Shackman et al.[119] conducted a cost-benefit analysis and found that the BHIVE model of integrated care required additional funding and resources to meet the demands of providing integrated care particularly when nonphysicians and providers render additional services ineligible for reimbursement from insurance payers. Although clinic costs may be higher on average, the cost savings across systems of care by delivering integrated treatments compared to providing either treatment individually emphasize the promise of integrating OUD and HIV services into primary care. The costs of adding resources without adequate financial compensation could function as a disincentive for primary care providers to integrate treatment for OUD and HIV services into primary care.[17,144]

National insurance policies governing reimbursement of HIV care use different formulas compared to substance abuse that present macro-level barriers to engaging people who use drugs in substance abuse and HIV care.[112] National policies governing insurance reimbursement for HIV care, especially those utilizing different formulas compared to treatments for OUD, must be changed. Rates of reimbursement of SBIRT by Medicare and other carriers of insurance do not promote utilization of SBIRT in primary care settings.[145] State and federal public health agencies must work with insurance carriers to develop rates of reimbursement for intensive services and resources needed to implement integrated OUD-HIV services in primary care.

Practices of the US criminal justice system create racial inequities in access to health-promoting resources that widen inequities in substance abuse and HIV treatment outcomes. The criminalization of drug use has led to disproportionate numbers of people who use drugs who are African American, Hispanic, and other minorities experiencing questioning by the police, arrest, and incarceration.[146–148] Incarceration disrupts HIV care and substance abuse treatment leading to interruptions in medication adherence and resulting in increases in viral load and risk of relapse to high-risk drug use.[149,150]

Access to integrated substance abuse treatment is integral during the periods of time immediately following incarceration and detention. The period immediately following incarceration is characterized by very high risk of overdose due to diminished tolerance and HIV infection from injection drug use and sexual risk behaviors.[151] Primary care clinics should work with local jails and prisons to enable intake and engagement of formerly incarcerated people with OUDs in HIV primary care. One administrative solution is to establish clinic policies to not terminate from treatment clients who become incarcerated and, upon incarceration, to establish communication of medical and medication history to the correctional facility to prevent lapses in treatment. Reforms are necessary to reduce aggressive policing and to improve service delivery of integrated substance abuse and HIV treatment among people who use drugs. Interventions to train the police to help people with OUD including reversal of overdose, providing referrals to healthcare providers, and diversion from arrest are fundamental to the success of integrated interventions in primary care.[152,153]

Gender-based violence and lack of women-specific treatment that address reproductive health care and childcare needs are macro-structural barriers that account for lower rates of women accessing and staying in substance abuse treatment.[122,154]

Conclusion

To increase engagement in treatment and care and to address the global opioid epidemic, this chapter provided an argument for responsive, appropriate, and convenient integrated HIV and substance abuse programs in primary care settings for individuals who use drugs. The integration and co-location of MAT and other substance abuse behavioral interventions in a package of comprehensive services in primary care is a promising structural intervention to address economic, political, and social barriers to accessing treatment among people who use drugs. This chapter provided a description of models of service delivery that integrate substance abuse treatment for OUD into HIV or regular primary care settings in the United States with implications to be used in other parts of the world. We identified three models integrating treatment for HIV and substance abuse: (a) clinical integration model with primary care providers, (b) service integration model with primary care providers and addiction specialists, and (c) clinical-service integration hybrid model. Integrated care addresses complex service needs and multiple behavioral outcomes to move patients along the HIV continuum of care and increase the likelihood of achieving viral suppression. We discussed the multilevel barriers and implementation of the models and provided structural strategies to address them.

Providing substance abuse treatment with a universal access to primary care is a fundamental step in fighting the HIV epidemic and is the most effective model to reducing HIV morbidity and mortality as well as the risk of transmission. Healthcare systems must remove multilevel social and structural barriers to allow the integration of treatment for substance abuse disorders and HIV in primary care settings. This integration of services is critically needed, given the severity of the opioid epidemic, and the AIDS epidemic, especially among people who use drugs.

References

1. Centers for Disease Control and Prevention. (2017, August 30). Understanding the epidemic. https://www.cdc.gov/drugoverdose/epidemic/index.html
2. Center for Behavioral Health Statistics and Quality. (2015). 2014 National Survey on Drug Use and Health: Detailed Tables. Rockville, MD: Substance Abuse and Mental Health Services Administration.

3. Substance Abuse and Mental Health Services Administration (2015). Opioid Use Disorders. https://www.samhsa.gov/disorders/substance-use

4. Centers for Disease Control and Prevention. (2017). HIV and Injection Drug Use. https://www.cdc.gov/hiv/risk/idu.html

5. El-Bassel, N., Shaw, S. A., Dasgupta, A., & Strathdee, S. A. (2014). Drug use as a driver of HIV risks: Re-emerging and emerging issues. *Current Opinion in HIV and AIDS, 9*(2), 150.

6. United Nations Office of Drugs Control (2014). World Drug Report. http://www.unodc.org/wdr2014/en/drug-use.html

7. Conrad, C., Bradley, H. M., Broz, D., Buddha, S., Chapman, E. L., Galang, R. R., . . . Duwve, J. M. (2015). Community outbreak of HIV infection linked to injection drug use of oxymorphone—Indiana, 2015. *MMWR: Morbidity and Mortality Weekly Report, 64* 443–444.

8. Rural Indiana struggles to contend with H.I.V. outbreak. (2015, May 6). *The New York Times.* https://www.nytimes.com/2015/05/06/us/rural-indiana-struggles-to-contend-with-hiv-outbreak.html

9. Altice, F. L., Bruce, R. D., Lucas, G. M., Lum, P. J., Korthuis, P. T., Flanigan, T. P., . . . Cajina, A. (2011). HIV treatment outcomes among HIV-infected, opioid-dependent patients receiving buprenorphine/naloxone treatment within HIV clinical care settings: Results from a multisite study. *JAIDS Journal of Acquired Immune Deficiency Syndromes, 56*(Suppl. 1), S22.

10. Gowing, L., Ali, R., & White, J. (2006). Buprenorphine for the management of opioid withdrawal. *Cochrane Database of Systematic Reviews, 2*(2).

11. Gowing, L., Farrell, M., Bornemann, R., Sullivan, L., & Ali, R. (2008). Substitution treatment of injecting opioid users for prevention of HIV infection. *Cochrane Database of Systematic Reviews, 2.*

12. Gowing, L. R., Farrell, M., Bornemann, R., Sullivan, L. E., & Ali, R. L. (2006). Brief report: Methadone treatment of injecting opioid users for prevention of HIV infection. *Journal of General Internal Medicine, 21*(2), 193–195.

13. Springer, S. A., Qiu, J., Saber-Tehrani, A. S., & Altice, F. L. (2012). Retention on buprenorphine is associated with high levels of maximal viral suppression among HIV-infected opioid dependent released prisoners. *PLoS One, 7*(5), e38335.

14. Springer, S. A., Chen, S., & Altice, F. L. (2010). Improved HIV and substance abuse treatment outcomes for released HIV-infected prisoners: The impact of buprenorphine treatment. *Journal of Urban Health, 87*(4), 592–602.

15. Strathdee, S. A., Shoptaw, S., Dyer, T. P., Quan, V. M., Aramrattana, A., & Substance Use Scientific Committee of the HIV Prevention Trials Network. (2012). Towards combination HIV prevention for injection drug users: Addressing addictophobia, apathy and inattention. *Current Opinion in HIV and AIDS, 7*(4), 320.

16. Sullivan, L. E., & Fiellin, D. A. (2005). Buprenorphine: Its role in preventing HIV transmission and improving the care of HIV-infected patients with opioid dependence. *Clinical Infectious Diseases, 41*(6), 891–896.

17. Volkow, N. D., Frieden, T. R., Hyde. P. S., & Cha, S. S. (2014). Medication-assisted therapies—tackling the opioid-overdose epidemic. *New England Journal of Medicine*, 370(22):2063–2066.

18. Petersen, Z., Myers, B., Van Hout, M. C., Plüddemann, A., & Parry, C. (2013). Availability of HIV prevention and treatment services for people who inject drugs: findings from 21 countries. *Harm Reduction Journal, 10*(1), 13.

19. Tkatchenko-Schmidt, E., Renton, A., Gevorgyan, R., Davydenko, L., & Atun, R. (2008). Prevention of HIV/AIDS among injecting drug users in Russia: Opportunities and barriers to scaling-up of harm reduction programmes. *Health Policy, 85*(2), 162–171.

20. Wolfe, D., Carrieri, M. P., & Shepard, D. (2010). Treatment and care for injecting drug users with HIV infection: A review of barriers and ways forward. *The Lancet, 376*(9738), 355–366.

21. Meyer, J. P., Althoff, A. L., & Altice, F. L. (2013). Optimizing care for HIV-infected people who use drugs: Evidence-based approaches to overcoming healthcare disparities. *Clinical Infectious Diseases, 57*(9), 1309–1317.

22. Volkow, N. D., & Montaner, J. (2011). The urgency of providing comprehensive and integrated treatment for substance abusers with HIV. *Health Affairs, 30*(8), 1411–1419.

23. Khalsa, J. H., Vocci, F., Altice, F., Fiellin, D., & Miller, V. (2006). Buprenorphine and HIV primary care: New opportunities for integrated treatment. *Clinical Infectious Diseases, 43*(4), S169

24. Substance Abuse and Mental Health Services Administration. (2015). Legislation, regulations and guidelines. https://www.samhsa.gov/medication-assisted-treatment/legislation-regulations-guidelines

25. Chaudhry, A. A., Botsko, M., Weiss, L., Egan, J. E., Mitty, J., Estrada, B., . . . BHIVES Collaborative. (2011). Participant characteristics and HIV risk behaviors among individuals entering integrated buprenorphine/naloxone and HIV care. *JAIDS Journal of Acquired Immune Deficiency Syndromes, 56*, S14–S21.

26. Drainoni, M. L., Farrell, C., Sorensen-Alawad, A., Palmisano, J. N., Chaisson, C., & Walley, A. Y. (2014). Patient perspectives of an integrated program of medical care and substance use treatment. *AIDS Patient Care and STDs, 28*(2), 71–81.

27. Samet, J. H., Friedmann, P., & Saitz, R. (2001). Benefits of linking primary medical care and substance abuse services: patient, provider, and societal perspectives. *Archives of Internal Medicine, 161*, 85–91.

28. Walley, A. Y., Palmisano, J., Sorensen-Alawad, A., Chaisson, C., Raj, A., Samet, J. H., & Drainoni, M. L. (2015). Engagement and substance dependence in a primary care-based addiction treatment program for people infected with HIV

and people at high-risk for HIV infection. *Journal of Substance Abuse Treatment*, *59*, 59–66.

29. Crepaz, N., Baack, B. N., Higa, D. H., & Mullins, M. M. (2015). Effects of integrated interventions on transmission risk and care continuum outcomes in persons living with HIV: Meta-analysis, 1996–2014. *AIDS*, *29*, 2371–2383.

30. Haldane, V., Cervero-Liceras, F., Chuah, F. L., Ong, S. E., Murphy, G., Sigfrid, L., . . . Buse, K. (2017). Integrating HIV and substance use services: A systematic review. *Journal of the International AIDS Society*, *20*(1).

31. Lansky, A., Finlayson, T., Johnson, C., Holtzman, D., Wejnert, C., Mitsch, A., . . . Crepaz, N. (2014). Estimating the number of persons who inject drugs in the United States by meta-analysis to calculate national rates of HIV and hepatitis C virus infections. *PLoS One*, *9*(5), e97596.

32. Centers for Disease Control and Prevention. (2012). HIV care continuum. Monitoring selected national HIV prevention and care objectives by using HIV surveillance data—United States and 6 US dependent areas—2010. Atlanta: Author.

33. Karch, D. L., Gray, K. M., Shi, J., & Hall, H. I. (2016). HIV infection care and viral suppression among people who inject drugs, 28 US jurisdictions, 2012–2013. *The Open AIDS Journal*, *10*, 127.

34. Grigoryan, A., Hall, H. I., Durant, T., & Wei, X. (2009). Late HIV diagnosis and determinants of progression to AIDS or death after HIV diagnosis among injection drug users, 33 US States, 1996–2004. *PLoS One*, *4*(2), e4445.

35. Crawford, T. N., Sanderson, W. T., & Thornton, A. (2014). Impact of poor retention in HIV medical care on time to viral load suppression. *Journal of the International Association of Providers of AIDS Care*, *13*(3), 242–249.

36. Nijhawan, A. E., Liang, Y., Vysyaraju, K., Muñoz, J., Ketchum, N., Saber, J., . . . Villarreal, R. (2017). Missed initial medical visits: Predictors, timing, and implications for retention in HIV care. *AIDS Patient Care and STDs*, *31*, 213–221.

37. Okeke, N. L., Ostermann, J., & Thielman, N. M. (2014). Enhancing linkage and retention in HIV care: A review of interventions for highly resourced and resource-poor settings. *Current HIV/AIDS Reports*, *11*(4), 376–392.

38. Platt, L., Easterbrook, P., Gower, E., McDonald, B., Sabin, K., McGowan, C., . . . Vickerman, P. (2016). Prevalence and burden of HCV co-infection in people living with HIV: A global systematic review and meta-analysis. *The Lancet Infectious Diseases*, *16*(7), 797–808.

39. Rockstroh, J. K., Mocroft, A., Soriano, V., Tural, C., Losso, M. H., Horban, A., . . . Lundgren, J. (2005). Influence of hepatitis C virus infection on HIV-1 disease progression and response to highly active antiretroviral therapy. *The Journal of Infectious Diseases*, *192*(6), 992–1002.

40. McArthur, J. C. (2004). HIV dementia: an evolving disease. *Journal of Neuroimmunology*, *157*(1), 3–10.

41. Bluespruce, J., Dodge, W. T., Grothaus, L., Wheeler, K., Rebolledo, V., Carey, J. W., . . . Thompson, R. S. (2001). HIV prevention in primary care: Impact of a clinical intervention. *AIDS Patient Care and STDs, 15*(5), 243–253.

42. Chander, G., Monroe, A. K., Crane, H. M., Hutton, H. E., Saag, M. S., Cropsey, K., . . . Boswell, S. (2016). HIV primary care providers—Screening, knowledge, attitudes and behaviors related to alcohol interventions. *Drug and Alcohol Dependence, 161*, 59–66.

43. Monroe, A. K., Fleishman, J. A., Voss, C. C., Keruly, J. C., Nijhawan, A. E., Agwu, A. L., . . . HIV Research Network. (2017). Assessing antiretroviral use during gaps in HIV primary care using multisite Medicaid claims and clinical data. *JAIDS Journal of Acquired Immune Deficiency Syndromes, 76*(1), 82–89.

44. O'Connor, P. G., Molde, S., Henry, S., Shockcor, W. T., & Schottenfeld, R. S. (1992). Human immunodeficiency virus infection in intravenous drug users: A model for primary care. *American Journal of Medicine, 93*, 382–386.

45. Aberg, J. A., Gallant, J. E., Ghanem, K. G., Emmanuel, P., Zingman, B. S., & Horberg, M. A. (2013). Primary care guidelines for the management of persons infected with HIV: 2013 update by the HIV Medicine Association of the Infectious Diseases Society of America. *Clinical Infectious Diseases, 58*(1), e1–e34.

46. Koenig, L. J., Lyles, C., & Smith, D. K. (2013). Adherence to antiretroviral medications for HIV pre-exposure prophylaxis. *American Journal of Preventive Medicine, 44*(1), S91–S98.

47. Underhill, K., Operario, D., Skeer, M., Mimiaga, M., & Mayer, K. (2010). Packaging PrEP to prevent HIV: An integrated framework to plan for pre-exposure prophylaxis implementation in clinical practice. *Journal of Acquired Immune Deficiency Syndromes, 55*(1), 8.

48. Martin, M., Vanichseni, S., Suntharasamai, P., Sangkum, U., Mock, P. A., Leethochawalit, M., . . . Kittimunkong, S. (2015). The impact of adherence to preexposure prophylaxis on the risk of HIV infection among people who inject drugs. *AIDS, 29*(7), 819–824.

49. Spector, A. Y., Remien, R. H., & Tross, S. (2015). PrEP in substance abuse treatment: A qualitative study of treatment provider perspectives. *Substance Abuse Treatment, Prevention, and Policy, 10*(1), 1.

50. Krakower, D., & Mayer, K. H. (2012). What primary care providers need to know about preexposure prophylaxis for HIV prevention: A narrative Review. *Annals of Internal Medicine, 157*(7), 490–497.

51. Centers for Disease Control and Prevention. (2013). Update to interim guidance for preexposure prophylaxis (PrEP) for the prevention of HIV Infection: PrEP for injecting drug users. *MMWR: Morbidity and Mortality Weekly Report, 62*(23), 463.

52. Günthard, H. F., Aberg, J. A., Eron, J. J., Hoy, J. F., Telenti, A., Benson, C. A., . . . Reiss, P. (2014). Antiretroviral treatment of adult HIV infection: 2014 recommendations of the International Antiviral Society–USA Panel. *JAMA, 312*(4), 410–425.

53. Baggaley, R. F., Irvine, M. A., Leber, W., Cambiano, V., Figueroa, J., McMullen, H., ... Hollingsworth, T. D. (2017). Cost-effectiveness of screening for HIV in primary care: A health economics modelling analysis. *The Lancet HIV, 4,* e465–e474.

54. Long, E. F., Brandeau, M. L., & Owens, D. K. (2010). The cost-effectiveness and population outcomes of expanded HIV screening and antiretroviral treatment in the United States. *Annals of Internal Medicine, 153*(12), 778–789.

55. Belani, H., Chorba, T., Fletcher, F., Hennessey, K., Kroeger, K., Lansky, A., ... O'Connor, K. (2012). Integrated prevention services for HIV infection, viral hepatitis, sexually transmitted diseases, and tuberculosis for persons who use drugs illicitly: Summary guidance from CDC and the US Department of Health and Human Services. *MMWR: Morbidity and Mortality Weekly Report, 61*(5), 1–43.

56. Guise, A., Seguin, M., Mburu, G., McLean, S., Grenfell, P., Islam, Z., ... Rhodes, T. (2017). Integrated opioid substitution therapy and HIV care: A qualitative systematic review and synthesis of client and provider experiences. *AIDS Care, 29,* 1119–1128.

57. Kinahan, J. C., Surah, S., Keating, S., Bergin, C., Mulcahy, F., Lyons, F., & Keenan, E. (2016). Effect of integrating HIV and addiction care for non-engaging HIV-infected opiate-dependent patients. *Irish Journal of Medical Science, 185*(3), 623–628.

58. Simeone, C., Shapiro, B., & Lum, P. J. (2017). Integrated HIV care is associated with improved engagement in treatment in an urban methadone clinic. *Addiction Science & Clinical Practice, 12*(1), 19.

59. Suthar, A. B., Rutherford, G. W., Horvath, T., Doherty, M. C., & Negussie, E. K. (2014). Improving antiretroviral therapy scale-up and effectiveness through service integration and decentralization. *AIDS, 28,* S175–S185.

60. Rotheram-Borus, M. J., Swendeman, D., & Chovnick, G. (2009). The past, present, and future of HIV prevention: Integrating behavioral, biomedical, and structural intervention strategies for the next generation of HIV prevention. *Annual Review of Clinical Psychology, 5,* 143–167.

61. Haddad, M. S., Zelenev, A., & Altice, F. L. (2015). Buprenorphine maintenance treatment retention improves nationally recommended preventive primary care screenings when integrated into urban federally qualified health centers. *Journal of Urban Health, 92*(1), 193–213.

62. Metzger, D. S., Woody, G. E., & O'Brien, C. P. (2010). Drug treatment as HIV prevention: a research update. *JAIDS Journal of Acquired Immune Deficiency Syndromes, 55*(Suppl. 1), S32.

63. Metzger, D. S., & Zhang, Y. (2010). Drug treatment as HIV prevention: Expanding treatment options. *Current HIV/AIDS Reports, 7*(4), 220–225.

64. Low, A. J., Mburu, G., Welton, N. J., May, M. T., Davies, C. F., French, C., ... Rhodes, T. (2016). Impact of opioid substitution therapy on antiretroviral therapy outcomes: A systematic review and meta-analysis. *Clinical Infectious Diseases, 63*(8), 1094–1104.

65. Stover, J., Bollinger, L., Izazola, J. A., Loures, L., DeLay, P., Ghys, P. D., & Fast Track Modeling Working Group. (2016). What is required to end the AIDS epidemic as a public health threat by 2030? The cost and impact of the fast-track approach. *PLoS One, 11*(5), e0154893.

66. MacArthur, G. J., Minozzi, S., Martin, N., Vickerman, P., Deren, S., Bruneau, J., . . . Hickman, M. (2012). Opiate substitution treatment and HIV transmission in people who inject drugs: Systematic review and meta-analysis. *BMJ, 345*, e5945.

67. American Society for Addiction Medicine. (2015). Practice guidelines. https://www.asam.org/docs/default-source/practice-support/guidelines-and-consensus-docs/asam-national-practice-guideline-supplement.pdf

68. Substance Abuse and Mental Health Treatment Services Administration. (2015). Methadone. https://www.samhsa.gov/medication-assisted-treatment/treatment/methadone

69. Marsch, L. A. (1998). The efficacy of methadone maintenance interventions in reducing illicit opiate use, HIV risk behavior and criminality: A meta-analysis. *Addiction, 93*(4), 515–532.

70. Metzger, D. S., Woody, G. E., McLellan, A. T., Druley, P., DePhillipis, D., O'Brien, C., . . . Abrutyn, E. (1993). HIV seroconversion among in and out of treatment intravenous drug users: An 18-month prospective follow-up. *AIDS, 6*(9), 1049–1056.

71. Lucas, G. M., Mullen, B. A., Weidle, P. J., Hader, S., McCaul, M. E., & Moore, R. D. (2006). Directly administered antiretroviral therapy in methadone clinics is associated with improved HIV treatment outcomes, compared with outcomes among concurrent comparison groups. *Clinical Infectious Diseases, 42*(11), 1628–1635.

72. Palepu, A., Tyndall, M. W., Joy, R., Kerr, T., Wood, E., Press, N., . . . Montaner, J. S. (2006). Antiretroviral adherence and HIV treatment outcomes among HIV/HCV co-infected injection drug users: The role of methadone maintenance therapy. *Drug and Alcohol Dependence, 84*(2), 188–194.

73. Reddon, H., Milloy, M. J., Simo, A., Montaner, J., Wood, E., & Kerr, T. (2014). Methadone maintenance therapy decreases the rate of antiretroviral therapy discontinuation among HIV-positive illicit drug users. *AIDS and Behavior, 18*(4), 740–746.

74. Substance Abuse and Mental Health Treatment Services Administration. (2015). Buprenorphine. https://www.samhsa.gov/medication-assisted-treatment/treatment/buprenorphine

75. Mello, N. K., & Mendelson, J. H. (1980). Buprenorphine suppresses heroin use by heroin addicts. *Science, 207*(4431), 657–659.

76. Guichard, A., Lert, F., Calderon, C., Gaigi, H., Maguet, O., Soletti, J., . . . Zunzunegui, M. V. (2003). Illicit drug use and injection practices among drug users on methadone and buprenorphine maintenance treatment in France. *Addiction, 98*(11), 1585–1597.

77. Korthuis, P. T., Fiellin, D. A., Fu, R., Lum, P. J., Altice, F. L., Sohler, N., . . .
    Flanigan, T. P. (2011). Improving adherence to HIV quality of care indicators in
    persons with opioid dependence: The role of buprenorphine. *JAIDS Journal of
    Acquired Immune Deficiency Syndromes, 56*(Suppl. 1), S83.

78. Substance Abuse and Mental Health Services Administration. (2015).
    Medication and counseling treatment. https://www.samhsa.gov/medication-
    assisted-treatment/treatment

79. Gibson, A. E., Doran, C. M., Bell, J. R., Lintezris, N. (2003). A comparison of
    buprenorphine treatment in clinic and primary care settings: A randomized
    trial. *The Medical Journal of Australia, 179*, 38–42.

80. Fiellin. D. A., Gooseneck, R. A., Kosten, T. R. (2001). Office-based treatment
    for opioid dependence: Reaching new patient populations. *American Journal of
    Psychiatry, 158*, 1200–1204.

81. Fiellin, D. A., & O'Connor, P. G. (2002). Clinical practice: Office-based treatment
    of opioid dependent patients. *New England Journal of Medicine, 347*, 817–823.

82. Fudala, P. J., Bridge, T. P., Herbert, S., et al. (2003). Office-based treatment of
    opiate addiction with a sublingual-tablet formulation of buprenorphine and nal-
    oxone. *New England Journal of Medicine, 349*, 949–958.

83. Fiellin, D. A., Moore, B. A., Sullivan, L. E., Becker, W. C., Pantalon, M. V.,
    Chawarski, M. C., . . . Schottenfeld, R. S. (2008). Long-term treatment with
    buprenorphine/naloxone in primary care: Results at 2–5 years. *The American
    Journal on Addictions, 17*(2), 116–120.

84. McMurphy, S., Shea, J., Switzer, J., et al. (2006). Clinic-based treatment for
    opioid dependence: a qualitative inquiry. *American Journal of Health Behavior,
    30*, 544–555.

85. Minozzi, S., Amato, L., Vecchi, S., Davoli, M., Kirchmayer, U., & Verster, A.
    (2011). Oral naltrexone maintenance treatment for opioid dependence. *Cochrane
    Database of Systematic Reviews, 4*.

86. Korthuis, P. T., Lum, P. J., Vergara-Rodriguez, P., et al. (2017). Feasibility and
    safety of extended-release naltrexone treatment of opioid and alcohol use dis-
    order in HIV clinics: A pilot/feasibility randomized trial. *Addiction, 112*,
    1036–1044.

87. Krupitsky, E., Nunes, E. V., Ling, W., Gastfriend, D. R., Memisoglu, A., &
    Silverman, B. L. (2013). Injectable extended-release naltrexone (XR-NTX)
    for opioid dependence: Long-term safety and effectiveness. *Addiction, 108*(9),
    1628–1637.

88. Krupitsky, E., Nunes, E. V., Ling, W., Illeperuma, A., Gastfriend, D. R., &
    Silverman, B. L. (2011). Injectable extended-release naltrexone for opioid de-
    pendence: a double-blind, placebo-controlled, multicentre randomised trial. *The
    Lancet, 377*(9776), 1506–1513.

89. Lee, J. D., Friedmann, P. D., Kinlock, T. W., et al. (2016). Extended-release nal-
    trexone to prevent opioid relapse in criminal justice offenders. *New England
    Journal of Medicine, 374*(13), 1232–1242.

90. Lee, J. D., Nunes, E. V., Bailey, G. L., Brigham, G. S., Cohen, A. J., Fishman, M., . . . May, J. (2016). NIDA Clinical Trials Network CTN-0051, extended-release naltrexone vs. buprenorphine for opioid treatment (X: BOT): Study design and rationale. *Contemporary Clinical Trials, 50,* 253–264.

91. Springer, S. A., Azar, M. M., Barbour, R., FL A, Di Paola, A. (2016). Extended-release naltrexone is associated with sustained virologic suppression among HIV+ prisoners with alcohol use disorders after release to the community. Late Breaker Abstract number: A-792-0201-10499. 21th International AIDS Conference, Durban, South Africa.

92. Springer, S., Barbour, R., Azar, M. M., et al. (2017). Results of a double blind placebo controlled randomized trial of extended-release naltrexone among HIV+ inmates with opioid dependence. Conference and Proceedings on Drug Dependence. Montreal, Canada.

93. Springer, S. A., Altice, F. L., Herme, M., & Di Paola, A. (2014). Design and methods of a double blind randomized placebo-controlled trial of extended-release naltrexone for alcohol dependent and hazardous drinking prisoners with HIV who are transitioning to the community. *Contemporary Clinical Trials, 37*(2), 209–218.

94. Substance Abuse and Mental Health Services Administration. (2015) Naltrexone. https://www.samhsa.gov/medication-assisted-treatment/treatment/naltrexone

95. Agerwala, S. M., & McCance-Katz, E. F. (2012). Integrating screening, brief intervention, and referral to treatment (SBIRT) into clinical practice settings: A brief review. *Journal of Psychoactive Drugs, 44*(4), 307–317.

96. Babor, T. F., McRee, B. G., Kassebaum, P. A., Grimaldi, P. L., Ahmed, K., & Bray, J. (2007). Screening, Brief Intervention, and Referral to Treatment (SBIRT) toward a public health approach to the management of substance abuse. *Substance Abuse, 28*(3), 7–30.

97. Bernstein, E., Bernstein, J., Feldman, J., Fernandez, W., Hagan, M., Mitchell, P., . . . Lee, C. (2007). An evidence-based alcohol screening, brief intervention and referral to treatment (SBIRT) curriculum for emergency department (ED) providers improves skills and utilization. *Substance Abuse, 28*(4), 79.

98. Finnell, D. S. (2012). A clarion call for nurse-led SBIRT across the continuum of care. *Alcoholism: Clinical and Experimental Research, 36*(7), 1134–1138.

99. Prendergast, M. L., & Cartier, J. J. (2013). Screening, Brief Intervention, and Referral to Treatment (SBIRT) for offenders: Protocol for a pragmatic randomized trial. *Addiction Science & Clinical Practice, 8*(1), 16.

100. McCance-Katz, E. F., & Satterfield, J. (2012). SBIRT: A key to integrate prevention and treatment of substance abuse in primary care. *The American Journal on Addictions, 21*(2), 176.

101. Pilowsky, D. J., & Wu, L. T. (2012). Screening for alcohol and drug use disorders among adults in primary care: A review. *Substance Abuse and Rehabilitation, 3,* 25.

102. Saitz, R., Palfai, T. P., Cheng, D. M., Alford, D. P., Bernstein, J. A., Lloyd-Travaglini, C. A., . . . Samet, J. H. (2014). Screening and brief intervention for drug use in primary care: the ASPIRE randomized clinical trial. *JAMA, 312*(5), 502–513.

103. Center for Community Collaboration. (2012). SBIRT for mental health and substance use screen, brief intervention, and referral to treatment implementation guide for HIV care service providers. Baltimore, MD: UMBC Psychology Department.

104. Levy, S. J., & Williams, J. F. (2016). Substance use screening, brief intervention, and referral to treatment. *Pediatrics, 138*(1), e20161211.

105. Madras, B. K., Compton, W. M., Avula, D., Stegbauer, T., Stein, J. B., & Clark, H. W. (2009). Screening, Brief Interventions, Referral to Treatment (SBIRT) for illicit drug and alcohol use at multiple healthcare sites: Comparison at intake and 6 months later. *Drug and Alcohol Dependence, 99*(1), 280–295.

106. National Institute on Drug Abuse. (2017). Evidence-based screening tools for adults and adolescents. https://www.drugabuse.gov/nidamed-medical-health-professionals/tool-resources-your-practice/screening-assessment-drug-testing-resources/chart-evidence-based-screening-tools-adults

107. Mitchell, S. G., Gryczynski, J., O'Grady, K. E., & Schwartz, R. P. (2013). SBIRT for adolescent drug and alcohol use: Current status and future directions. *Journal of Substance Abuse Treatment, 44*(5), 463–472.

108. Substance Abuse and Mental Health Services Administration. (2017). SBIRT. https://www.samhsa.gov/sbirt

109. Gryczynski, J., Mitchell, S. G., Peterson, T. R., Gonzales, A., Moseley, A., & Schwartz, R. P. (2011). The relationship between services delivered and substance use outcomes in New Mexico's Screening, Brief Intervention, Referral and Treatment (SBIRT) initiative. *Drug and Alcohol Dependence, 118*(2), 152–157.

110. Roy-Byrne, P., Bumgardner, K., Krupski, A., Dunn, C., Ries, R., Donovan, D., . . . Joesch, J. M. (2014). Brief intervention for problem drug use in safety-net primary care settings: A randomized clinical trial. *JAMA, 312*(5), 492–501.

111. Tempalski, B., Cleland, C. M., Pouget, E. R., Chatterjee, S., & Friedman, S. R. (2015). Persistence of low drug treatment coverage for injection drug users in large US metropolitan areas. *Substance Abuse Treatment, Prevention and Policy, 5*, 23.

112. Basu, S., Rohrberg, D. S., Bruce, R. D., & Altice, F. L. (2006). Models for integrating buprenorphine therapy into the primary HIV care setting. *Clinical Infectious Diseases, 42*(5), 716–721.

113. Sylla, L., Bruce, R. D., Kamarulzaman, A., & Altice, F. L. (2007). Integration and co-location of HIV/AIDS, tuberculosis and drug treatment services. *International Journal of Drug Policy, 18*(4), 306–312.

114. Weiss, L., Netherland, J., Egan, J. E., et al. (2011). Integration of buprenorphine/naloxone treatment into HIV clinical care: Lessons from the BHIVES collaborative. *JAIDS Journal of Acquired Immune Deficiency Syndromes, 56*(Suppl. 1), S68–S75.

115. Altice, F. L., Bruce, R. D., Lucas, G. M., Lum, P. J., Korthuis, P. T., Flanigan, T. P., . . . Finkleman, R. (2011). BHIVES Collaborative. HIV treatment outcomes among HIV infected, opioid-dependent patients receiving buprenorphine/ naloxone treatment within HIV clinical care settings: Results from a multisite study. *JAIDS Journal of Acquired Immune Deficiency Syndromes*, 56(Suppl. 1), S22–S32.

116. Egan, J. E., Netherland, J., Gass, J., Finkelstein, R., Weiss, L., & Collaborative B. Patient perspectives on buprenorphine/naloxone treatment in the context of HIV care. *JAIDS Journal of Acquired Immune Deficiencies*, 56(Suppl. 1), S46–S53.

117. Finkelstein, R., Netherland, J., Sylla, L., et al. (2011). Policy implications of integrating buprenorphine-naloxone treatment and HIV Care. *JAIDS Journal of Acquired Immune Deficiencies Syndromes*, 56, S98–S104.

118. Weiss, L., Egan, J. E., Botsko, M., Netherland, J., Fiellin, D. A., & Finkelstein, R. (2011). The BHIVES collaborative: Organization and evaluation of a multisite demonstration of integrated buprenorphine/naloxone and HIV treatment. *JAIDS Journal of Acquired Immune Deficiency Syndromes*, 56, S7–S13

119. Schackman, B. R., Leff, J. A., Botsko, M., Fiellin, D. A., Altice, F. L., Korthuis, P. T., . . . Gass, J. (2011). The cost of integrated HIV care and buprenorphine/ naloxone treatment: results of a cross-site evaluation. *JAIDS Journal of Acquired Immune Deficiency Syndromes*, 56(Suppl. 1), S76.

120. Degenhardt, L., Mathers, B., Vickerman, P., Rhodes, T., Latkin, C., & Hickman, M. (2010). Prevention of HIV infection for people who inject drugs: Why individual, structural, and combination approaches are needed. *The Lancet*, 376(9737), 285–301.

121. Abdul-Quader, A. S., & Collins, C. (2011). Identification of structural interventions for HIV/AIDS prevention: The concept mapping exercise. *Public Health Reports*, 126(6), 777–788.

122. Auerbach, J. (2009). Transforming social structures and environments to help in HIV prevention. *Health Affairs*, 28(6), 1655–1665.

123. Sumartojo, E. (2000). Structural factors in HIV prevention: concepts, examples, and implications for research. *AIDS*, 14, S3–S10.

124. Strathdee, S. A., Hallett, T. B., Bobrova, N., Rhodes, T., Booth, R., Abdool, R., & Hankins, C. A. (2010). HIV and risk environment for injecting drug users: The past, present, and future. *The Lancet*, 376(9737), 268–284.

125. Blankenship, K. M., Bray, S. J., & Merson, M. H. (2000). Structural interventions in public health. *AIDS*, 14, S11–S21.

126. Blankenship, K. M., Friedman, S. R., Dworkin, S., & Mantell, J. E. (2006). Structural interventions: Concepts, challenges, and opportunities for research. *Journal of Urban Health*, 83 (1), 59–72.

127. Blankenship, K. M., Reinhard, E., Sherman, S. G., & El-Bassel, N. (2015). Structural interventions for HIV prevention among women who use drugs: A

global perspective. *JAIDS Journal of Acquired Immune Deficiency Syndromes, 69,* S140–S145.

128. Gupta, G. R., Parkhurst, J. O., Ogden, J. A., Aggleton, P., & Mahal, A. (2008). Structural approaches to HIV prevention. *The Lancet, 372*(9640), 764–775.

129. Latkin, C. A., & Knowlton, A. R. (2005). Micro-social structural approaches to HIV prevention: A social ecological perspective. *AIDS Care, 17*(Suppl. 1), 102–113.

130. Remme, M., Vassall, A., Lutz, B., Luna, J., & Watts, C. (2014). Financing structural interventions: Going beyond HIV-only value for money assessments. *AIDS, 28*(3), 425–434.

131. Hankins, C. A., & de Zalduondo, B. O. (2010). Combination prevention: A deeper understanding of effective HIV prevention. *AIDS, 24,* S70–S80.

132. Beyrer, C., Malinowska-Sempruch, K., Kamarulzaman, A., Kazatchkine, M., Sidibe, M., & Strathdee, S. A. (2010). Time to act: A call for comprehensive responses to HIV in people who use drugs. *The Lancet, 376*(9740), 551–563.

133. Rhodes, T., Singer, M., Bourgois, P., Friedman, S. R., & Strathdee, S. A. (2005). The social structural production of HIV risk among injecting drug users. *Social Science & Medicine, 61*(5), 1026–1044.

134. Shannon, K., Kerr, T., Allinott, S., Chettiar, J., Shoveller, J., & Tyndall, M. W. (2008). Social and structural violence and power relations in mitigating HIV risk of drug-using women in survival sex work. *Social Science & Medicine, 66*(4), 911–921.

135. Strathdee, S. A., Lozada, R., Martinez, G., Vera, A., Rusch, M., Nguyen, L., . . . Patterson, T. L. (2011). Social and structural factors associated with HIV infection among female sex workers who inject drugs in the Mexico-US border region. *PLoS One, 6*(4), e19048.

136. Ryan White HIV/AIDS Program. (2015). Annual client-level data report. Ryan White HIV/AIDS Program Services Report. https://hab.hrsa.gov/sites/default/files/hab/data/datareports/2015rwhapdatareport.pdf

137. Bowen, E. A., Canfield, J., Moore, S., Hines, M., Hartke, B., & Rademacher, C. (2017). Predictors of CD4 health and viral suppression outcomes for formerly homeless people living with HIV/AIDS in scattered site supportive housing. *AIDS Care, 29,* 1468–1472.

138. Metraux, S., Metzger, D. S., & Culhane, D. P. (2004). Homelessness and HIV risk behaviors among injection drug users. *Journal of Urban Health, 81*(4), 618–629.

139. Katz, I. T., Ryu, A. E., Onuegbu, A. G., Psaros, C., Weiser, S. D., Bangsberg, D. R., & Tsai, A. C. (2013). Impact of HIV-related stigma on treatment adherence: Systematic review and meta-synthesis. *Journal of the International AIDS Society, 16*(3Suppl 2).

140. Miller, N. S., Sheppard, L. M., Colenda, C. C., & Magen, J. (2001). Why physicians are unprepared to treat patients who have alcohol-and drug-related disorders. *Academic Medicine, 76*(5), 410–418.

141. Davis, C. S., & Carr, D. H. (2017). The law and policy of opioids for pain management, addiction treatment, and overdose reversal. *Indiana Health Law Review, 14,* 1.

142. Rosenblatt, R. A., Andrilla, C. H. A., Catlin, M., & Larson, E. H. (2015). Geographic and specialty distribution of US physicians trained to treat opioid use disorder. *The Annals of Family Medicine, 13*(1), 23–26.

143. Padwa, H., Urada, D., Antonini, V. P., Ober, A., Crèvecoeur-MacPhail, D. A., & Rawson, R. A. (2012). Integrating substance use disorder services with primary care: The experience in California. *Journal of Psychoactive Drugs, 44*(4), 299–306.

144. Greenfield, B. L., Owens, M. D., & Ley. D. (2014). Opioid use in Albuquerque, New Mexico: A needs assessment of recent changes and treatment availability. *Addiction Science & Clinical Practice, 9,* 10.

145. Fussell, H. E., Rieckmann, T. R., & Quick, M. B. (2011). Medicaid reimbursement for screening and brief intervention for substance misuse. *Psychiatric Services, 62*(3), 306–309.

146. Wildeman, C., & Wang, E. A. (2017). Mass incarceration, public health, and widening inequality in the USA. *The Lancet, 389*(10077), 1464–1474.

147. DeBeck, K., Cheng, T., Montaner, J. S., Beyrer, C., Elliott, R., Sherman, S., . . . Baral, S. (2017). HIV and the criminalisation of drug use among people who inject drugs: A systematic review. *The Lancet HIV, 4*(8), e357–e374.

148. Maher, L., & Dixon, T. C. (2017). Collateral damage and the criminalisation of drug use. *The Lancet HIV, 4*(8), e326–e327.

149. Meyer, J. P., Cepeda, J., Taxman, F. S., & Altice, F. L. (2015). Sex-related disparities in criminal justice and HIV treatment outcomes: A retrospective cohort study of HIV-infected inmates. *American Journal of Public Health, 105*(9), 1901–1910.

150. Meyer, J. P., Zelenev, A., Wickersham, J. A., Williams, C. T., Teixeira, P. A., & Altice, F. L. (2014). Gender disparities in HIV treatment outcomes following release from jail: Results from a multicenter study. *American Journal of Public Health, 104*(3), 434–441.

151. Degenhardt, L., Larney, S., Kimber, J., Gisev, N., Farrell, M., Dobbins, T., . . . Burns, L. (2014). The impact of opioid substitution therapy on mortality post-release from prison: Retrospective data linkage study. *Addiction, 109*(8), 1306–1317.

152. Beletsky, L., Cochrane, J., Sawyer, A. L., Serio-Chapman, C., Smelyanskaya, M., Han, J., . . . Sherman, S. G. (2015). Police encounters among needle exchange clients in Baltimore: Drug law enforcement as a structural determinant of health. *American Journal of Public Health, 105*(9), 1872–1879.

153. Strathdee, S. A., Beletsky, L., & Kerr, T. (2015). HIV, drugs and the legal environment. *International Journal of Drug Policy, 26*, S27–S32.

154. Gilbert, L., Raj, A., Hien, D., Stockman, J., Terlikbayeva, A., & Wyatt, G. (2015). Targeting the SAVA (substance abuse, violence and AIDS) syndemic among women and girls: A global review of epidemiology and integrated interventions. *JAIDS Journal of Acquired Immune Deficiency Syndromes, 69*(2), S118.

155. Kresina, T. F., Conder, L. D., & Lapidos-Salaiz, I. F. (2016). The impact in low and middle income countries of screening and management of substance-related and addictive disorders in HIV care. *Res HIV Retroviral Infect, 1*(3).

9

Structural-Level Approaches for HIV Prevention and Care in US Prisons

Robert E. Fullilove

Overview: HIV in Prison

Since the inception of the HIV/AIDS pandemic in the United States, the role of incarceration has had a major impact on the dynamics of this pandemic in poor communities of color. As has been frequently noted in research on health disparities and health inequities, high rates of incarceration have made the nation's jails and prisons reservoirs for individuals struggling with mental illness, substance abuse, and infectious diseases, including HIV and hepatitis C.[1-3] According to the US Department of Justice's Bureau of Justice Statistics (BJS),

- In 2011–2012, an estimated 40% of state and federal prisoners and jail inmates reported having a current chronic medical condition while about half reported ever having a chronic medical condition.
- Twenty-one percent of prisoners and 14% of jail inmates reported ever having tuberculosis, hepatitis B or C, or other sexually transmitted diseases (excluding HIV or AIDS).
- Both prisoners and jail inmates were more likely than the general population to report ever having a chronic condition or infectious disease. The same finding held true for each specific condition or infectious disease.[4]

The estimated rate of HIV infection in both federal and state prison facilities, as reported by the BJS in 2015, was reported at 1,297 per 100,000,[5] a rate that is substantially greater than the 14.5 per 100,000 rate reported by the US Centers for Disease Control and Prevention for the general population of the United States.[16] The BJS notes that 2015 marks the year with the lowest rate observed since 1991, when rates of HIV/AIDS were first reported, and is markedly less than the peak rate of 2,471 per 100,000 that was recorded in 1992.[5]

The War on Drugs has been a significant factor in both general increases in the incarcerated population of the United States as well as in the HIV infection rates reported for those in prison.[17] As has been noted elsewhere, the incarceration of injection drug users in increasing numbers since the 1970s was tantamount to placing individuals who were at substantial risk for exposure to the virus behind bars.[7,8] Moreover, national and state policies that limit condom distribution in these facilities as well as the failure to make HIV treatments easily available to incarcerated persons are also important contributing factors to the impact of HIV in prisons.

In the United States, New York State is of particular significance because of its unique position in the HIV/AIDS pandemic.[6] Since the 1980s New York City, an important epicenter of HIV infection in the United States, has been the home community for the majority of men and women incarcerated in state prison facilities in the state. In addition to having one of the largest populations of individuals living with HIV, New York State prison facilities have continually held the largest group of incarcerated persons living with HIV in the nation since the beginning of the epidemic.[7,8] In 2010, for example, the number of incarcerated persons in New York State facilities living with HIV was 3,080 compared with 2,920 in Florida, 2,394 in Texas, and 1,235 in California.[4]

In recognition of these rates, the New York State AIDS Advisory Council empaneled the Criminal Justice Subcommittee in 1999 to review the state's inmate HIV services. Its report represents an important commentary on the need to provide improved HIV/AIDS services to the population of incarcerated individuals. It notes in its summary report,

Inadequate health care is not a condition of punishment. The state has particularly stringent obligations to provide access to health information, prevention measures, and medically appropriate treatment to people who are confined and unable to seek other medical opinions or health care providers. People with HIV in prisons should be accorded treatment that meets the same standards of care as people with HIV in any other setting.[9]

Significantly, the report concluded with a far-reaching recommendation: that the New York State Department of Health should assume overall responsibility for correctional health and for the provision of health care services. The report noted that such a shift in oversight and management would ensure that HIV care in these facilities would be "consistent with statewide standards."[9] The standard of care in the state and the requirements for the provision of HIV care stand in stark contrast to what the report notes was the norm for correctional facilities at that time; norms that often lacked the means to deliver care and prevention services effectively.

This recommendation, had it been implemented, would have been an important structural intervention for HIV/AIDS care in prisons. More importantly, it would have been unique. At the time the report was written in 1999, a survey of 19 State Department of Health HIV directors that had been undertaken by the report's authors revealed that not one of the states surveyed was responsible for medical care in prisons.[9]

At this writing, no changes have occurred in provision of HIV services that would place them under the jurisdiction of a state department of health. The Pew Foundation's 2014 report, *State Prison Health Care Spending*, observes that many states have some, often modest, Department of Health involvement. Psychiatric services in New York State prisons, for example, are managed by the state's Office of Mental Health,[10] but correctional health in the United States remains a system of care apart from the management efforts of state departments of health.

The state of New York under a mandate from Governor Mario Cuomo created the End the Epidemic Program in 2014, an ambitious initiative that committed the state to reduce new HIV infections by 2020 from 3,000 to 750. According to the initiative's webpage, End the Epidemic

1. Identifies persons with HIV who remain undiagnosed and links them to healthcare.
2. Links and retains persons diagnosed with HIV in healthcare to maximize virus suppression so they remain healthy and prevent further transmission.

3. Facilitates access to pre-exposure prophylaxis (PrEP) for high-risk persons to keep them HIV negative.

Ending the Epidemic in New York State will maximize the availability of life-saving, transmission-interrupting treatment for HIV, saving lives and improving the health of New Yorkers. It will move New York from a history of having the worst HIV epidemic in the country to a future where new infections are rare and those living with the disease have normal lifespans with few complications (https://www.health.ny.gov/diseases/aids/ending_the_epidemic/).

Significantly, the major focus here is on HIV prevention, care, and treatment and represents a *medicalized* approach to the HIV/AIDS pandemic. In this context, a medicalized approach is less concerned with the social determinants of HIV and much more focused on the factors that limit the creation of adequate and appropriate medical care. However, as is evident in the chapters in this volume, if the HIV/AIDS pandemic is to be eradicated, structural factors that influence the conditions in which people live and work must be confronted and dramatically improved. Structural interventions for HIV prevention typically involve at least one of the following: effecting policy or legal changes; enabling environmental changes; shifting harmful social norms; catalyzing social and political change; and empowering communities and groups.[11]

How might such an approach be undertaken in correctional facilities? What can be done, for example, to empower inmates to be the change agents working to end the epidemic? As will be proposed in subsequent sections of this chapter, peer education programs that are created, managed, and administered by incarcerated persons have significant and often unrecognized potential.

Peer Education Programs and HIV Prevention in Prison

One of the most comprehensive reviews of the literature on HIV prevention efforts for incarcerated persons was conducted by Underhill and colleagues.[12] The authors followed the Cochrane Collaboration procedures in the conduct of their systematic review of HIV prevention programs for systematic review of HIV prevention programs in carceral and or community settings. Their efforts focused on randomized and quasi-randomized controlled trials of "any behavioral, social, biomedical, structural, or HIV-testing intervention designed to reduce HIV-related risk."[12]

Perhaps the most important contribution from this review is to point out the paucity of well-controlled studies on this that have been published to date. Although a database search by the authors initially identified more than 40,000 articles, only 37 studies met inclusion criteria. The strength of this review was in its attempt to identify factors that might exhibit causal relationships between program inputs and behavioral/clinical outputs, between actions and results. The weakness of the approach is that there is tremendous variation across state prisons systems and their inmates. Thus generalizing from one setting to another or from one prison population to another in such studies becomes almost impossible.

Although the outcome measures that were of greatest interest in this study are of great importance, variables that include getting tested for HIV and retaining patients in care, this extensive review ultimately is best used as a template for the design of studies that use randomization to assess the impact of prison and community-based interventions.[12] The interventions that have the possibility of being expanded as structural interventions in HIV prevention, treatment, and care were not a prominent feature of the study's findings.

Nonetheless, Underhill and colleagues identified one study examining peer education as an effective behavioral intervention and that study was conducted as a doctoral dissertation.[12] The focus was on reducing high-risk behavior among urban, crack cocaine using women and focused on promoting the development of personal empowerment to make wise choices about sex and drug use.[13] This theme of personal empowerment and the focus on creating personal agency to reduce HIV risk is not a dominant theme in much HIV intervention research, but it merits further examination.

Empowering individuals at risk for or struggling with the impact of HIV infection serves to resist the temptation to regard them as "victims." Victims, by definition, are individuals who are often helpless in the face of the struggles in which they are engaged. Victims must depend on others for assistance. By contrast, any policy, program, or intervention that promotes a sense of personal agency has the potential to transform victims into effective actors capable of working to reverse the disadvantages confronting them.

Among the interventions that show significant promise to transform the lives of incarcerated individuals and strengthen personal agency, those programs that train and educate those in prison show the greatest promise. Moreover, two books—*College in Prison: Reading in an Age of*

Mass Incarceration by Daniel Karpowitz and *Liberating Minds: The Case for College in Prison* by Ellen Condliffe Lagemann—make a compelling case for the manner in which higher education creates the type of empowerment that transforms the lives of inmates in prison and transforms their options for remaining in the community upon their return to the community. Both scholars were important leaders of the Bard Prison Initiative (BPI), an innovative program formed in 1999 at Bard College, a liberal arts institution in New York State. The program has been repeatedly identified as one of the most significant education interventions in US correctional facilities with an enviable track record of success. Informal results associated with this program include a 2016 study by BPI staff demonstrating that the recidivism rate among BPI graduates was 2.5% in 2015.[14]

Bard students serving time in three New York prison facilities have also had exposure to the principles, practices, and research methods of public health. Since 2011, a BPI Concentration in Public Health has been offered that closely resembles the undergraduate degree programs in this field that are offered in many mainstream US colleges and universities.[14] BPI students taking public health courses have made the HIV pandemic one of their primary foci, and they have contributed leadership and technical assistance to an intervention of considerable significance, the Prisoners for AIDS, Counseling and Education (PACE) program, which was active and in operation in 28 state prison facilities in New York in 2017.

The PACE program seeks to accomplish a number of important objectives in organizing inmate peer educators in each facility to "provide HIV/AIDS general education to various inmate groups at each facility and provide referrals, advocacy, counseling and support for inmates who are HIV infected."[15] The direction of the program and its mission reflect one of the key needs highlighted in the AIDS Advisory Council's 1999 report:

> It is not possible to adequately address HIV in the prison system without acknowledging the interdependence of many aspects of the problem. A great many inmates with HIV are not receiving care because they don't know their HIV status. They don't know their status because they don't believe they are at risk, fear loss of confidentiality, are not informed about the benefits of treatment, or don't think they will get adequate care if they are positive. Effective treatment therefore starts with education and testing.[9]

The exact year that PACE was organized is not entirely clear. Different community-based agencies support and fund the program depending on the region (called a "Hub") in which a facility is located. Bard students are active in PACE in the "Sullivan Hub," for example, in the two facilities (Woodbourne and Eastern) where BPI programs have been established since 1999.

The connection between BPI and PACE is important. I have been teaching or lecturing in these two facilities since 2010 and has been a participant in many of the initiatives organized by BPI students and PACE organizers. These programmatic efforts have involved a conscious effort to imagine and plan HIV/AIDS-centered community organizing programs in the neighborhoods to which PACE staff and trainees will ultimately return. PACE qualifies as a structural HIV intervention precisely because of its emphasis on empowering program participants and committing them to return to their communities to work with the large number of returning citizens who are HIV-positive and who struggle to achieve the continuity of HIV care that is essential for their survival.

At the end of 2017, significant numbers of returning citizens with PACE training—and in many instances, armed as well with undergraduate degrees awarded through the auspices of BPI—had been hired as community outreach workers, patient navigators, and HIV/AIDS peer counselors in AIDS service programs in the New York City boroughs of Manhattan, the Bronx, and Brooklyn. In 2017, HIV/AIDS service programs such as Harlem United and a number of clinical centers such as Brooklyn's Interface Medical Center had eagerly employed returning PACE workers for community HIV/AIDS prevention and treatment programs.

The impact of these hires on the multitude of problems that community AIDS organizations must confront has not yet been evaluated, but the potential that they represent is evident. Neighborhoods with historically high rates of HIV incidence and prevalence are also home to large numbers of individuals who have been released from prison. According to the Bureau of Justice Statistics, in 2015 more than 4.6 million persons in the United States were on parole or probation in their home communities,[16] and estimates from the Mayor's Office of Criminal Justice, New York City, are that 45,000 persons are returned to neighborhoods in New York City from prison each year.[17]

Outreach to formerly incarcerated persons is often best accomplished when those who have served time themselves are in charge of efforts to do outreach and engagement in care.[18] PACE staff are ideal candidates for such posts, and their interest in organizing community HIV/AIDS programs can have a dramatic impact on future efforts to contain and ultimately eliminate HIV in their home communities. This potential is particularly evident in the course of World AIDS Day events organized by PACE programs at three New York prison facilities between 2014 and 2017. I was an observer and a presenter at these events, and an account of what was observed is a useful example of the structural interventions that currently and formerly incarcerated persons are uniquely positioned to create and administer.

World AIDS Day in Prison: Fishkill, Eastern, and Woodbourne State Correctional Facilities

World AIDS Day was first celebrated nationally and internationally in 1988. At present, it serves as one of the World Health Organization's eight official global public health campaigns. Its objective is to raise awareness and consciousness of HIV/AIDS and to enjoin individuals, governments, and communities to commit to efforts to end the pandemic and to provide the resources needed to make such an ending a reality.

World AIDS Day events universally identify the need to confront HIV stigma as a vital, necessary step in promoting an AIDS-free world. This is especially relevant for incarcerated populations. In prisons, many incarcerated persons often have the same stigmatized view of HIV and of those who are living with it as are found in the general US population. Many of these beliefs are based on stereotypes or erroneous beliefs about the pandemic, among them being the notion that HIV is contagious or that it is a routinely fatal condition or that it is an illness that all gay men have.[20]

World AIDS Day events in prison that are organized by PACE staff are directed at identifying these stigmatized attitudes and confronting them directly with facts about the HIV pandemic. Participants at these events are exposed to personal testimonials about the importance of being personally aware of HIV-related risk behaviors and a call to action to be united as a community to prevent the transmission of the virus. Participants are also encouraged to commit to assist those—both in prison and back in the community—who are engaged in the struggle to eliminate AIDS.

What frequently strikes the outside observer who has the opportunity to participate in these World AIDS Day events in prison is the large number of participants in attendance. I have been a speaker in AIDS Day events in Black and Latino communities in New York City, for example, where speakers at an event typically outnumber the community members in attendance. During six such events, in three different New York state prisons between 2014 and 2017, average attendance exceeded 100 persons, comprising 10% to 15% of each facility's population.[19]

Participants typically hear rousing oratory, poetry, and personal testimony from those who have suffered personally because of HIV, followed by invitations to become active in promoting PACE programs and trainings. Each event has acknowledged the existence of HIV stigma and has detailed how such attitudes have prevented an effective, unified community response to the threat of HIV. As one speaker at an event in 2016 noted,

> Nothing keeps us from effectively stopping AIDS like our inability to talk to each other about this epidemic. If we can't speak of it, how can we be organized to fight it? Brothers, we have the power to teach our home communities how to become informed, organized, and prepared to help those at risk as well as those who are suffering. We have to take what we do back home! We got to do it right here on 'the inside,' then we got to move heaven and earth to see that our families, our friends, and our neighbors follow our lead!

PACE staff are acutely aware of the fact that the training they have received and the effectiveness of their PACE efforts in the facility will quite possibly translate to a job on the outside when they are released. Former PACE staff often returns to the prisons from which they are released to do technical assistance workshops to keep PACE staff on the inside abreast of changes in the policies and practices in HIV/AIDS care and treatment. The passage of the Affordable Care Act and the constant changes in benefits and programs for those who are exiting prison with HIV have, for example, been an important part of the transitional planning that is provided to incarcerated persons at the point they leave prison. PACE's commitment to assist with prerelease planning for its staff and for those who are in HIV care in prison creates continuity in programming offered on the inside as well as to that made available on the outside.

Without question, however, the most important message from PACE staff in the course of a World AIDS Day commemoration is the sense that being incarcerated is not the same as being helpless. One speaker summed this up as he noted, "If we are the group that is the target for this virus, we are also the group that is best placed to do something concrete to improve our condition. But to do this, we have to be informed, we have to believe, and we have to know that we have the power to transform!"

Implications and Conclusions

Much of the literature on structural interventions for HIV/AIDS concentrates on the social drivers of the epidemic in marginalized communities. One of the messages that come through clearly is that changing and/or eliminating the conditions that create HIV risk will ultimately translate into significantly reducing the numbers of people who are exposed to and will ultimately become infected with HIV. Thus, confronting racism, sexism, homophobia, and poverty become priorities for the development of programs, policies, and interventions.

Structural interventions directed at incarcerated individuals, it has been argued here, can include efforts that create agency and power for inmates to become actively engaged in the struggle to eliminate HIV/AIDS. Incarcerated individuals are easily seen as in need of services and assistance, but viewing them as agents of change and empowering them to make changes must be considered. As noted here, the PACE program is a little known but very significant structural intervention. PACE strategies and techniques can be adapted for use in other many prison settings, with willingness to make the requisite structural-level changes the only stipulation.

I have been engaged in HIV/AIDS programming and research since 1986 and would rank PACE as the most easily implemented, cost-effective approach for directly confronting the conditions rendering prisons as significant reservoirs of HIV/AIDS. PACE has additionally provided prison staff members with public health training. Of special significance is the fact there has been a growing number of BPI/PACE workers who have been released from prison and who have gone on to become public health professionals.[21] The PACE story serves, in many respects, as the classic example of an innovation whose time has come.

References

1. Golembeski C, Fullilove RE (2005) Criminal (in)justice in the city and its associated health consequences. Am J Public Health: 95:170+1–1706.
2. Massoglia M, Pridemore WA (2015) Incarceration and health. Annu Rev Sociol: 41:291–310.

3. Wilderman C, Wang EA (2017) Mass incarceration, public health, and widening inequality in the USA. *Lancet*: 389:1464–1474.

4. Maruschak LM, Berzofsky M, Unangst J (2015) Medical problems of state and federal prisoners and jail inmates, 2011–12. US Department of Justice, Bureau of Justice Statistics. Retrieved December 27, 2017 at https://www.bjs.gov/content/pub/pdf/mpsfpji1112.pdf

5. Maruschak LM, Bronson J (2017) HIV in prisons, 2015—Statistical tables. US Department of Justice, Bureau of Justice Statistics. Retrieved December 27, 2017 at https://www.bjs.gov/index.cfm?ty=pbdetail&iid=6026

6. Centers for Disease Control and Prevention (2017, July) HIV Surveillance Supplemental Report, Monitoring Selected National HIV Prevention and Care Objectives by Using HIV Surveillance Data, Vol. 21, No. 4.

7. Fullilove RE (2011) Mass incarceration in the United States and HIV/AIDS: cause and effect? *Ohio State J Crim Law* 9:353–361.

8. Fullilove RE (2006) African Americans, health disparities and HIV/AIDS. National Minority AIDS Council. Retrieved December 28, 2017 at https://www.prisonlegalnews.org/news/publications/nmac-report-on-hiv-among-minorities-condoms-in-prison-2006/

9. New York State AIDS Advisory Council (1999) HIV/AIDS services in New York state correctional facilities. Retrieved December 27, 2017 at https://www.health.ny.gov/diseases/aids/providers/workgroups/aac/docs/servicescorrectional.pdf

10. Pew Charitable Trust (2014) State prison health care spending: An examination. Retrieved December 30, 2017 at http://www.pewtrusts.org/~/media/assets/2014/07/stateprisonhealthcarespendingreport.pdf

11. Adimora AA, Auerbach JD (2010) Structural interventions for HIV prevention in the United States. *J Acquir Immune Defic Syndr*, 55:S132–S135.

12. Underhill K, Dumont D, Operario D (2014) HIV prevention with adults with criminal justice involvement: A systematic review of HIV risk-reduction interventions in incarceration and community settings *Am J Public Health*; 104:e27–e53.

13. Callahan C (2008) *The association of criminal justice system involvement on change in high-risk behaviors among urban, crack-cocaine using women* [doctoral thesis]. St Louis, MO: George Warren Brown School of Social Work, Graduate School of Arts and Sciences of Washington University.

14. Bard Prison Initiative (2017) By the numbers. Retrieved December 27, 2017 at: https://bpi.bard.edu/

15. Hudson Valley Community Services (2016) Prison services. Retrieved December 30, 2017 at: http://www.hudsonvalleycs.org/prison-services/

16. Kaeble D, Bonczar TP (2016) Probation and parole in the US, 2015. US Department of Justice, Bureau of Justice Statistics. Retrieved December 30, 2017 at: https://www.bjs.gov/content/pub/pdf/ppus15.pdf

17. Mayor's Office of Criminal Justice (2016) Mayor's Office of Criminal Justice to develop targeted interventions that improve public safety and reduce the number of people who enter and return to jail. Retrieved January 2, 2018 at: https://www1.nyc.gov/site/criminaljustice/news/ReEntry%20Release%204-28-16.page

18. Portillo S, Goldberg V, Taxman FS (2017) Mental health peer navigators: Working with criminal justice-involved populations. *Prison J*; 97:318–341.

19. New York State Department of Health: End the epidemic in New York State web page. Retrieved December 28, 2017 at: https://www.health.ny.gov/diseases/aids/ending_the_epidemic/

20. Derlega V, Winstead BA, Gamble KA, Kelkar K, Khuanghlawn P (2010) Inmates with HIV, stigma, and disclosure decision-making. *J Health Psychol*; 15:258–268.

21. Sandoval E (2017, May 8) Former Queens gang member and prison inmate set to graduate from Columbia University; "Education rehabilitated me." *New York Daily News*. Retrieved January 10, 2017 at: http://www.nydailynews.com/new-york/queens-gang-member-finds-redemption-columbia-degree-article-1.3145934

10

Getting to 40!

STRUCTURAL APPROACHES IN ENGLAND TO REDUCING HIV INCIDENCE IN MEN WHO HAVE SEX WITH MEN

Will Nutland

Overview

This chapter explores the role of a broad range of structural and educational interventions that contributed to the availability of HIV pre-exposure prophylaxis (PrEP) among men who have sex with men (MSM) in England. Those interventions lead to the formation of a clinical trial, making PrEP available to 10,000 people. However, before that trial commenced, interventions instigated by a movement of grassroots activism led to thousands of people obtaining generic formulations of PrEP via the Internet. This availability of PrEP, outside of a formal health system, along with initiatives to enhance frequent HIV testing and the early treatment of people diagnosed with HIV, led to a reported 40% reduction in HIV diagnoses, within just one year, among MSM in London.

This chapter explores how a range of interventions contributed to "getting to 40," including innovative collaborations between community activists and clinician activists, working within the national health system, framing more traditional forms of advocacy alongside newer methods of activism (termed "Activism 2.0"). Further, the chapter provides insights into how these methods might also be transferred to other settings and other health conditions.

HIV in the United Kingdom

HIV infection resulting from sex between men accounts for the majority of UK-acquired HIV diagnoses.[1] HIV diagnoses among MSM have risen steadily each year since 2001 and, despite a leveling-off during 2007–2009, increased each year until the end of 2015. In 2016, 54% of HIV diagnoses reported in England were among MSM. HIV prevalence in MSM in 2016 in England was estimated to be 77 per 1,000 population, compared with an estimated England general population prevalence of 1.6 per 1,000. It was higher still in MSM in London (128 per 1,000), compared to MSM in the rest of England (57 per 1,000). Of key significance are the large geographical variations: in 2016, almost half of the HIV diagnoses in MSM were made in London.[1]

With early diagnosis of HIV infection and significant improvements in HIV antiretroviral treatments, HIV infection in the UK is thought to have an insignificant impact on longevity of life. Mathematical models suggest that a nonsmoking, 30-year-old gay man who receives a prompt diagnosis after infection has a life expectancy of 78 years, compared to a life expectancy of 82 for a man who does not have HIV.[2] However, the long-term impacts of HIV infection and HIV medication are uncertain; stigma and discrimination against people with HIV—in personal and sexual relationships, in medical settings, and from wider society—exist and can impact on the mental, sexual, and physical health of a person with HIV;[3-5] and the costs of HIV medication, treatment, and care have a significant impact on the National Health Service, with the lifetime costs of HIV treatments alone estimated to be between £280,000 and £360,000 per person.[6] As such, measures to prevent primary HIV infection remain essential, with a particular need to prioritize the prevention of HIV infection amongst MSM.

Over the last three decades, significant activity has been undertaken to reduce HIV infection in the UK. Strategies for reducing HIV acquisition amongst MSM in England have focused on the concept of "best sex with least harm" and have included raising awareness of HIV status and diagnosis of HIV; raising awareness, diagnosis and treatment of STIs; interventions that increase MSM's knowledge of HIV, as well as its prevention and treatment; interventions that increase men's skills to negotiate and have the sex they want; and interventions that facilitate increased awareness of risk reduction in environments where men meet for sex—such as the provision of information or condoms and lubricant.[7]

There have been notable successes in HIV prevention activity, not least those that have been connected to increased levels of HIV testing.[8] Systematic reviews have identified evidence of behavioral interventions—including interpersonal skills training, multimethod interventions, and multiple interventions over durations of a minimum of three weeks—that have been shown to impact on HIV risk on an individual, group, or community level.[9–12] Yet these interventions are costly to implement on a population level, and resources to adequately scale-up these interventions have not been forthcoming. Indeed, structural impediments to implementing behavioral interventions, including opposition to school-based sex education and complex reorganization of health service, have further impacted upon behavioral implementation.[13] Additionally, behavioral-only interventions have been shown to be less acceptable, appropriate, or feasible with many MSM, with international bodies, such as UNAIDS, making a strong case for combination prevention: prevention that combines behavioral, biomedical, and structural interventions.[14,15]

PrEP in the United Kingdom

The last decade has witnessed significant scientific developments with regard to preventing HIV transmission using medical technologies. Antiretroviral therapy, once thought of only in terms of maintaining the well-being of those already infected with HIV, is now emerging as a central component of HIV *prevention* efforts. Early treatment of people with HIV with antiretrovirals has been found to lower HIV viral load (a measure of the amount of HIV in an individual's body fluids) and reduce onward transmission of HIV by up to 97%, thus rendering them effectively uninfectious.[16] This has led to a reconstruction of antiretroviral therapy as Treatment as Prevention,[17–19] as exemplified in the recent international undetectable = untransmittable (U = U) movement.[20]

In addition to the use of antiretroviral therapy to reduce viral load of those already with HIV, the same medication has been used to reduce the likelihood of HIV transmission to uninfected individuals who are exposed to HIV. This "post-exposure prophylaxis" (PEP) for individuals exposed to HIV has been used in medical settings following needle-stick and surgical injuries with protocols on occupational use developed internationally.[21] Guidelines for the prescription of PEP for individuals who have been sexually exposed to HIV were introduced in England in 2006,[22] along with a raft of health promotion interventions to increase knowledge and access to PEP among at-risk MSM.[23]

Further to the notion of "Treatment as Prevention" and PEP, there has been significant development of antiretroviral medication that can be used *prior* to HIV exposure to prevent an HIV-negative individual from becoming infected. PrEP is a biomedical technology that allows HIV-uninfected individuals to control their susceptibility to HIV prior to exposure. Current scientific research is being undertaken that explores the safety and efficacy of PrEP in in a range of different formats including:

- **Oral PrEP**—taken as a tablet either daily or intermittently
- **PrEP in a topical gel or foam** format—inserted vaginally or rectally (often termed "microbicides")
- **PrEP in an injectable** format—either for short periods of time or in a long-acting formulation, similar to slow-release contraceptive methods
- **PrEP in an insertable format**—such as cervical rings, for use by women during sex with men

How Many People Are Using PrEP?

Although, as it is outlined later, access to generic online PrEP started to become increasingly common beginning in October 2015, it is hard to accurately establish how many people were using PrEP. The PROUD trial provided PrEP to over 500 MSM in England, and there was gradual attrition of PrEP users accessing PROUD trial drugs once the trial was halted in October 2014. Although community education initiatives began to increase in the autumn of 2014 and into summer of 2015, including activities that publicized the availability of online PrEP, it is unlikely that significant numbers of individuals were accessing online PrEP at this time. The launch of community websites in October of 2015 most likely served as the catalyst that facilitated access to online PrEP. Attempts were made to engage with online sellers to gauge the broad numbers of individuals purchasing from each site (along with attempts to engage with sellers to predict "stock outs" or any other supply issues). Those attempts were unsuccessful, with sellers predictably being unwilling to share confidential sales data that might become available to competitors. It was not until

January 2017, with the launch of a new online supplier, founded by a PrEP user and community advocate, that any indication of reliable sales data could be established. Using sales data from this new seller, along with user information established from a community survey undertaken in the summer of 2017,[28] extrapolated data estimated that there might be between 8,000 and 10,000 people in the UK buying generic online PrEP by the close of summer 2017.

Reductions in HIV Incidence

In December 2016, a small number of HIV clinics in London started to report significant reductions, of around 40%, in HIV diagnoses, compared with the previous year. This was initially reported by Dean Street, based in the heart of Soho and one of Europe's busiest sexual health clinics. Days later, the nearby Mortimer Market Centre issued data reporting similar reductions in diagnosis, and other central London clinics then reported similar drops.[24] These sharp falls were seen only in MSM, with the falls in London being much more significant than those outside of the capital. This data was reported across the world, albeit with a degree of caution, as being driven by the widespread use of generic online purchased PrEP, and figures released in proceeding months indicated ongoing drops in HIV diagnoses and incidence.[25]

There remains a lack of consensus about the extent to which PrEP played in these dramatic and stunning declines in HIV incidence.[26] Commentators have noted that there have been stark improvements in combination prevention in the UK over the past decade, and in recent years in particular. For instance, an individual receiving an HIV-positive diagnosis will be offered free HIV treatment within days, if not hours, of that diagnosis. There have been substantial increases in the numbers of HIV tests offered, in part due to changes in HIV testing technologies, and in approaches to where HIV tests are offered, including substantial increases in the use of self-sampling and home-testing. For instance, it is not uncommon to encounter HIV testing services in entertainment settings such as bars and clubs, as well as in community and other business settings. There is compelling data to show that HIV diagnoses amongst MSM, especially in London, was starting to fall—even if not at the sudden and huge level as it did in from October 2015—before the broad use of PrEP.[27]

The Relative Impact of PrEP on HIV Incidence

While it is not possible to accurately establish the relative impact of various structural-level and education-based initiatives on the observed declines in HIV incidence, three possibilities exist: (a) increases in HIV testing, (b) early treatment of people diagnosed with HIV, and (c) access to PrEP. It *is* possible, however, to establish that a significant and growing number of people were accessing and using generic PrEP by September 2017. This access probably started on a relatively small scale during 2015, accelerating from the autumn of 2015, and increased to many thousands of individuals by the close of 2017. While this PrEP use was probably the driver for the sudden and sharp fall in HIV diagnoses, its relative impact will probably never be established.

This significant use and uptake of PrEP (and the impact on HIV diagnoses) happened before any central government-funded resourcing for PrEP education and before the availability of PrEP on UK clinical trials (other than the relatively small PROUD trial). These successes happened despite a failure of bureaucrats within National Health Service (NHS) England to provide PrEP (even given compelling international evidence of its efficacy); despite there being no clear and articulate government or NHS policy to champion, resource, and prioritize PrEP (despite it being recommended in the United States in 2012); and despite a broad lack of leadership from within community organizations (including some international institutions) to promote and champion PrEP. It is to this issue that this chapter now turns.

Slow Progress in PrEP Implementation

Several possible reasons exist as to why the observed level of resistance to PrEP may have occurred. First, there was a sense that England needed to better understand the potential uptake and use of PrEP outside of a randomized control trial and there was a reluctance to move toward commissioning of PrEP until the PROUD trial had reported its conclusions. Second, 2012 Health and Social Care Act—a major piece of legislation that transferred the provision of public health functions, including sexual health, to local authorities—illuminated confusion about which body is responsible for commissioning PrEP (itself the subject of the court case that took place in August 2016 as outlined later). Third, a reluctance from some of the UK's HIV sector leaders to embrace PrEP as an HIV prevention technology should be considered. This is exemplified in this response in July 2014 when the World Health Organization made a statement recommending that PrEP be made available to all MSM. This quote, given to the BBC, from the (then) chief executive of the Terrence Higgins Trust (THT; the UK's largest and arguable most influential HIV and sexual health charity):

> The idea of treatment as prevention is not new, but the idea of extending treatment to HIV-negative people from high-risk groups is. Pre-exposure prophylaxis is an exciting approach, and likely to be one of a number of ways in which we can reduce the spread of HIV in the future. However, we need to evaluate how effective it will be in preventing HIV among gay men.[29]

This very measured response suggests that a sense of urgency to implement PrEP for MSM in the UK was not present at that time. Despite the leading body responsible for global health making a recommendation that PrEP should be available, the leader of the UK's most influential HIV charity stated publicly that PrEP might be appropriate in the future (and not now) and that its effectiveness needed evaluating (despite findings from international research demonstrating its efficacy and effectiveness). It is unclear why this position was taken; however, several possibilities exist. For example, it is plausible that a tension existed between THT's role as the main contractor of a national HIV program, funded through the England Department of Health. Also, it could be that advocating for PrEP before it could be made widely available was an issue.

A fourth reason for the rather slow movement involves a fragmented HIV sector that had been forced to compete for limited funding across a number of years contributed to a reluctance to work toward a common goal. Although a community consensus statement on PrEP was driven by community-based organizations from as early as 2014, and further collaborative work was driven by RESHAPE in 2014, it is hard to conclude that there was a clear and unambiguous shared goal about PrEP, its benefits, and the role it might play in future combination prevention (in part, exacerbated by the preceding factors, outlined earlier).

A final possible reason involves frontline staff reporting they were unable or unwilling to be seen to be promoting a technology that was not approved and thus not formally available. This included concerns about responses from funders (including statutory funders and pharmaceutical donors); concerns from managers or board members; concerns about the legal implications of providing information that might be seen to be quasi-legal, such as buying PrEP online; questions about efficacy, adverse side effects or unintended consequences of PrEP use; and, in some instances, an individual or organizational reluctance to "move beyond condoms" as an HIV prevention approach.

A New Movement

The new movement of HIV prevention activism has been termed "HIV activism 2.0,"[30] and it positions a new wave of activism alongside, rather than in opposition to, more traditional forms of HIV activism. Whilst those traditional methods have taken the form of street activism, legal action, and educational activities (such as outreach) funded through HIV prevention contracts, HIV Activism 2.0 has galvanized new methods of doing HIV prevention. This has included establishing buyers' clubs for the importation of generic formulations of PrEP, establishing "do-it-yourself" educational websites by those who are seeking or using PrEP themselves (as opposed to websites created by more formal and long established nongovernmental organizations), and establishing innovative supply chains for accessing PrEP (such as using parcel forwarding services to get around border restrictions within Europe on the direct importation of HIV medications).

Arguably, there have been four key factors that have come together in a synergistic manner that have contributed to a marked increase in access to PrEP.

- The leadership of a new wave of HIV activists, including people who have had no formal HIV prevention training and have had scarce contact with HIV organizations.
- Access to global generic markets, including drugs that are often nine times (or more) cheaper than the patented versions in the countries were they are being used.
- Innovative supply chains (as outlined earlier) have emerged.
- Use of social media and the Internet, which has facilitated peer-driven communication and advice about where to access PrEP, how to use it, and the legal implications of self-importation and use of generic imported pharmaceuticals.

The Development of a New PrEP Movement in England

In addition to the work of RESHAPE, an independent think-tank formed to respond to the crisis in sexual health, (that facilitated the formation of the United4PrEP coalition from 2015), and the community consensus statement (as outlined earlier), a small handful of HIV prevention advocates started to organize a series of community-based PrEP awareness events towards the end of 2014. In the absence of any coordinated PrEP education activity these events were initially focused around the queer Fringe! Film Festival in the east of London in the fall of 2014 and included a PrEP forum coordinated by Act Up London in coalition with local health advocates. Community-led educational activities continued through spring and summer of 2015, including the showing of Nicholas Feustel's short documentary on the England PrEP PROUD study at venues across England. These community forums included the first public discussions on the safety and ethics of purchasing online generic PrEP.

During the early summer of 2015, four London-based HIV advocates (including those involved in the aforementioned community-based educational activities) met to coordinate a broader and more comprehensive educational and advocacy strategy. This group included individuals who were using PrEP (through the England PROUD trial), PrEP seekers, and gay men with HIV. The result of this strategizing was an intervention called *PrEPster*: a project that sought to both educate and agitate for PrEP access in England and beyond. Formally launched in October 2015, the project aimed to build upon, rather than duplicate, existing HIV prevention programs, by providing accessible "top-level" educational information about PrEP. The PrEPster website served as an initial reference point about PrEP that outreach workers and front-line staff could use to refer people to (something that was lacking, based on reports by front-line staff). In addition, the website provided clear and tangible actions that individuals and communities could take to advocate for increased PrEP access (such as writing to their government representatives, lobbying Gilead—the manufacturer of Truvada, the patented version of PrEP—to lower the price of their drug, contacting their local authority's director of public health and asking for details of how PrEP might be implemented in the future).

PrEPster positioned *action* about how to educate and agitate for PrEP at the core of their ethos. By creating a set of tangible, relatively simple actions that individuals and communities could take, PrEPster sought to build activism in people who had previously not known *where* or *how* to advocate or agitate for PrEP access. The intervention sought to draw-in a new demographic of people who had not previously been involved in HIV advocacy. Crucially, PrEPster framed a debate that said individuals and communities *themselves* are the most productive forces in forging and facilitating change. That is, PrEPster said to people they encountered that "you are the greatest resource there is to educate and agitate for PrEP: by talking to a peer, sex partner, or family member about PrEP; being out as a PrEP user; by talking about how PrEP can make sex more pleasurable and increase intimacy, and how it can reduce stress and anxiety, as well as reducing HIV." Of great importance, PrEPster featured the power of one-to-one education as well as community peer education. Both forms of education were suggested as one of the tangible "actions" that people could take in becoming a highly effective PrEP advocate. This type of informal advocacy proved to be crucial.

In addition, PrEPster positioned diversity at its core, ensuring that not just the imagery used on the website and other materials was representative of the key populations that might most benefit from PrEP but by taking concerted actions to include, involve, and reach communities that would not ordinarily be targeted with PrEP education and advocacy.

From its inception, PrEPster undertook activity under an ethos of "DIY kitchen table activism." This activism was characterized by implementing HIV prevention education regardless of the budget and resources available, and without having an infrastructure or bureaucracy to support its work (often working from each other's kitchen tables). As such, initial activity included condom and lubricant packs with written PrEP information inside (counterintuitively, providing PrEP information alongside condoms, in part to counter concepts that PrEP replaces condoms); building capacity to potential PrEP advocates and educators through training, support, and resourcing, especially within communities underserved by PrEP education; commissioning a film "PrEP17" that portrayed the fight for PrEP in England, that was taken across the UK and seen by thousands of people; training dozens of community advocates in media skills, so that they could confidently face the media and discuss PrEP; and doing the "hard graft" of talking to hundreds and hundreds of influencers, decision-makers and potential PrEP users through community events, workshops, meetings, seminars, conferences, and outreach.

Key to all of this activity was bringing people who use PrEP, potential PrEP users, and those who had recently sought PrEP (and for whom it was too late), right to the forefront of every activity. As such, the work of PrEPster was crucially seen as being done *by* and *with* target communities, rather than being done *by* health professionals *to* communities of concern. That meant, for example, rather than audiences hearing about research-reported side effects of PrEP, audiences learned first-hand from PrEP users about their own experience of side effects *in addition* to research-reported instances.

Meanwhile, and unbeknown to PrEPster, two other HIV prevention activists were developing a new website—iwantPrEPnow (IWPN). The individuals building IWPN previously had no experience within the HIV prevention sector and were driven by their own experience of using or seeking PrEP. One had, in the summer of 2015, used PrEP whilst in New York City and returned to London to find it to be unavailable. The other, having heard about PrEP from friends, had sought PrEP but had found out that he was already infected with HIV when he went for his pre-PrEP HIV test. IWPN sought to facilitate access to cheap generic versions of PrEP by providing details of online pharmacies that were selling PrEP from countries such as India and Thailand. Providing a basic website with easy-to-understand information about PrEP, IWPN became another example of "DIY kitchen table activism" as they developed the website in the late summer of 2015.

Both websites launched within a week of each other and, despite the very different backgrounds and experiences of the individuals involved in each project, made a decision to work collaboratively. That first collaboration involved providing a level of consumer standard review for the generic PrEP becoming available online and, while IWPN was not a direct seller of PrEP, the listings of sellers on the website was sometimes seen as an endorsement of those products. Three standards were developed and then tested, by both projects working together and with "clinician activists" from a number of central London sexual health clinics. The first standard sought to establish that buyers were not being "ripped off" by sellers (e.g., not having their debit or credit cards used for other sales, or having monies withdrawn from their bank accounts); the second to ensure that sales, once made, were being delivered to the stated address; and third, and most importantly, to ensure that the generic PrEP being purchased online was genuine. Both websites worked together to undertake test purchases of current listed sellers (and then any new sellers went through the same scrutiny), with a number of volunteers acting as "guinea pigs" to physically trial drugs purchased from sellers, and to have a therapeutic drug monitoring (TDM) performed (a test taken after starting a drug that tests blood for the product).

In essence, by the start of 2016, a reliable and regular supply chain of cheap generic PrEP was being tested and, over time, users were able to access "wrap around" support from sexual health clinics that would provide initial HIV tests, kidney function tests, and ongoing PrEP support. In effect, this created a semi-NHS service, where the drug (that the NHS would not provide) was being self-funded by individuals, and the clinical support services were being provided by the NHS (albeit at the start in an unofficial or "rogue" way). Over time, as more individuals started to seek and purchase online PrEP, NHS sexual health services came under increasing pressure to offer PrEP support services to those users. Key activist clinicians sought legal guidance and advice from their trade unions on the implications of providing advice and support for a drug that was not yet available for HIV prevention from the NHS.

Meanwhile, two London clinics started to offer TDM tests as part of their PrEP support service to establish whether the online purchased drugs were genuine, thereby offering reassurance to those who were considering accessing PrEP via this route. Both London's Mortimer Market Centre sexual health clinic and 56 Dean Street offered TDMs to limited numbers of people who were using PrEP, building a database of the main sources of where PrEP was being bought. Data on 234 samples was presented at a conference in October 2016,[31] showing that there was no evidence of fake drugs in the samples tested between February and September 2016. Nneka Nwokolo, who led the study at Dean Street, highlighted that the TDM testing initiative was

> an important collaboration between clinic patients, community activists and clinicians—it is a verification that online pharmacies are genuine and results can be made available, and adds to the testimonies from PrEP users. As long as PrEP is unavailable from the National Health Service, it is crucial that it is accessible to those who need it.[32]

Essentially, when PrEPster and IWPN were launched, both websites saw themselves a as a "stop gap" to PrEP provision until NHS England commissioned a full roll out of PrEP in the first half of 2016. In September 2014 NHS England had established, as with the commissioning of any new health technology, a process to establish the efficacy, need, and cost-effectiveness of PrEP. NHS England had also established a full public consultation process on its possible commissioning of PrEP. The availability of PrEP was broadly expected, albeit with possible caveats about who might be able to access PrEP under a full commissioned service. Although there were ongoing debates about the relative responsibilities of different parts of the health service to commission different aspects of PrEP provision, broad consensus was apparent. NHS England would be the body responsible for providing the drugs itself and local authorities would, although reluctantly, become the bodies responsible for the costs of wrap-around services for PrEP users, such as HIV testing, from their public health budget allocations. These initial plans were shattered in March of 2016 when a dramatic reversal occurred.

The "U Turn"

The process that NHS England had established in September 2014 had been based upon these very principles, and an assumption by all involved in that process that this was the established model for how PrEP would be commissioned in England.

In March of 2016 NHS England announced the reversal on their understanding of the commissioning process. In a statement released to an unwitting HIV prevention sector,[33] NHS England established that it was the remit of local authorities to commission HIV prevention services and that PrEP was not their responsibility. Astonished advocates could not understand why NHS England's own consultation processes had been allowed to progress for so long and, then at the eleventh hour, a phenomenal U-turn had been performed.[34] For advocates campaigning for several years for PrEP provision, this decision came as a substantial blow. Protests and demonstrations were held outside of the headquarters of NHS England, questions were raised in Parliament, and the Secretary of State for Health was lobbied.

Subsequent Court Cases

NHS England argued that PrEP was a preventative treatment and they were not legally the body that should provide PrEP. Instead, PrEP should be funded by local councils, through their public health budgets. In response, National AIDS Trust, the UK's HIV policy organization, led a court case against NHS England, taking the case to a judicial review. In August 2016, the High Court ruled that NHS England did indeed have the power to fund PrEP, and NHS England appealed this ruling.[35]

The appeal was heard in November 2016, and the judges in that appeal found in favor of National AIDS Trust. The court case cost NHS England in excess of £100,000 and, after the first ruling NHS England announced that it would not be able to guarantee to commission a range of other treatments that were also being considered for funding. This announcement led to a series of newspaper headlines pitching PrEP against other health conditions, with *The Times* reporting that the court ruling would lead to other care being "put at risk."[36]

Soon after the appeal ruling, NHS England and Public Health England announced a three-year trial (later called the IMPACT Trial) that would provide PrEP to over 10,000 people in England. This example of PrEP access in England is intriguing given the two very distinct factions involved. On the one hand, grassroots activism had lobbied for longer term access to PrEP, albeit through a clinical trial. On the other hand, an altogether different form of grassroots activism opened up access to generic formulations of PrEP. Throughout this period of activism there was an acknowledgment that there were at least two parallel processes that sometimes intertwined: one that sought full provision of PrEP for free on the NHS and another that sought to get PrEP into the bodies of people who needed it, as soon as possible, regardless of free NHS provision. Most activists involved in these discussions recognized that free NHS provision must be the ultimate goal (not least because of the widespread belief in the ethos that NHS services should be free at the point of access) and that providing access to PrEP outside the NHS was a stop-gap. The inadequacies of that stop-gap provision have been highlighted by an understanding that some PrEP users have not made use of "wrap-around" PrEP services, such as regular HIV testing and renal function monitoring, and that online PrEP has broadly been accessed by those with the most economic and social capital and the ability to navigate (sometimes quite complex) buying and delivery processes, further exacerbating existing health inequalities.

The collective activism of a large and motivated body of individuals and groups to access an otherwise unavailable medication, and to influence— or at least substantially contribute to—the largest ever fall in HV diagnosis in England, makes such "stop-gap" provision worthy of further consideration. There is a field of thought that says that provision of health services outside of our current NHS provision lets the providers and commissioners of existing (funded) services "off the hook": why would a health service invest in a new technology or service when the "problem" is already being resolved externally?

Yet this stop-gap provision has in essence provided a "testing ground" for future NHS PrEP provision: the early PrEP clinical support services that were developed in coalition by early PrEP adopters and clinician activists have provided the model for establishing future PrEP clinical services. At a time when popular discourse has painted gay men as complacent about HIV and their sexual health, and as activism being something left behind from the 1980s and 1990s, this recent galvanization of thousands of gay men—who took it upon themselves to take care of their own HIV prevention needs at a time when health services bureaucrats ignored those needs—has demonstrated the willingness of thousands of people to "do something" in the face of inaction.

A possible unintended outcome of this scenario is that HIV prevention activists are realizing that there are elements of what they have learned about navigating PrEP access that might be translated to other settings and other health conditions. A generation of activists have navigated the complexities of international patent laws, understood national and regional laws on (generic) drug importation, and become more attuned to the politics of global pharmaceutical research and development. As such, some PrEP activists are building newer coalitions, not only with HIV prevention activists globally, but with those are addressing the same issues around access to lifesaving or life-changing drugs including hepatitis C and cancer drugs.

Conclusion

This chapter has outlined how a broad coalition of community-based and clinical advocates worked together to facilitate access to HIV PrEP in England, while working outside and alongside established and formal health systems. These events suggests that a new form of activism ("Activism 2.0") that comprises of a new wave of activist leadership (often not associated with the HIV sector), alongside radical and innovative access to generics pharmaceuticals, facilitated through social media, has resulted in access to PrEP to tens of thousands of people. More "traditional" forms of activism– especially with regard to legal action—has played a key role in securing longer term (and free, at least for those who can access a trial) access to PrEP. Widespread access to PrEP, alongside increased testing and "Treatment as Prevention" has had a significant impact on HIV incidence. A broad range of structural interventions have contributed to this success and thus suggests that such approaches might also be applied in other settings experiencing HIV epidemics among gay men.

References

1. Brown, A.E., Kirwan, P.D., Chau, C., Khawam, J., Gill, O.N., & Delpech, V.C. (2017, November) Towards the elimination of HOV transmission, AIDS and HIV-related deaths in the UK—2017 report. London: Public Health England.

2. Nakagawa, F. (2011) Projected life expectancy of people with HIV according to timing of diagnosis. *AIDS*, 26(3) [Online edition].

3. Smit, P., Brady, M., Carter, M., et al. (2012) HIV-related stigma within gay communities: a literature review. *AIDS Care*, 24, 405–412.

4. Bourne, A., Hickson, F., & Keogh, P. (2012) Problems with sex among gay and bisexual men with diagnosed HIV in the United Kingdom. *BMC Public Health*, 12, 916.

5. Bourne, A., Dodds, C., Keogh, P., Weatherburn, P., & Hammond, G. (2009) Relative safety II—risk and unprotected anal intercourse among gay men with diagnosed HIV. London: Sigma Research.

6. Select Committee on HIV and Aids in the United Kingdom (2011) No vaccine, no cure: HIV and AIDS in the United Kingdom—1st Report of Session 2010– 12. London: House of Lords.

7. Chaps Partnership. (2011) Making it count: a collaborative planning framework to minimise the incidence of HIV during sex between men. 4th ed. London: Sigma.

8. Brown, A.E., Mohammed, H., Ogaz, D., Kirwan, P.D., Yung, M., Nash, S.G., et al. (2017). Fall in new HIV diagnoses among men who have sex with men (MSM) at selected London sexual health clinics since early 2015: Testing or treatment or pre-exposure prophylaxis? *Eurosurveillance*. 22, 30553.

9. Herbst, J., Beeker, C. & Mathew, A. (2007) The effectiveness of individual, group, and community-level HIV behavioral risk-reduction interventions for adult men who have sex with men: a systematic review. *American Journal of Preventative Medicine*, 32, S38–S67.

10. Herbst, J., Sherba, R., & Crepaz, N. (2005) The HIV/AIDS Prevention Synthesis Team: a meta-analysis review of HIV behavioral interventions for reducing sexual risk taking behavior of men who have sex with men. *Journal of Acquired Immune Deficiency Syndromes*, 39, 228–241.

11. Johnson, W., Hedges, L., & Ramirez, G. (2002) HIV prevention research for men who have sex with men: a systematic review and meta-analysis. *Journal of Acquired Immune Deficiency Syndromes*, 30, S118–S129.

12. Johnson, W., Holtgrave, D., & McClellan, W. (2005) HIV intervention research for men who have sex with men: a 7-year update. *AIDS Education and Prevention*, 17, 568–589.

13. Select Committee on HIV and Aids in the United Kingdom (2011) No vaccine, no cure: HIV and AIDS in the United Kingdom—1st Report of Session 2010–12. London: House of Lords.

14. Tatoud, R. (2011) HIV combination prevention: ingredients and recipes for a success. Available at: http://www.incidenceo.org/2011/05/10/combination-hiv-prevention- ingredients-recipes-for-a-success/

15. UNAIDS (2010) Combination HIV prevention: tailoring and coordinating biomedical, behavioural and structural strategies to reduce new HIV infections. Geneva: UNAIDS.

16. Cohen, M., Chen, Y., McCauley, M., et al. (2011) Antiretroviral treatment to prevent the sexual transmission of HIV-1: results from the HPTN 052 multinational randomized controlled trial. Paper presented at the Sixth IAS Conference on HIV Pathogenesis, Treatment and Prevention. Rome.

17. Das Douglas, M., & Chu, P. (2010) Decreases in community viral load are associated with a reduction in new HIV diagnoses in San Francisco. Paper presented at the 17th Conference on Retroviruses and Opportunistic Infections. San Francisco.

18. Lima, V., Johnson, K., Hogg, R., et al. (2008) Expanded access to highly active antiretroviral therapy: a potentially powerful strategy to curb the growth of the HIV epidemic. *Journal of Infectious Diseases*, 198, 59–67.

19. UNAIDS (2011) Groundbreaking trial results confirm HGIV treatment prevents transmission of HIV. Geneva: UNAIDS.

20. United States Prevention Action Campaign: Consensus statement. Available at: https://www.preventionaccess.org/consensus

21. Rey, D., Den Diane, M., & Moatti, J. (2000) Post-exposure prophylaxis after occupational exposure to HIV: overview of the policies implemented in 27 European countries. *AIDS Care*, 12, 263–265.

22. Fisher, M., Benn, P., & Evans, B. (2006) UK guidelines for the use of post-exposure prophylaxis for HIV following sexual exposure. *International Journal of STD & AIDS*, 17, 81–92.

23. Terrence Higgins Trust. (2006) Post-exposure prophylaxis micro-site. Available at: http://www.pep.chapsonline.org.uk/

24. Wilson, C. (2017, January 9) Massive drop in London HIV rates may due to Internet drugs. *New Scientist*. Available at: https://www.newscientist.com/article/2117426-massive-drop-in-london-hiv-rates-may-be-due-to-internet-drugs/

25. Public Health England. (2017) HIV in the United Kingdom: decline in new HIV diagnoses in gay and bisexual men in London, 2017 report. *Health Protection Report*, 11(35).

26. Gill, N. (2017, October) What is happening with new HIV diagnoses in gay men in England and why? Paper presented during Session PS11, Understanding our Evolving Epidemic, 16th European AIDS Conference. Milan.

27. Public Health England. (2017) HIV in the United Kingdom: decline in new HIV diagnoses in gay and bisexual men in London, 2017 report. *Health Protection Report*, 11(35).

28. Cairns, G. (2017, August 4) PrEP demand in England is rapidly accelerating and most will want to join the trial. London: NAM Publications. Available at: https://www.aidsmap.com/

29. Mundasad, S. (2014, July). Healthy gas men urged to take HIV drugs—WHO. BBC News. Available at: http://www.bbc.co.uk/news/health-28264436

30. Nutland, W. (2018, February 9) The state of PrEP activism in Europe and worldwide. 1st European PrEP Summit. Amsterdam.

31. Wang, X., Nwokolo, N., Boffito, M. et al. (2016, October) InterPrEP: Internet-based pre-exposure prophylaxis (PrEP) with generic tenofovir DF/emtricitabine (TDF/FTC) in London—analysis of pharmacokinetics, safety and outcomes. Paper presented at the International Congress on Drug Therapy in HIV Infection. Glasgow.

32. Cairns, G. (2016, October 26) Tests of online PrEP purchases by London clinic find no fakes and adequate drug levels. London: NAM Publications. Available at: http://www.aidsmap.com/

33. Update on commission and provision of pre exposure prophylaxis (PREP) for HIV prevention. (2016, March 21). NHS England. Available at: https://www.england.nhs.uk/2016/03/prep/

34. Peabody, R. (2016, March 22) England's PrEP policy in disarray after NHS U-turn. London: NAM Publications. Available at: http://www.aidsmap.com/

35. NHS can fund "game-changing" PrEP HIV drug, court says. (2016, August 2). *The Guardian*. Available at: https://www.theguardian.com/society/2016/aug/02/nhs-can-fund-game-changing-prep-hiv-drug-court-says

36. Anonymous. HIV drug puts other care at risk, warns NHS. The Times. August 2, 2016. Available at: https://www.thetimes.co.uk/article/victory-for-hiv-campaigners-means-nhs-could-pay-for-prevention-drug-zzhvmn6x9.

11

Community Mobilization as an HIV Prevention Strategy

THE POLITICAL CHALLENGES OF CONFRONTING THE AIDS EPIDEMIC IN BRAZIL

Richard Parker, Jonathan Garcia, Miguel Muñoz-Laboy, Laura Rebecca Murray, and Fernando Seffner

Overview

Over the course of nearly four decades, Brazil has struggled to control the HIV and AIDS epidemic as one of its most significant national public health challenges. As in most countries, the Brazilian government had a slow start in responding to the epidemic in the 1980s. Thanks in large part to the political mobilization of civil society, beginning in the early 1990s, the federal Brazilian government began to adopt a pioneering, rights-based approach to HIV and AIDS. Central to its response, the government prioritized community mobilization and the empowerment of key affected populations and communities. Over the course of the 1990s and the 2000s, this emphasis was translated into a commitment to addressing the structural determinants of HIV and AIDS and allowed Brazil to build what is widely recognized as one of the most successful multilevel responses to the epidemic that any country (whether in the global North or the global South) had developed.[1-3] But by the end of the third decade of the epidemic, as the result of a range of political changes taking place in the country, Brazil's focus on the structural dimensions of HIV and

AIDS began to wane, and increasing biomedicalization of the Brazilian response to epidemic began to unravel earlier successes.[4]

This chapter seeks to analyze both the important accomplishments of the Brazilian response to the structural dimensions of the HIV and AIDS as well as the political challenges to sustaining that response over time. It documents the ways in which a focus on community mobilization and empowerment succeeded in implementing timely and effective HIV prevention programs in key affected communities such as sex workers and gay men, bisexual men, and other men who have sex with men (MSM). It analyzes the ways in which this strategy made it possible to address many of the structural drivers of HIV in these communities. But it also highlights the extent to which addressing these structural forces depended on a favorable political context capable of supporting and nurturing such approaches.

Our overarching goal in the chapter is thus twofold. On the one hand, we try to highlight the important lessons that can be learned from HIV prevention community mobilization case studies based on the Brazilian experience. On the other hand, we seek to analyze the ways in which community mobilization strategies, their effectiveness and sustainability, are shaped by broader political ecology of the country and by the ways in which this ecology may change over time.

The Brazilian Response to HIV

In its "golden years," from the early 1990s into the late 2000s, the Brazilian response to HIV and AIDS became widely recognized as a model for best practices for integrating prevention, care, and treatment programs in a developing country. The political and social response to HIV in Brazil was shaped by the democratization movement, driven by human rights and solidarity at the interface of politics and public health, and was set against a backdrop of a culture of solidarity and of a positive celebration of sexual diversity that values eroticism as key to prevention. The period when Brazil was considered a model in its response to HIV and AIDS provides a strong contrast to the current period of reactionary conservatism described later in this chapter.

Principles of citizenship, solidarity, and human rights framed social mobilization for democracy and became central to the Brazilian response to HIV and AIDS. Citizenship defined the relationship between the Brazilian people and the state (through its democratic institutions);

solidarity, and respect for human rights defined the relationship among the people.[5-7] Post-dictatorship, this redemocratization movement built political parties, trade unions, and nongovernmental organizations (NGOs) throughout the 1980s and culminated in a demand for elections for a new and free Congress. Democratic elections were initially held only at the municipal and state levels. The negotiation and promulgation of the new democratic Constitution, passed in 1988, included the reinstitution of free national elections as of 1990. Since its original proclamation of independence in 1822, Brazil has had no fewer than seven constitutions: in 1824, 1891, 1934, 1937, 1946, 1967, and most recently in 1988. But it was only in the constitutions of 1946 and 1988 that the constitutional processes took place with more intense participation on the part of the broader society. This was especially true in 1988, taking place after 20 years of authoritarian military rule, which permitted the incorporation of popular amendments as the result of social movement organizing, which could directly demand the insertion of legal provisions into the constitutional text. Because of this, the 1988 constitution became known as the "citizen's constitution" due to the incorporation into its text of a large range of social rights and political liberties.

Taking place shortly after the beginning of the AIDS epidemic in the country, and as a result of the growing vigor of social movements with an important impact on the fight against the epidemic—such as the lesbian, gay, bisexual, and transgender (LGBT) and feminist movements, as well as the AIDS movement itself—the 1988 constitution was especially important in creating a legal foundation for a rights-based approach to the epidemic. Social movements benefited from the spirit of the Federal Constitution of 1988 and succeed in impacting both its constitutional principles and its goals for reaching society. Several examples are:

- the declaration of human dignity as a basic right of life guaranteed to any Brazilian citizen and defined as a human right in the 1988 constitutional text;
- the equality of rights thought of as a suitable terrain for life in society and with social justice and as a duty of guarantee by the state and public policies;
- the recognition and appreciation of differences and diversity, implying an analytical debate of each context and adoption of legal mechanisms that take into account the different social markers of difference that may lead to situations of inequality;

- the secularity of the state, a constitutional principle expressed in the Federal Constitution of 1988, which seeks to ensure that the state does not promote any religion in particular but will ensure that each one can profess the faith that seems to him or her most appropriate, in harmony with secular liberties (such as freedom of conscience, freedom of expression, and freedom of belief, all of which are contained in the charter);
- the compulsory exercise of democratic management in public education policies, which must also be expressed in the daily school life and which is guaranteed both in the constitutional text and in the ordinations of the National Education Plan;
- the guarantee of the widest freedom of individual and social expression;
- the guarantee of the construction of public systems of health, education, and social security.

In this environment of democratic reconstruction legally reinforced by the Federal Constitution of 1988, discourses and actions in the field of human rights were strengthened in ways that were crucial for structuring the national response to HIV and AIDS. In 1996, under the government of Fernando Henrique Cardoso, the country created the first version of the National Human Rights Program, which had its third version in the first term of the Lula government. Examining the three editions of the program, it is possible to perceive an effort to create public policies and strategies of government in themes that connect directly or transversally with the construction of the national response to AIDS.

Over the second half of the 1980s, a vibrant rebirth of civil society (linked to the political processes that produced the *"citizen's constitution"* in 1988) led to the formation of NGOs focused on HIV and AIDS in key cities and states around the country.[8,9] This coalition of NGOs and community-based initiatives, led by a critical number of gay men and human rights activists, hemophiliacs, as well as men and women infected or affected by HIV, openly confronted HIV stigma, demanding that the rights of people living with AIDS be respected by the government and by their fellow citizens.[10] Working together with progressive state and municipal health departments, they pressured the federal government to create a National AIDS Program (NAP), and then continued to pressure the new NAP to adopt progressive policies aimed at confronting stigma and discrimination and building a rights-based approach to the epidemic.[11] These factors combined to create an early response to HIV that was based on solidarity and inclusion rather than stigma, moral sanitation of sexual expressions, quarantine, direct and indirect neglect, and exclusion.[12]

This mobilization process, in which many diverse social movements made up of Brazilian citizens came together in a common struggle for democracy, was the basis for a sense of social solidarity across many traditional societal divisions.[13] This should not be idealized or romanticized: Brazil was and is a nation with great disparities of wealth, has a long history of social discrimination based on skin color, and is marked by oppressive gender relationships, all of which had (and continue to have) a longstanding negative impact on the health of the Brazilian population.[14] Despite these very real differences in power and prestige, however, social solidarity built up out of common suffering and the struggle for democracy and citizenship became a countervailing force to the stigma surrounding the emergence of HIV.[15]

Perhaps one of the clearest examples of a broadly implemented structural intervention, the Brazilian constitution created both a moral and a legal basis for the demand for comprehensive treatment for people living with HIV/AIDS (PLWHA).[16] However, it must be recognized that, at least until the mid-1990s, the government itself rarely took the initiative to expand services for PLWHA. AIDS advocacy groups developed legal aid programs and brought a series of successful class action suits focused on specific programmatic issues (e.g., free viral resistance testing, expanded drug formulary) that have operationalized the constitutional right to health.[17] These lawsuits, in turn, created a public venue where PLWHA could assert their rights as Brazilian citizens and function as protagonists in their own struggle for life.[18]

Even through a succession of different presidential administrations, the NAP sustained a consistent commitment to strengthening resources in previously marginalized communities, to defending their rights, and to articulating respect for diversity as key components of official government policy. It has been characterized by an active collaboration between government agencies and NGOs, as well as by the mobilization of activist political support and commitment within the machinery of the state itself, particularly on the part of local service providers in the public health system. Organizations representing sex workers, drug users, LGBT populations, PLWHA, and other groups affected by the epidemic received significant funding from the government.[19] Support has been provided for more than a decade now for legal aid work carried out by NGOs working on behalf of PLWHA.[18]

The commitment to human rights, and the early emphasis placed on solidarity as central to the response to HIV/AIDS in Brazil, while articulated as a response to the military authoritarian regime and social inequality, is clearly also deeply rooted in a long-standing emphasis on solidarity in Brazilian culture. Principles of solidarity and reciprocity have long been understood as central to the moral economy of the poor in Brazilian society.[20] Solidarity among family members and neighbors is a key element of the survival strategies traditionally employed by poor people with little access to services and social welfare benefits in Brazil. These same principles have been extremely important to critical societal institutions, such as the Catholic Church and the Brazilian state apparatus.[21,22] This same principle of solidarity has clearly resonated in response to the plight of PLWHA.

Just as moral principles of solidarity in Brazilian culture have been central to the foundation of a national response to HIV and AIDS, sexuality and sexual expression are also an integral part of Brazilian culture and have facilitated the development of an effective response to the epidemic.[23-25] Certainly, there is more than one discourse about sexuality in Brazil—a point that we return to later in discussing recent setbacks in AIDS-related policymaking. But an important part of Brazil's initial successes in mobilizing affected communities in response to the epidemic can be linked to the capacity for HIV prevention programs to address sexuality more openly than in most other countries.[26] Openness about sexuality and the diversity of gender and sexual identities that exist in a community have helped to break down the stigma surrounding both homosexuality and HIV.

Nowhere is the importance of sexual culture in Brazil as clear as in the ways in which prevention programs there were able to address sexuality, focusing consistently on condom promotion with sex-positive messaging, while also combating stigma and discrimination. The public service announcements sponsored by the NAP were among the most explicit of any governmental information campaign anywhere in the world. This was most visibly evident in public health campaigns that featured erotic, naked bodies and that promoted condom use as sexy. Condom use was promoted relentlessly, female as well as male condoms were widely distributed by the Brazilian government, and studies of sexual behavior have demonstrated significant increases in the actual adoption of condom use across population groups (especially among young people).[27] It is notable that a national survey of sexual behavior published in 2000 showed that condom sales and distribution had risen dramatically in the general population over the course of the 1990s, and these data also showed that condom use among HIV-infected people had increased as well.[28] Public information campaigns also focused on the need to combat stigma and support sexual diversity, with one campaign focusing on the need for parents to accept and support children who are homosexual (without even referring specifically to HIV). These mass media approaches went hand-in-hand with significant levels of government support for community-based prevention programs among MSM, sex workers, young people, and other populations perceived to be at elevated risk of HIV infection.

In many countries, HIV prevention has been blocked by societal and governmental leaders claiming that discussion of sexuality is antithetical to traditional culture. This assumes that culture is static, unresponsive to changing conditions or focused intervention. Although the Brazilian NAP acknowledged that reducing numbers of sexual partners can reduce an individual's risk of infection, it has also recognized that many people, especially women, are not always able to control the multiple relations of their primary partners. Throughout the 1990s and over the course of the 2000s, the NAP was therefore firm in promoting condom use at the center of its program[3,29]—a position that caused tension with some international agencies, such as the United States Agency for International Development (USAID). Indeed, the Brazilian government's refusal to adopt USAID's "ABC" (Abstinence, Be faithful, Condoms) prevention strategy, together with its very public refusal to accept the contractual clause referred to as the "anti-prostitution pledge," implemented as a part of US President George W. Bush's Emergency Plan for AIDS Relief Program (PEPFAR), led to the discontinuation of US-funded AIDS prevention activities in Brazil after 2003.[30]

Addressing the Needs of Key Affected Communities and Populations

Over the course of the first three decades of the HIV and AIDS epidemic in Brazil, this combination of contextual factors linked to both politics and culture helped to provide a supportive environment for ongoing community mobilization efforts as the core focus of the Brazilian government's attempt to address the structural dimensions of the epidemic. It is worth examining the development of community mobilization in relation to two key populations that were the central focus for the Brazilian government's efforts in this regard: (a) sex workers and (b) gay men, bisexual men, and other MSM.[1]

Sex Workers

The first HIV prevention project with sex workers in Brazil was called PREVINA. Developed in the late 1980s by the recently formed NAP, the project also targeted prisoners and drug users. The director of the NAP at the time, Dr. Lair Guerra, invited leaders of Brazil's *Rede Brasileira de Prostitutas* (RBP; Portuguese for the National Network of Prostitutes) to collaborate in designing the project. The RBP was founded in 1987 to fight police violence against sex workers and defend sex workers' right to work. Against the backdrop of the emerging AIDS epidemic, RBP quickly focused its attention on fighting the stigma attached to being categorized as a "risk group." PREVINA was initially designed by Ministry of Health technocrats as a morally charged clinical intervention, condemning sex work and promiscuity and promoting exiting sex work while also administering the initially available AIDS medical treatments and distribution of condoms. But the dialogue between the NAP and the RBP transformed the program into a groundbreaking initiative, building a civil society-government partnership and sex-positive approach to sexuality and sex work.[31]

This sex-positive approach to prevention, which included sex workers as protagonists in developing and implementing HIV outreach, education, and treatment programs, would go on to shape federally funded AIDS programs during the 1990s. Federal and state government AIDS programs and sex worker rights organizations grew rapidly during this period with financial support from loans from the World Bank, the Brazilian government for AIDS prevention and control programs, and international foundations for civil society organizations.[5] From 1993 to 1997, the NAP funded projects developed by 181 AIDS NGOs nationally[32(p.176)] and 52

---

1. We originally intended to also include transgender women as a third case study, but in reviewing the history of prevention initiative we found that until very recently trans populations have been addressed as a subcategory in programs designed for either sex workers or MSM. The space available for this chapter does not permit a detailed analysis of the problems that this created in seeking to address the needs of transgender women in particular.

projects with male, female, or transgender sex workers, with the majority (44) for female sex workers.[33] From 1998 to 2003, the Brazilian government funded the national project *Esquina da Noite* (Portuguese for Street Corner of the Night). Implemented as part of the second World Bank loan for AIDS prevention, the project covered 50 municipalities throughout the country. In this expansion of prevention for sex workers, the focus centered on increasing the number of sex worker-led organizations working in HIV prevention in rural areas and interior cities (i.e., noncoastal areas) where the epidemic was spreading rapidly. The widespread success and rapid adoption of *Esquina da Noite* can be attributed to its timely implementation, because it coincided with the Federal Ministry of Health's decentralization initiatives.

Maria Sem Vergonha (Portuguese for Maria Without Shame) was launched in 2002, marking one of the most important and victorious years for the Brazilian sex workers' movement. This national prevention campaign, run by the Federal Ministry of Labor, recognized *profissionais do sexo* (literally, sex professionals, translated to sex workers in English) as an official occupation within the Brazilian Occupation Classification System (CBO). Having a CBO qualification allows for federal government labor protections, including retirement benefits and health and social services assistance in case of work-related illness. Although third-party involvement (e.g., "pimps," "madams," or others who administer the work of sex workers) in prostitution remains illegal under the Brazilian penal code (Articles 228, 229, 231-A), the recognition of sex work as an occupation gave the movement an important basis from which to advocate for full decriminalization and recognition of sex work as a legitimate form of labor. Respect for sex work as a profession was the fundamental basis for the *Maria Sem Vergonha* campaign. It consisted of radio spots and educational print materials focusing on three main slogans: (a) No shame in being a prostitute, (b) No shame in valuing your work, and (c) Respect is good and I like it. In 2002, the sex workers movement's demands paralleled the rights- and citizenship-based approach of the NAP, creating a powerful overlap of pro-human rights approaches to addressing the Brazilian HIV and AIDS epidemic. This collective, intersectional pro-human rights approach to health started to change in 2005.

As mentioned, in January 2003, as part of the US PEPFAR Program, a contractual clause referred to as the "anti-prostitution pledge" was introduced to all financial contracts involving US government funds. This stipulated that organizations must have a clause within their organizational statute explicitly opposing prostitution. At the time the clause was introduced, a large prevention project was being implemented in Brazil with vulnerable population groups, including sex workers, through a bilateral agreement with the US government. In 2005, the Brazilian government, in partnership with the RBP, refused to implement the anti-prostitution pledge mandate, rejecting nearly US$40 million in HIV prevention funds that had been allocated to the country. Brazil's decision was heralded by the international community and applauded by sex worker activists globally.[1]

Sex worker organizations continued to advocate for rights-based approaches to HIV and increasingly lobbied for other branches of the government, such as the national Secretariats of Human Rights and Women's Policies, to join the Ministry of Labor in the fight for sex worker rights. A victory for the movement came in 2009 when sex workers were finally included in the revised version of the Secretariat of Women's Policies and Ministry of Health's joint Integral Plan to Confront the Feminization of the AIDS Epidemic and other STDs. The goal of the plan was to address the increasing prevalence of HIV among women in Brazil. The revised plan included a series of what were called *agendas afirmativas* (affirmative agendas) for specific populations, including sex workers. The Affirmative Agenda for Prostitutes contained 34 recommendations on how to confront HIV among sex workers in Brazil, all highlighting the need for intersectorial partnerships to address the various social and structural dimensions of HIV.

The Affirmative Agenda for Prostitutes was considered to be a victory by the sex worker movement when it was launched; however, it was never implemented in practice.[34] The RBP called on the federal government to support sex workers as women with equal needs and rights as other women, beyond the context of HIV; however, this did not happen.[35] In 2011, the RBP made the decision to no longer apply for federal funding for AIDS projects. The decision was made at the RBP network's regional conference in Belém, in a statement that began with the phrase, "We are professional sex workers, not [representatives of] the government."[31] The statement made various references to the difficulties organizations had encountered with federal and state funding and reporting mechanisms, and, while it recognized the importance of the RBP's partnership with the National AIDS Program, it expressed the RBP's dissatisfaction with the new policy orientation of the NAP. In particular, the statement articulated a sense that the "risk group mentality" that sex workers had fought so vehemently against in the late 1980s and the 1990s had returned through projects that "reinforce prostitutes as spreaders of disease and distributors of condoms."[35]

Two years later, in 2013, the extent to which the Ministry of Health's approach to HIV prevention had changed became even clearer with the censorship of a campaign developed by the National STD and HIV/ AIDS Department in collaboration with sex workers for International Sex Worker Rights Day. The most controversial of the posters, which featured a sex worker with the sentence "I'm happy being a prostitute," provoked immediate and angry reactions from conservatives in Brazil's Congress, forcing it to be removed and leading to punitive actions toward those responsible. The director of the STD and HIV/AIDS Department in the Ministry of Health was fired, and the entire campaign was taken offline just two days after its release.[35] An altered campaign was put up in its place, and only the posters with phrases about condom use were retained. At this time, the NAP had been incorporated within the broader structure of the Ministry of Health as a department, leading the AIDS program to lose the political and budgetary freedom it had as a separate bureaucratic institution. This shift in the AIDS program's location within the health bureaucracy in Brazil may have had some benefits internally but also made HIV and AIDS programming more politically fragile and dependent on the sway of conservative factions and trends toward biomedical prevention.

It was the third time in 18 months that materials referring to HIV prevention and sexuality had been censored by units and legislators of the state and federal governments. Activists argued this was a return to stigma, censorship, and solely biomedical approaches to prevention— which many of them had fought against in the AIDS social movement. Sex worker organizations responded with strong statements and public actions. As the Association of Prostitutes in Pernambuco stated at the time: "Once more, what was supposed to be a triumph for human rights has turned into a violation of those rights: the suspension of the right to affirm prostitution as a dignified and happy profession."[35]

Several months after the campaign censorship, the Ministry of Health introduced the Live Better Knowing [your HIV status] program, a "test and treat" project directed at sex workers, MSM, and people who use drugs. The Live Better Knowing project is emblematic of the AIDS program's move away from social mobilization and community empowerment approaches toward almost exclusively biomedical HIV prevention and treatment (and an emphasis on what has increasingly been described as "combination prevention"). Although the Ministry of Health has supported important events for sex workers, such as the VI National Meeting marking the 30th anniversary of the movement in 2017, biomedical approaches such as testing and pre-exposure prophylaxis (PrEP), have become the dominant focus of HIV programming and funding.

Indeed, the protagonist role that sex workers had played in the development of the earliest HIV prevention projects and the focus on pleasure and rights that made them a global reference are no longer central components of the current federally funded actions. While the development of the diverse plans and programs during the 2000s had a strong symbolic effect and reflected participatory processes, challenges posed by decentralization and the increasing power of religious conservative (and especially the Evangelical block in the Brazilian Congress) made implementing them nearly impossible, as fewer and fewer ministries and secretariats were willing to defend sex worker rights. Parallel to these processes, biomedical approaches such as PrEP, antiretroviral treatment as prevention, and "test and treat" gained steam on the global health landscape, providing programmatic justification, and funding, for a shift in approaches.[36]

Gay and Bisexual Men and Other MSM

Although prevention programs for sex workers were initiated at a very early stage, in the late 1980s, through the PREVENA Project described earlier, at that stage even though there was clear recognition of gay and bisexual men and other MSM as one of the communities at great risk of HIV infection in Brazil, there were initially no comparable prevention programs implemented for these men. At least in part, this was justified as due to the concern that to implement such projects would potentially increase stigma and discrimination against the gay community, which was widely perceived as the highest risk population in the country and was seriously stigmatized because of this association (Lair Guerra, personal communication). But this justification was also immediately questioned by AIDS activists and representatives of the LGBT community,[23] who argued that not developing programs for an at-risk community was itself a form of stigma. Key nongovernmental AIDS organizations in major cities around the country, such as Fortaleza, Porto Alegre, Rio de Janeiro, Salvador, and São Paulo, began to organize local community-based programs to reach gay and bisexual men and other MSM.[23] These programs initially had only limited support primarily from private philanthropic organizations but were nonetheless important in calling attention to the needs of gay men. At ABIA (the Brazilian Interdisciplinary AIDS Association) in Rio de Janeiro, for example, with support from the Ford Foundation, prevention education materials with homoerotic imagery modeled on gay icons such as Tom of Finland were used to try to reach gay-identified men with HIV prevention information. In Forteleza, at GAPA-CE (the AIDS Prevention and Support Group in the state of Ceará), also with support from the Ford Foundation, a very different strategy was employed, with informational pamphlets about sex with men (but no reference to gay identity or culture) designed to reach non-gay-identified men—as project coordinators described it, the goal was specifically to have material in the pocket of a man's clothes without "incriminating" him as being gay in case it was found by his mother or his wife (Rogério Godim, personal communication).

In another example of such work, beginning in 1991 (and continuing for an extended period going forward), in Porto Alegre, GAPA-RS (the AIDS Prevention and Support Group in the state of Rio Grande do Sul) initiated an HIV prevention program for prisoners in the Presídio Central (Central Prison) in Porto Alegre, focusing on both the gay-identified and transgender populations as well as homosexually-active (but not necessarily gay-identified) prisoners. With financial support from an organization linked to the Franciscan Order of the Catholic Church in Germany, they created a manual describing their work, illustrated by the prisoners themselves in cartoon-style drawings to disseminate prevention information. The central figure in this pamphlet was a prisoner named Lampadinha (literally, Street Lamp), a name chosen by the prisoners to designate someone with good, illuminating ideas. Written in the kind of jargon and slang used by the prisoners themselves and illustrated with drawings that represented their daily lives, it was widely accepted as especially effective among the prison population.

In 1992, when the NAP was reorganized and initial negotiations with the World Bank for a major loan to support HIV prevention and control began to take place, one of the authors of this chapter (RP) served as the chief of the Prevention Unit, and MSM were incorporated into the strategic plan for prevention that would be supported by the World Bank as well as by other important donors at the time, such as the USAID AIDSCAP Project in Brazil. Beginning in 1993, when the first major loan from the World Bank went into effect, and continuing over the course of the 1990s and the 2000s, literally hundreds of community-based prevention programs and interventions implemented by NGOs and focusing on MSM were supported by the Brazilian government with funds provided by the bank.

Although it is was not explicitly stated in the World Bank's own evaluation of its series of loans in Brazil how many of the 444 prevention projects funded during the first loan (from 1993 to 1998) were designed for each of the risk group categories, all of the projects funded necessarily had to prioritize commercial sex workers, injecting-drug users, or MSM. During the second loan (from 1999 to 2003), the total number of projects supported jumped to 1,664 projects, with 486 projects focusing on MSM, covering more than 3 million men. Even more striking, the number of projects supported for MSM increased from 17 in 1999, 30 in 2000, 57 in 2001, 138 in 2002, and 234 in 2003.[37]

The design and focus of these projects were highly variable, with no real attempt to systematize or impose a top-down model for prevention interventions. On the contrary, it would be more accurate to say that there was an emphasis on "letting a thousand flowers bloom" and on respecting the value of approaches rising from the ground up in the work of community-based organizations—as well as resisting the imposition of intervention models designed outside of Brazil and imported in by external donors. To give a better example of the content of such intervention programs, we briefly describe a number of projects developed in cities such as Porto Alegre and Rio de Janeiro, although dozens of other examples from other major urban centers around the country could also serve to illustrate this work.

In Rio de Janeiro, for example, social and behavioral intervention projects had been initiated beginning in the early 1990s, primarily with support from nongovernmental sources. From 1993 to 1997, ABIA (the Brazilian Interdisciplinary AIDS Association), together with the Grupo Pela Vidda-RJ (the Pela Vidda Group-Rio de Janeiro, the first organization of people living with HIV and AIDS to have been formed in Brazil) implemented a large-scale intervention program for community mobilization and empowerment of gay and bisexual men and other MSM.

In its first phase of work the program was funded primarily by the USAID AIDSCAP Project, with additional funding provided by the Ford Foundation, the John D. and Catherine T. MacArthur Foundation, and a range of smaller donors. The project was built around three key assumptions: (a) that high risk practices continue in spite of widespread knowledge about HIV; (b) among MSM, this is closely linked to their social isolation and their experience of prejudice and discrimination; and (c) responding to this wider context of sexual oppression would require the construction of "safer sex as a community practice" in ways that respect the broader culture of sexuality and erotic meanings in the gay community.[38] This program used a range of different strategies, including cultural activism through the performing arts and graphic arts, behavioral intervention workshops, theater workshop, cinema festivals, counseling services, community-based research, monitoring and evaluation, and other approaches to create what it described as a "multidimensional intervention" for gay community mobilization. After approval of the World Bank loan by the Brazilian government, the continuation of project activities by ABIA was supported primarily through funding from the Ministry of Health and executed through a series of targeted projects for diverse sectors of the broader community of gay and bisexual men and other MSM—young gay men, men involved in male sex work, transgender youth, and older (senior) MSM—developing into the longest-running program of HIV prevention anywhere in the country, for 25 years and counting as of 2018. During the most of this period, through 2012, the majority of these activities were supported by a series of short-term projects (normally 12 to 18 months) from government sources—primarily the federal government in Brasília but, in later years, as the World Bank-funded program began to be decentralized to states and municipalities, also through the State Secretariat of Health in Rio de Janeiro. But, after the early 2010s, funding opportunities from government sources for intervention projects by NGOs and CBOs was severely curtailed. The limited support that was available was directed to biomedical prevention programs based on a "test and treat" model, and national funds for the program were no longer available when the NAP was incorporated into the broader structure of the Ministry of Health. Since 2013, funding for the most recent focus of the project, serving sexually and gender-diverse youth, has relied entirely on support from the MAC AIDS Fund, with no support from governmental sources.[39]

In Porto Alegre, to offer another example from another region of the country, the main information and prevention actions aimed at gay and bisexual men and other MSM over the years have been made by the CBO Nuances in partnership with GAPA-RS, with various sources funding but from the Ministry of Health. Nuances began its AIDS activism trajectory through partnerships with GAPA-RS, and based on the notion of solidarity, as early as 1992. The emphasis was to promote a sense of solidarity that extended beyond simple "compassion" for those with AIDS and for it to be perceived as a strategy of union against the prejudice that the disease accentuates, especially in relation to the gay population. In tune with broader activist approaches, Nuances' projects emphasized the subject of sexual pleasure as especially important in times of AIDS, with safer sex (and the erotization of condoms) as the primary strategy. Nuances understood that the moment was one of coming "out of the closet"—and that AIDS could represent, in the lives of many homosexually active men, the permanence of life inside the closet—and that as a result it was important to link its activism to the broader international movement denouncing silence as equal to death.

Of the many projects that Nuances developed over the years, perhaps the main project that articulated its AIDS prevention in the gay population was developed beginning in 1995 and was called *POA NOITE HOMENS* (POA NIGHT MEN), a good-humored way of playing with the almost homonymous expression "good night," using the acronym (POA) of the city. The project involved a partnership with the GAPA-RS and aimed at what was then called "behavioral intervention for safer sex practices"—with the production of informational materials and direct distribution of condoms for gay men and male sex workers in bars, nightclubs, saunas, video rental shops, and other catchment sites around the city. In order to stimulate contact with the project agents, condoms were distributed with the words "use in the event of a *hard* time" and in dialogue with the project peer educators, who circulated at night in cruising areas and gay venues. A "condom carrying case" was also created, with the phrase "do not go to bed without a condom." The project had a strong presence in the city between 1995 and 1998, with high visibility in the media, and drew critical reactions from conservative sectors, since it worked to fight against two related stigmas: AIDS and homosexuality. It also generated a spin-off project starting in 1997 known as the *HOMENS SEXO HOMENS* (MEN SEX MEN) Project, which approached HIV prevention in relation to themes such as sorodiscordance, bisexuality, and relationships outside of marriage. Some years later, this in turn generated another intervention, known as the *Pegação Segura* (Safe Cruising) project.

The daring mark of these projects (and others like them that were developed in cities around the country from the late 1990s through the 2000s, primarily supported through funds from the Ministry of Health to NGOs and CBOs) was the use of direct and open language in terms of sexuality and the defense of pleasure and sex without moralism. One of the most controversial issues over time was the fight against the idea of "reduction of [the number of] partners" as the focus of prevention strategies, consistently defending a pleasurable sexual life, with numerous partners if that were the person's desire, and with the use of condoms and adoption of other prevention harm reduction strategies. Another source of friction with the conservative press was the defense of sex work and paid sex for those that so wished, practiced with care in relation to prevention and without sacrificing sexual pleasure.

While community mobilization interventions such as the ones described here (and the hundreds of others funded by the Ministry of Health with funds provided through the World Bank loans) lay at the heart of the Brazilian government's strategy for HIV prevention among gay and bisexual men and other MSM, these interventions were integrated within a broader rights-based approach to the affirmation and empowerment of gay communities. Nowhere was this clearer than in the extensive support that the Ministry of Health provided over more than a decade for the realization of gay pride parades in cities around the country. Beginning in 2000, at the end of President Fernando Henrique Cardoso's second government, the Ministry of Health began funding the LGBT Pride Parade in São Paulo (the first, and always the largest, of the gay pride parades) as part of a strategy of simultaneously disseminating HIV prevention information and strengthening the gay community.[40] By 2005, during the first Lula administration, support from the Ministry of Health had grown to include 32 organizations responsible for organizing gay pride parades in different cities around the country, covering 22 (out of 26) states as well as the Federal District in Brasília.[41] In 2006, the total amount of support from the Ministry of Health for gay pride parades doubled from the 2005 amount, totaling R$1 million distributed around the country.[42] Support for gay pride parades continued consistently from 2000 to 2010, at the end of the second Lula administration, but was the object of severe criticism from religious conservatives and was discontinued at the start of the first Dilma Rousseff administration in 2011.[43] From that time on, support for the parades became a constant focus of political arm-wrestling between conservative religious forces and the LGBT movement, with more limited support (R$600,000) again being provided by the Ministry of Health in 2014 but then discontinued again in 2015.[44]

This broad-based approach to building gay communities and promoting gay community mobilization as the overarching strategy for confronting the epidemic in these communities, especially over the course of the 2000s, was also evident in the elaboration and publication of the *Plano Nacional de Enfrentamento da Epidemia de Aids e DST entre Gays, outros Homens que fazem Sexo com Homens (HSH) e Travestis* (the National Plan for Confronting the AIDS and STD Epidemic among Gays, Other Men Who Have Sex with Men [MSM] and Transvestites).[45] Based on an extensive consultation with civil society organizations involved in responding to the epidemic among these populations, followed by a national meeting commissioned by the Ministry of Health and organized by ABIA and the Grupo Pela Vidda-São Paulo, outlined an extremely detailed and comprehensive plan of action for confronting the epidemic in gay and trans* communities. It created the platform for the most explicit yet also broad-based national communication and consciousness-raising campaign, launched by the Ministry of Health in 2008 through all of the most important mass media venues in the country, as well as through the major AIDS NGOs and NGO networks (for copies of the campaign's various educational materials, see http://www.aids.gov.br/pt-br/campanha/plano-nacional-de-enfrentamento-da-epidemia-de-aids-e-das-dst-entre-gays-hsh-e-travestis). This, in turn, was followed in 2009 by the publication of the *Guia de Advocacy e Prevenção em HIV/AIDS: Gays e outros Homens que fazem Sexo com Homens* (the Guide for Advocacy and HIV/AIDS Prevention: Gays and Other Men Who Have Sex with Men),[46] again based on a national consultation, in this case coordinated by a network of gay activist organizations led by the Grupo Dignidade in Curitiba. The partnership between the Ministry of Health, networks of AIDS-service and advocacy organizations, and LGBT activist organizations that came together to develop these documents and campaigns marked in many ways the high point of the Brazilian response to HIV in communities of gay and bisexual men and other MSM, as well as the fullest inclusion of transgender communities recognized as a distinct population requiring their own affirmative agenda for advocacy and action.

In spite of these significant accomplishments, and the generally very positive political partnership between the LGBT movement and the Worker's Party governments during President Lula's two terms, following the election of Lula's hand-picked successor, Dilma Rousseff, in 2010, the relationship between the federal government and both AIDS and gay activists began to deteriorate rapidly after Rousseff took office at the start of 2011. Precisely because President Rousseff was seen as far weaker politically than Lula, the conservative religious coalition in Congress almost immediately began to exert pressure on her to withdraw support for policies and programs that were seen to promote sexual and gender diversity, threatening to withdraw support for key legislation related to economic issues if the government failed to roll back the programs implemented during earlier Partido dos Trabalhadores (PT, Workers Party) governments that promoted the so-called gay agenda.

The difference in strategy was already evident inside the Ministry of Health as early as 2011. Brazil had become known internationally over the course of the 1990s and the 2000s for its refusal to accept international pressure—such as the World Bank's resistance to universal treatment access and the US government's demands concerning the Prostitution Pledge. On the contrary, Brazil had championed its own strategies, and in particular its emphasis on a rights-based approach to the epidemic, as a model that other countries should follow. In a remarkable change of course, following the election of President Rousseff, the new regime in the Ministry of Health and its staff in the HIV/AIDS Department began to design many of its key activities using models imported from abroad. This was already evident starting in 2011, when the major program documents for how to reach key populations with prevention interventions began to be modeled on the US Centers for Disease Control and Prevention's (CDC) Diffusion of Effective Behavior Intervention program. For the first time in the nearly 30-year history of the Brazilian government's response to the epidemic, Ministry of Health guidelines for prevention were based on models developed in the global North, translated and tailored for application in Brazil with support from both the CDC and the US PEPFAR program.[47] While described as an extension of the Brazilian National Plan for Confronting the AIDS and STD Epidemic among Gays, Other Men Who Have Sex with Men [MSM] and Transvestites, this new wave of programs for MSM were explicitly based on US behavioral interventions such as the Popular Opinion Leader intervention, the Many Men, Many Voices intervention, and the MPowerment intervention.[48] This emphasis on behavioral interventions, as opposed to community mobilization and empowerment models, was extended further beginning in 2013 and 2014, as Brazil adopted the "test and treat" approach promoted by UNAIDS as its primary initiative to bring HIV-positive people into treatment and to effectively use Treatment as Prevention, even enlisting the help of President Dilma Rousseff to send out messages on her Twitter account encouraging HIV testing for key populations to commemorate World AIDS Day in 2013.[49–51] The Ministry of Health continued to invest its primary prevention resources in biomedical approaches, planning its traditional Carnival prevention campaign in 2015 around messages promoting HIV testing disseminated through cell phone apps such as Tinder e Hornet.[52]

This remarkable conversion from its traditional emphasis on structural interventions using community mobilization and empowerment approaches to behavioral and biomedical prevention strategies that played itself out within the ambit of the Ministry of Health and its various partners over the course of the 2010s, however, was only one part of the shifting scene in relation to the HIV response for gay and bisexual men and other MSM. As was the case in terms of programs for sex workers, programs direct to gay men and their communities would also become the focus for serious negative criticism on the part of conservative politicians in the Brazilian Congress, who used their position and their increasing numbers to pressure Dilma Rousseff's government. In 2011, for example, after very visible protests on the part of Evangelicals from the House of Representatives, Rousseff agreed to halt the distribution of educational materials to schools through the Brazil Without Homophobia Program (referred to by the media as the "anti-homophobia kit" or "gay kit").[53] Although this program was based in the Ministry of Education, it had been developed in close dialogue with the Ministry of Health's AIDS Department, and it was enthusiastically supported by the AIDS movement as an extension of the conviction that a rights-based approach to the HIV epidemic demanded confronting structural stigma, especially in relation to gay men. The ending of the Brazil Without Homophobia Program was thus seen as a major setback not only to the fight against homophobia in schools but to the fight against HIV and AIDS as well. The declining relationship between the federal government and the LGBT and AIDS movements took another turn for the worse in 2012, when conservative politicians again pressured the government, this time focusing on the Ministry of Health's HIV prevention for Carnival, which had been designed to target gay and transgender youth. The campaign was severely criticized as promoting homosexuality rather than preventing HIV and was again suspended in the midst of significant controversy, substituted by a campaign that generically targeted youth and avoided any reference to sexual or gender diversity.[54] Although the leadership of the LGBT movement continued to support Rousseff on through to her impeachment (ironically, in part led by the conservative evangelical political forces who had succeeded so effectively in pressuring her to move to the right), more grassroots activists and a significant part of the AIDS activist movement largely abandoned its support for the government, and, in return, the government largely abandoned its support for nonbiomedical prevention interventions, events such as the gay pride parades, and the other activities that had marked its approach to community mobilization as its primary strategy for addressed the vulnerability of gay and bisexual men and other MSM.

The Political Challenges of Sustainability

As both of these case studies illustrate, albeit in slightly different ways, following a long period of important success in using community mobilization and collective empowerment strategies as the key to a broader rights-based framework to HIV prevention over the course of the 1990s and the 2000s, a series of new challenges began to emerge that have called into question the long-term sustainability of the Brazilian response to the epidemic. This chapter analyzes the ways in which Brazil was able to build rights-based approach to HIV/AIDS, which served as the foundational base for the development of structural interventions and community mobilization programs developed in partnership with civil society. This commitment made it possible to address many of the structural drivers of HIV in affected communities, as well as the intersectionality of structural forces responsible for vulnerability to HIV. But it also highlights the extent to which addressing these structural forces depended on a favorable political context capable of supporting and nurturing such approaches—and it emphasizes the ways in which key aspects of the Brazilian response to the epidemic have increasingly fragmented and disintegrated as the broader base of political support for a rights-based response to structural determinants of HIV and AIDS has been lost.

The reasons for these developments are neither simple nor one dimensional, and they cannot be fully analyzed in the space of a single chapter. But it is nonetheless crucially important to try to develop an interpretation of some of the causes for these changes, as they may offer important insights into the challenges of sustaining the AIDS response not only in Brazil but potentially in other countries as well.

One important factor in this regard has to do with the complex relationship between the state and civil society. Beginning in 2008, during the second term of President Lula (whose two terms ran 2003–2006 and 2007–2010), Brazil's emphasis on structural interventions and on community mobilization for key vulnerable populations—which depended heavily on nongovernmental civil society organizations as the key social

actors who would be responsible for mobilizing affected communities—
began to suffer from the effects of this prolonged period during which civil
society leaders had joined government institutions (at the federal, state,
and municipal levels), leading to a gradual loss of autonomy for NGOs.
This process included both voluntary participation on the part of NGOs
and deliberate cooptation of them by the government. Civil society thus
increasingly came to be seen as the executor of actions defined by public
policies, essentially supporting the government's initiatives rather than
helping to generate them. As a result, NGOs lost financing for activities
involving social control and for developing pilot demonstration projects,
both of which had been key aspects that had linked innovation to sustainability in earlier decades of the response to the epidemic in Brazil.

This process has combined with a second one: the emergence of
a more outspoken conservative critique of previous successful AIDS
policies, which are often created based primarily on moral objections.
These critiques have been led by strong social actors such as Brazil's Neo-
Pentecostal churches, which have established caucuses within congress,
drawing on their media power and ability to recruit individuals. These conservative players are also courted by the federal executive branch which,
following the logic of "coalitional presidentialism" that has marked Brazil's
republican life for some time now, can no longer count on a majority in
Congress.[55] The progressive agendas involved in the struggle against
AIDS and in human rights advocacy for different sexual orientations and
diverse genders have become currency of exchange in political deals made
in the name of "governability."

A third factor has been the gradual cooptation of key social movements,
essential to the response to AIDS, through the strategy of inclusion via
consumption rather than to citizenship. This has been the case of the
LGBT movement, for example. The international economic market provided an argument that negatively affected the budgets of AIDS programs
based on human rights. The result of these changes has been a resurgence
of increasing HIV infection in key populations and the demobilization of
the broader society in relation to the challenges.

The Brazilian experience offers important lessons about how, under
the right circumstances, structural interventions, community mobilization approaches, and empowerment of affected populations can combine to create a powerful positive, sustainable response to the AIDS
epidemic. Further, it teaches us a great deal about how much effective
responses to HIV depend upon larger macro-economic and political

processes, as well as cultural conditions that can either reinforce or undermine policies, interventions, and programs aimed at confronting the epidemic. The Brazil experience raises important concerns about the sustainability of the global response to the epidemic, as well as about the directions that this response has moved in recent years as a result of its increasing commitment to biomedical solutions (rather than social transformation) as the most effective approach to AIDS prevention and control.

References

1. Okie S. Fighting HIV—Lessons from Brazil. *The New England Journal of Medicine.* 2006;354:1977–1981.

2. Oliveira-Cruz V, Kowalski J, McPake B. The Brazilian HIV/AIDS "success story"— Can others do it? *Tropical Medicine & International Health.* 2004;9(2):292–297.

3. Seffner F. *Targets and Commitments Made by Member States at the United Nations General Assembly Special Session on HIV/AIDS UNGASS—HIV/AIDS Brazilian Response 2008, 2009 Country Progress Report.* 2010.

4. ABIA (Associação Brasileira Interdisciplinar de AIDS) Myth vs. Reality about the Brazilian Response to the AIDS epidemic in 2016. Accessed at: http://abiaids.org.br/wp-content/uploads/2016/07/Mito-vs-Realidade_HIV-e-AIDS_BRASIL2016.pdf (accessed on 31 January 2018).

5. Berkman A, Garcia J, Muñoz-Laboy M, Paiva V, Parker R. A critical analysis of the Brazilian response to HIV/AIDS: lessons learned for controlling and mitigating the epidemic in developing countries. *American Journal of Public Health.* 2005;95(7):1162–1172.

6. Parker R. *A Construção da Solidariedade: AIDS, Sexualidade, e Política no Brasil.* Rio de Janeiro: Editora Relume-Dumará; 1994.

7. Parker R, Passarrelli CA, Terto V, Pimenta C, Berkman A, Muñoz-Laboy M. The Brazilian response to HIV/AIDS: assessing its transferability. *Divulgação em Saúde para Debate.* August 2003.

8. Parker R. Building the foundations for the response to HIV/AIDS in Brazil: the development of HIV/AIDS policy, 1982–1996. *Divulgação em Saúde Para Debate.* 2003;27:143–183.

9. Galvão J. As respostas das organizações não-governamentais brasileiras frente à epidemia de HIV/AIDS. In: Parker R, ed. *Políticas, Instituições e AIDS: Enfrentando a Epidemia no Brasil.* Rio de Janeiro: ABIA; 1997:67–108.

10. Galvão J. AIDS e Activismo: o Surgimento e a Construção de Novas Formas de Solidariedade. In: Parker R, Bastos C, Galvão J, Stalin Pedrosa J, eds. *A AIDS No Brasil.* Rio de Janeiro: ABIA; 1994:341–350.

11. Parker R. Introdução. In: Parker R, ed. *Políticas, Instituições e AIDS: Enfrentando a Epidemia no Brasil.* Rio de Janeiro: ABIA; 1997:7–15.

12. Teixeira PR. Políticas públicas em AIDS. In: Parker R, ed. *Políticas, Instituições e AIDS: Enfrentando a Epidemia no Brasil.* Rio de Janeiro: ABIA; 1997:43–68.

13. Parker R. Introdução. In: Parker R, ed. *Políticas, Instituições e AIDS: Enfrentando a Epidemia no Brasil.* Rio de Janeiro: ABIA; 1997:7–15.

14. Parker R, Rochel de Camargo Jr K. Pobreza e HIV/AIDS: aspectos antropológicos e sociológicos. *Cadernos de Saúde Pública.* 2000;16(Supp. 1):89–102.

15. Parker R, ed. *Políticas, Instituições e AIDS: Enfrentando a Epidemia no Brasil.* Rio de Janeiro: ABIA; 1997.

16. National Coordination for STD and AIDS. *The Brazilian Response to HIV/AIDS.* Brasília: Ministry of Health; 2000.

17. Rich J, Garrison J. Brazil's virtuous alliance: how the grassroots and the government joined forces against AIDS. *Inter-American Foundation Grassroots Development Journal.* Available at:https://www.iaf.gov/resources/publications/grassroots-development-journal/2013-focus-the-iaf-s-investment-in-young-people/brazil-s-virtuous-alliance-how-the-grassroots-and-the-government-joined-forces-against-aids.

18. Ventura M. Strategies to promote and guarantee the rights of people living with HIV/AIDS. *Divulgação em Saúde Para Debate.* 2003;27:239–246.

19. Galvão J. *AIDS no Brasil.* São Paulo: Editora 34; 2000.

20. Zaluar AM. Exclusion and public policies: theoretical dilemmas and políticas alternatives. *Revista Basileira de Ciências Sociais.* 2000;1:25–42.

21. Zaluar AM. *Condomínio do Diabo.* São Paulo: Editora Brasiliense; 1996.

22. Fonseca C. Mãe é uma só?: Reflexões em torno de alguns casos brasileiros. *Psicologia USP.* 2002;13(2):49–68.

23. Daniel H, Parker R. *Sexuality, Politics and AIDS in Brazil: In Another World?* London: Falmer Press; 1993.

24. Parker R. *Na contramão da AIDS: sexualidade, intervenção, politica.* Rio de Janeiro: ABIA; 2000.

25. Parker R. *Bodies, Pleasures and Passions: Sexual Culture in Contemporary Brazil.* Boston: Beacon Press; 1991.

26. Paiva V. Beyond magic solutions: prevention of HIV and AIDS as a process of psychosocial emancipation. *Divulgação em Saúde Para Debate.* 2003;27:192–203.

27. Parker R, TertoJr V, eds. *Entre Homens: Homossexualidade e AIDS no Brasil.* Rio de Janeiro: ABIA; 1998.

28. Berquó E. *Comportamento Sexual da População Brasileira e Percepções do HIV/AIDS.* Brasília: Ministério da Saúde; 2000.

29. World Bank. Project Appraisal Document on a Proposed Loan in the Amount of US $165 Million; 1998. Report No. 18338-BR.

30. Agência de Notícias de AIDS. Estados Unidos cancelam grande programa de combate à AIDS no Brasil. Available at: www.agenciaaids.com.br.

31. Murray LR. *Not fooling around: The politics of sex worker activism in Brazil* (PhD dissertation). Sociomedical Sciences Department, Columbia University, New York; 2015.

32. Nunn A. *The politics and history of AIDS treatment in Brazil*. New York: Springer; 2009.

33. Rossi L. *Prevencao das DST/Aids e a prostitucao feminina no Brasil*. Brasília: Ministeiro de Saude: Coordenacao Nacional de DST e Aids; 1998.

34. Associacao Braseleira Interdiscipliner de AIDS and Davida. *Analysis of prostitution contexts in terms of human rights, work, culture, and health in Brazilian Cities*. Rio de Janeiro: ABIA; 2013. Available at: www.sxpolitics.org/ptbr/wp-content/uploads/.../analise_contexto_abia-davida.pdf.

35. Leite, G., Murray, L. R., & Lenz, F. (2015). The peer and non-peer: the potential of risk management for HIV prevention in contexts of prostitution. *Revista Brasileira de Epidemiologia*. 2015;15(Suppl 1):7–25. doi:10.1590/1809-4503201500050003

36. Nguyen VK, Bajos N, Dubois-Arber F, O'Malley J, Pirkle CM. Remedicalizing an epidemic: from HIV Treatment as Prevention to HIV treatment is prevention. *AIDS*. 2011;25(3):291–293.

37. Beyrer C, Gauri V, Vaillancourt D. *Evaluation of the World Bank's Assistance in Responding to the AIDS Epidemic: Brazil Case Study*. Washington, DC: World Bank; 2005.

38. Parker R, Quemmel R, Guimarães K, Mota M, Terto Jr V. AIDS prevention and gay community mobilization in Brazil, *Development*. 1995;2:49–53.

39. Parker RG, Veriano T. *Solidariedate: A ABIA na Virada do Milenio*. ABIA. Rio de Janeiro; 2001.

40. Faria A. Ciências Sociais Uninove, 4ª Parada Gay da cidade de São Paulo, Publicado em 6 de junho de 2017. Available at https://sociaisuninove.com.br/2017/06/06/4a-parada-gay-da-cidade-de-sao-paulo/

41. Mott L. Ministério da Saúde Divulga Resultado de Financiamento para Paradas GLBT, 21/4/2005, Centro de Mídia Independente. Available at: https://midiaindependente.org/pt/blue/2005/04/315188.shtml.

42. Éboli E. Governo Lula dá mais R$ 1 milhão para parada gay. *Por Brasil*, CMI Brasil, June 17, 2006. Available at: https://midiaindependente.org/pt/red/2006/06/356002.shtml.

43. A invenção da "homolesbotransfobia"—Seu dinheiro financia a Parada Gay. Cruz Glorioso. May 5, 2014. Available at: http://www.cruzgloriosa.com.br/Pagina/4407/A-invencao-da-homolesbotransfobia-Seu-dinheiro-financia-a-Parada-Gay.

44. GGB lamenta falta de patrocínio e editais para Parada Gay: "Qual problema de nos financiar?" Correio 24 Horas, February 23, 2015. Available at: http://www.correio24horas.com.br/noticias/categoria/salvador/.

45. Ministério da Saúde, por intermédio do Programa Nacional de DST e Aids. *Plano Nacional de Enfrentamento da Epidemia de Aids e DST entre Gays, outros Homens que fazem Sexo com Homens (HSH) e Travestis*. 2007. Available at: http://bvsms.saude.gov.br/bvs/publicacoes/plano_enfrentamento_epidemia_aids_hsh.pdf.

46. Associação Paranaense da Parada da Diversidade. *Guia de Advocacy e Prevenção em HIV/AIDS: Gays e outros Homens que fazem Sexo com Homens*. 2009. Available at: http://www.grupodignidade.org.br/wp-content/uploads/2015/11/guia-advocacy-aids.pdf.

47. Ministério da Saúde, Programa Nacional de DST e Aids. January 12, 2013. Available at: http://www.brasil.gov.br/saude/2013/11/brasil-e-lider-no-tratamento-a-pacientes-soropositivos.

48. Ministério da Saúde do Brasil, Secretaria de Vigilância em Saúde, Departamento de DST, Aids e Hepatites Virais, Líder De Opinião Popular LOP: Estratégia de Prevenção para as DST-HIV. Available at. http://bvsms.saude.gov.br/bvs/publicacoes/lider_opiniao_popular_prevencao_dst_hiv.pdf.

49. Ministério da Saúde divulga ação em aplicativo de relacionamento para prevenção à aids. UNA-SUS. Avaiable at: https://www.unasus.gov.br/noticia/ministerio-da-saude-divulga-acao-em-aplicativo-de-relacionamento-para-prevencao-aids 01/02/2015.

50. Lançada campanha para prevenção, teste e tratamento da Aids: No Dia Mundial de Luta contra a Aids, o Ministério da Saúde lançou uma campanha para prevenção, teste e tratamento da doença. Portal Brasil. Available at: http://www.brasil.gov.br/saude/2014/12/lancada-campanha-para-prevencao-teste-e-tratamento-da-aids. 02/12/2014.

51. Tratamento como prevenção apresenta primeiros resultados na epidemia da aids Available at: http://www.blog.saude.gov.br/index.php/570-perguntas-e-respostas/34812-tratamento-como-prevencao-apresenta-primeiros-resultados-na-epidemia-da-aids 01/12/2014

52. Ministério da Saúde divulga ação em aplicativo de relacionamento para prevenção à aids. UNA-SUS. Available at: https://www.unasus.gov.br/noticia/ministerio-da-saude-divulga-acao-em-aplicativo-de-relacionamento-para-prevencao-aids. 01/02/2015

53. McLoughlin B. Brazil gay rights progress highlights deep divisions. BBC News. June 25, 2011. Available at: http://www.bbc.com/news/world-latin-america-13890258

54. Carneiro JD. Brazil HIV/AIDS strategy needs new focus, campaigners say. BBC News. July 26, 2012. Available at: http://www.bbc.com/news/world-latin-america-18980108

55. Power TJ. Optimism, pessimism, and coalitional presidentialism: debating the institutional design of Brazilian democracy. *Bulletin of Latin American Research* 2010;29(1):18–33. Available at http://scholar.harvard.edu/files/levitsky/files/power_0.pdf.

12

Evaluating Structural Interventions

Bernadette Hensen, Stefanie Dringus, Robyn Eakle,
Michelle Remme, and James Hargreaves

Overview

In this book, a host of scholars have discussed structural factors affecting HIV risk and described interventions developed and implemented to address these factors. Evaluating structural interventions to understand whether they are effective, for whom, and in what context is critical. A comprehensive evaluation effort can support policymakers and programmers in deciding whether, where, and how to deliver structural interventions at scale. Such an effort will include three main components:

1. evaluation of the impact of structural interventions on their intended and unintended outcomes;
2. process evaluation to understand implementation of the intervention, pathways, and mechanisms through which an intervention creates change, and any contextual factors that influenced them; and
3. economic evaluation to assess their value for money.

In this chapter, we first describe methods for evaluating the impact of structural interventions using a number of key terms (Table 12.1). We describe key features of structural HIV prevention interventions and show that, despite these features, structural interventions are amenable to

Table 12.1 Definitions of Terms

Confounding	The "mixing" between the intervention, the outcome, and a third variable termed a confounder, that independently affects the risk of the outcome and is imbalanced across intervention and control groups in a CRT[2]
Coefficient of between cluster variation	A measure of the variation in the outcome between clusters, this measures a similar concept to the intra-cluster correlation coefficient[3]
Disability-adjusted life year (DALY)	One lost year of "healthy" life. The sum of DALYs across the population, or the burden of disease, is often considered a measurement of the gap between current health status and an ideal health situation where the population lives to an advanced age, without disease and disability[4]
Intracluster correlation coefficient	A measure of the correlation in the primary outcome between individuals in the same clusters, relative to individuals in another cluster (see coefficient of between cluster variation)[3]
Pair-matched randomization	In a pair-matched CRT, clusters are matched to another cluster with similar characteristics that are important risk factors for the outcome, for example, population size. Within the matched pair, one cluster is randomly allocated to the intervention
Opportunity cost	The benefits forgone or harm caused as a result of spending limited resources on one intervention and not on another
Power	The ability of a study to detect an intervention effect if one exists. Power is dependent on the sample size, the hypothesized size of the effect of the intervention that the study aims to detect, and how common the outcome is before the intervention is implemented
Quality-adjusted life year (QALY)	A measure of the state of health of a person or group in which the benefits, in terms of length of life, are adjusted to reflect the quality of life. One QALY is equal to 1 year of life in perfect health[5]
Restricted randomization	A method to constrain randomization of clusters. The number of possible allocations of clusters to intervention or control group is restricted to those that are balanced with regards to important risk factors for the outcome[3]
Sample size	The number of people included in a trial or study
Utility	An economic concept of the "satisfaction" an individual derives from the consumption of a good or a service

Note: CRT = cluster randomized trial.

evaluation using adaptation of the gold-standard randomized controlled trial (RCT) design. Where randomization is not feasible, alternative designs to evaluate effectiveness are proposed. Next, we provide guidance to those designing and conducting a process evaluation. We then describe economic evaluation methods for comparing the costs and consequences of alternative investments.

Throughout the chapter, we illustrate our approach to comprehensive evaluation through discussion of an applied example that included these three evaluation components: the Intervention with Microfinance for AIDS and Gender Equity (IMAGE) study (Box 12.1).[1] In addition to IMAGE, we draw on other evaluations as further examples of methods used to evaluate structural HIV prevention interventions.

BOX 12.1

Components of the IMAGE Study[1]

The IMAGE intervention targeted gender inequalities and IPV as structural drivers of HIV risk. The intervention included two main components, one focused on a microfinance initiative for poverty alleviation and the second on gender-based training and community mobilization to reduce IPV.

Poverty alleviation: The Small Enterprise Foundation implemented microfinance services, which were targeted exclusively at women and facilitated by one field worker in every village. The intervention included borrowing and repayment of loans over 10- or 20-week periods and eight group meetings every two weeks with 40 women per group. Loans were used for income-generating activities and were guaranteed by the groups of 40 women, who repaid loans together to be able to receive additional loans.

Gender and HIV training program: A team of trainers facilitated a program called *Sisters for Life*, which included two phases: In Phase 1, 10 sessions of structured training on gender roles, gender and HIV, and knowledge were delivered. In Phase 2, the focus was on community mobilization, including election of leaders from within each of the groups of women, training for these leaders, and the development of action plans responding to local priorities.

Key Features to Consider in Designing an Evaluation of a Structural Intervention

As described in Chapter 2, structural interventions are complex interventions that aim to change the physical, social, cultural, economic, legal, or policy environments that influence vulnerability to HIV infection. As such, structural interventions are usually allocated to groups of individuals or social organizations (termed "clusters"), as opposed to individuals themselves. Although allocated to clusters, the direct HIV prevention benefits may be targeted at specific subgroups of individuals within clusters (e.g., young women or older men).[6,7] The allocation of structural interventions to clusters raises key issues for the design of an impact evaluation, as it requires consideration of how to define the "cluster" that will receive the intervention, who the intended HIV prevention beneficiaries are, and how and among which target population to measure outcomes.[8]

By altering *macro-level structures*, structural interventions often involve multiple sectors, which contribute to the complexity of how structural interventions are implemented and operate.[9] For example, a structural intervention to reduce HIV among sex workers and their clients may involve a change to the legality of selling sex. Modelling studies suggest that decriminalization of sex work could have a large impact on HIV epidemics in concentrated and generalized epidemic settings.[10] Decriminalization of sex work would involve a number of stakeholders and alter numerous factors that influence HIV risk, including improved access to health services, reduced violence from partners and police, and greater control of how women sell sex.[11] By modifying distal structures that influence HIV risk, structural factors and interventions to address these affect HIV risk through long causal pathways.[12] This is in contrast with interventions traditionally termed behavioral in the HIV prevention literature that directly change an individual's behaviors through individual counseling or training on prevention, for example.[8,13] A theory of change that defines the intervention components and maps the expected causal pathways should be developed to guide a process evaluation in measuring how the intervention works, for whom, and any contextual factors that influence intervention implementation or outcomes.

Features of structural interventions also have important implications for design of the economic evaluation. For one, their costs and effects may also be dependent on context, and because most costs are derived from small-scale or pilot studies, there are concerns around their generalizability.[14]

Moreover, structural interventions that only operate at the community level may have uncertain scale-up pathways and would therefore be particularly challenging to model in terms of cost-effectiveness of optimal delivery and budget impact. In addition, the upstream and *multisectoral* nature of structural interventions means that they often have multiple effects that cut across (sub)sectors and payers.

The Cluster Randomized Trial for Evaluating the Effectiveness of Structural Interventions

In medicine, RCTs are the "gold-standard" design for evaluating the cause–effect relationship between an intervention and an outcome of interest.[2] In an RCT, individuals are prospectively randomized to receive either the intervention or the currently available best standard of care (control). After a predetermined time period, the outcomes of interest are compared between the two groups. If designed and conducted well, RCTs provide strong evidence of the probability of the causal relationship between intervention and outcome. This is because random allocation removes bias with regards to which individuals receive the intervention and which individuals receive control. By removing this bias, and where there are sufficient numbers of individuals randomized, randomization should ensure that intervention and control groups are comparable in observed and unobserved factors that could influence the primary outcome, termed *confounders*.

A modification of the RCT called the *cluster randomized trial* (CRT), in which clusters of individuals rather than individuals themselves are randomized to the intervention, are increasingly being used to evaluate complex public health interventions.[15] Like the RCT, a CRT design provides an estimate of the probability that any difference in the primary outcome between intervention and comparison groups is due to the intervention.[16] CRTs of complex public health interventions, such as structural HIV prevention interventions, implemented in real-world settings add complexities to conducting RCTs traditionally designed to evaluate the efficacy of medicines in highly controlled settings. Moreover, features of structural interventions mean randomization may not always be feasible, practical, or ethical—considerations which have, to date, limited the use of randomization in the evaluation of structural interventions.[13,17]

Critics of the CRT design for the evaluation of complex interventions argue that limitations inherent to the CRT, whose design is founded on methods of RCTs for drugs and vaccines, make them inappropriate.[18,19] A key criticism is that the CRT fails to account for, or even ignores, interactions between complex interventions and social environments.[20] As such, findings from a CRT are considered nongeneralizable across place and time; CRTs are considered too time-limited and focused on quantitative outcomes and thereby are unable to identify complex causal pathways, and contamination of the intervention, which occurs when the intervention components are inadvertently delivered in or spill-over to the control clusters to clusters not allocated the intervention, is considered inevitable as individuals are part of social networks lacking geographical boundaries inherent to a "cluster" in a CRT.[19]

Critics argue that measuring the impact of an intervention on a primary outcome simplifies the complexity of behavior change, and trying to control for confounding and minimizing contamination removes the social realities that influence how people behave and the very nature of what an intervention is aiming to modify.[19] Central to this *realist evaluation* is the notion that interventions interact with context; thus understanding how an intervention works requires observations of context-mechanism-outcome configurations within different settings.[18] Realists similarly argue that CRTs fail to recognize the critical role of social contexts and that use of comparison group removes the social realities that complex interventions are dependent on.[18,20] Further, realists also argue that CRTs are devoid of theory regarding how an intervention works and for whom.[18,20]

We argue that, where practical, feasible, and ethical, well-designed CRTs can provide rigorous evidence of intervention effectiveness while accounting for complex social dynamics within and across clusters. When a CRT is coupled with a clearly articulated theoretical framework of how and for whom the intervention is expected to work is bolstered by measures of implementation, the result is improved inquiry into the mechanisms of change and contextual factors that may affect implementation. This inquiry can be greatly improved through the inclusion of ongoing process evaluation). This allows for an evaluation that provides a strong and comprehensive evidence base. The use of randomization, rather than ignoring social realities that influence HIV risk and whether and how an interventions works, recognizes these as critical. As such, randomization seeks to balance these factors across groups that receive and do not receive the intervention to allow for a better understanding of whether the intervention works within these real-world settings.[20]

Key Design Features

Key features of a CRT design that require consideration when designing an impact evaluation include:

1. choosing and defining the cluster to be included in the trial;
2. determining the number of clusters required to be able to detect a difference in the primary outcome at the end of the trial;
3. randomization of clusters to intervention or comparison group; and
4. determining what primary and secondary outcomes to measure, among which population to measure these outcomes, and how to select this population.

Cluster Definition and Number of Clusters

Determining what the cluster is in a CRT will depend on where and how the intervention is being delivered. Examples of clusters targeted with structural interventions include geographical areas, such as villages or census enumeration areas, health facilities or schools, or networks of vulnerable populations including female sex workers (FSW), injecting drug users or men who have sex with men.[3] In IMAGE, the clusters included in the trial were villages (Box 12.2). A further example is the evaluation of the SASA! community mobilization intervention to reduce intimate partner violence (IPV) and HIV in Kampala, Uganda (Table 12.2).[21,22] In SASA!, the target population for the intervention consisted of entire communities within two larger administrative divisions of Kampala; trial clusters were defined as "sites" that were delineated based on population size, geographical area, socioeconomic characteristics, and accessibility to the offices of the organization delivering the intervention.[21] A CRT of a cash transfer program to keep girls in school in Zomba district, Malawi, randomized 176 enumeration areas within three strata: urban, rural close to, and rural far from Zomba city, to the cash transfer program or control (Table 12.2).[23]

In an RCT, the number of individuals required in the study, termed the *sample size*, needs to be large enough for the trial to have the *statistical power* to detect a difference in the primary outcome if one exists.[2] Power

The IMAGE Evaluation[1]

IMAGE was evaluated using a pair-matched cluster-randomized trial. The clusters included in the trial were existing villages in Limpopo province, South Africa. Eight villages were pair-matched on estimated size and accessibility. Within each pair, one village was blindly selected during an implementation team meeting. The IMAGE intervention was allocated to each randomly selected village within a pair.

Decisions to include eight villages in the trial were determined by:

1. The *feasibility* of implementing the intervention over large geographical areas;
2. The *time* required to recruit the target population into a cohort and follow up on this population;
3. *Ethical concerns* about withholding the intervention from the comparison group.

Primary outcomes of the trial were:

- experience of physical or sexual IPV in the past 12 months among loan recipients;
- unprotected sexual intercourse at last once in the past 12 months with a nonspousal partner among loan recipients, and among young people living in the households of loan recipients; and
- HIV incidence in the community as a whole.

The primary outcomes were measured among cohorts of women who applied for a loan in the intervention villages and cohorts of control women matched on village, age, and sex (cohort 1), cohorts of individuals aged 14 to 35 who resided in a household where someone applied for a loan or in the household of a matched woman in a control village (cohort 2), and cohorts of individuals aged 14 to 35 who were residents in randomly selected households in intervention and control villages (cohort 3). For cohorts 2 and 3, and cohort 1 in the control villages, populations to be followed up in the three cohorts were individuals residing in randomly selected households within the villages.

Table 12.2 Key Design Features of CRT of Structural HIV Prevention Interventions

| | Key Features of the CRT Design | | | |
Trial Name/ Description	Intervention under Evaluation	Number and Type of Clusters Included	Randomization	Primary Outcome Measurement	Population for Outcome Measurement
SASA[21]	Community mobilization to change norms, attitudes and behaviors that underlie power imbalances between men and women	Eight communities (four intervention, four control)	Pair-matched randomization	Acceptability of IPV; acceptability that a woman can refuse to have sex; past year experience of physical/sexual violence from a partner; appropriate response to women experiencing physical and/or sexual IPV in past year; past year concurrent sexual partners	Males and females aged 18–49 who lived in the village for ≥1 year

(continued)

Table 12.2 Continued

Key Features of the CRT Design

Trial Name/ Description	Intervention under Evaluation	Number and Type of Clusters Included	Randomization	Primary Outcome Measurement	Population for Outcome Measurement
The Zomba trial[23]	Cash transfers to females aged 13–22 to support them to stay in school, Zomba, Malawi	176 enumeration areas (defined by National Statistics Office of Malawi; 88 intervention, 88 control)	Randomization within geographical stratum (Zomba city, near rural, far rural areas); further randomization to conditional or unconditional cash transfer within the intervention group	HIV and HSV-2 prevalence at 18 months, collected by home-based voluntary testing and counseling	Never married females aged 13–22

Intervention	Description	Sample	Randomization	Outcome measure	Data collection
Samvedana Plus[26]	Multilevel intervention targeting FSW, their intimate partners, sex worker community-based organizations, and the general population. Interventions include workshops, counseling training, India	47 villages (24 intervention; 23 wait-list control, to receive intervention after trial completion)	Villages stratified by village population size and number of FSW and intimate partners, randomization within these strata	The % of FSW experiencing physical or sexual partner violence and the proportion who report consistent condom use in intimate relationship in the past six months	Surveys with FSW and their intimate partners
Community Mobilization to Change Gender Norms and Reduce HIV Risk[17]	Workshops to increase awareness about the relationship between gender inequities and HIV risk; community activities (including door-to-door visits, soccer events and theatre), South Africa	22 communities (11 intervention, 11 control)	Restricted on population size, average education, number of working residents, number of foreign residents, % temporary migrants and % female-headed household	Gender norms (as measured using Gender Equitable Men's Scale)	Baseline and endline population based survey with adults aged 18–35

(continued)

Table 12.2 Continued

	Key Features of the CRT Design			
Trial Name/ Description	Intervention under Evaluation	Number and Type of Clusters Included	Randomization	Primary Outcome Measurement	Population for Outcome Measurement
Samata[27]	Multicomponent intervention to reduce school drop-out, child marriage and entry into sex work among adolescent girls in Karnataka state, India	80 village clusters that included one "main" village with ≥high schools and neighboring villages with children who attended school in the "main" village (20 intervention; 20 wait-list control, to receive intervention after trial completion).	1:1 randomization	Four coprimary outcomes: % entering 8th standard; % completing standard 10; % married before age 15, and % experiencing first sex before age 15	Two sequential cohorts of low-caste girls who have completed standard 7th; cohorts recruited 1 year apart

Note: CRT = cluster randomized trial; IPV = intimate partner violence; HSV-2 = herpes simplex virus 2; FSW= female sex worker.

is dependent on the number of individuals in the study, how common the outcome is, and the hypothesized effect that the intervention will have on this outcome. In the absence of sufficient power, a trial may incorrectly conclude that an intervention is not effective. A trial is generally considered sufficiently powered if it has 80% power to detect a difference in the primary outcome.[24] This principle is true in a CRT. After determining how a cluster will be defined, a sample size calculation specific to CRTs is required to determine how many clusters are needed and how many individuals will be recruited to the study from within these clusters.[3] Sample-size calculations for CRTs need to take into account that individuals in a cluster are more likely to be similar to each other, including in the primary outcome, than they are to individuals from another cluster, known as *intracluster correlation* (ICC) or the coefficient of between cluster-variation (k).[25] This similarity between individuals in the same cluster is due to shared characteristics, for example socioeconomic status, or exposure to similar external factors within clusters, such as available clinical services.[24] Estimates of the ICC are generally not available for an outcome at a particular time and place, as such estimates of the ICC are made using data from previous studies to allow for an accurate sample size calculation. Samvedana Plus is a CRT of an intervention to reduce IPV and increase consistent condom use among FSW and their partners in Karnataka state, India.[26] An initial assessment of IPV found that the prevalence of IPV in the previous 12 months was 47%; using this estimate, different hypothesized levels of k, a narrow range of possible effect sizes of the intervention, and a 5% level of probability (p-value) that any observed effect would be due to chance, simulations were conducted to estimate the power of the study.[26] The simulations suggested that the trial would have 80% power to detect an 11% difference in IPV.[26]

Randomization Procedures

For randomization to reduce confounding, an adequate sample size is required. Reducing confounding in a CRT is more challenging compared to an RCT, as fewer clusters than individuals are generally available for randomization, particularly in trials where the clusters are large geographical areas. To make clusters more similar with regards to potential confounders, cluster randomization is restricted to being conducted within clusters that are matched on confounding factors or by randomizing the intervention within strata of factors likely to differ across clusters.[3] In a *matched CRT,* clusters are matched on characteristics considered important risk factors for the primary outcome and, within the matched paired, are randomized to intervention or control.[3] In the IMAGE trial (Box 12.1), villages were pair-matched on estimated size and accessibility.[1] Within each pair, one village was randomly selected to be allocated the intervention. In Samvedana Plus, the unit of randomization was villages, with 47 villages stratified by population size and the number of FSW with less than or more than 12 intimate partners, as measured during mapping and enumeration of FSW within the trial villages (Table 12.2).[26] Within these groups, the 47 villages were randomized to intervention or control.

A further approach to randomization is restricted randomization. In restricted randomization, all possible allocations of the intervention are initially explored. Subsequently, balance in measures considered likely to influence the primary outcome is examined across all possible allocations, and the number of allocations that are balanced across important characteristics are extracted.[3] In a CRT of a community mobilization intervention to change gender norms and thereby reduce HIV risk in South Africa, randomization was restricted by community characteristics reported in the 2011 Agincourt Health and Socio-Demographic Surveillance System, including population size, average education, number of employed residents and of foreign residents, and proportion of temporary migrants and of female-headed households (Table 12.2).[17] After applying restrictions, 50 allocations were randomly selected from the list of restricted allocations and one allocation randomly selected during a community meeting.

Alongside an adequate number of clusters to achieve statistical power, physical distance between clusters should be considered to minimize contamination. For example, contamination of comparison clusters might occur in a CRT examining community mobilization among FSWs if communities are contiguous and FSW are socially networked and highly mobile across intervention and control clusters. In *Samata*, a *multicomponent intervention* to reduce school drop-out, child marriage, and entry into sex work among adolescent girls in Karnataka state, India, components of the intervention involved schools and school staff, village clusters (defined as a "main" village with one or more high schools and neighboring villages; Table 12.2), rather than schools were randomized to the intervention to minimize contamination across schools within the same village.[27] After randomization, the study team concluded that there was risk of contamination as some village clusters were in close proximity to a village cluster in another study arm.[27] Contamination can affect power of the study to detect a difference in the outcome by making the clusters more alike to each other in the outcome. To increase study power, additional village clusters were randomly allocated to intervention or control.[27]

Defining Target Populations and Outcomes

Designing an impact evaluation includes defining the outcomes that the intervention is expected to change, measurement of these outcomes among a well-defined target population, and identification and selection of a sample of individuals from this population among whom to measure the outcomes. Structural interventions for HIV prevention aim to reduce new HIV infections by altering the environment within which HIV risks occur.[9] In IMAGE, HIV incidence was measured among randomly selected cohorts of males and females aged 14 to 35 years old in intervention and control villages (Box 12.2).[1] Measuring incident HIV infections is, however, challenging as new HIV infections are relatively rare and the timing of infection is difficult to pinpoint. Measuring HIV incidence therefore requires a large sample of individuals. In addition to sample size, time is required for a structural intervention to have an impact on HIV risk-related behaviors and thereby reduce new HIV infections.

Financial and logistical constraints limit the feasibility of including a large sample size over a long period of time; therefore, few CRTs of structural interventions have included HIV incidence as the primary outcome.[13] As an alternative, evaluations include intermediary outcomes, including self-reported sexual behaviors or HIV prevention–related knowledge, to determine whether an intervention was effective. Self-reported outcomes and measures of knowledge have numerous limitations. More robust primary outcomes as proxies for the potential cause–effect relationship between an intervention and HIV are other biological outcomes, including HIV prevalence (particularly among younger populations more likely to have been recently infected) and rates other sexually transmitted infections herpes simplex virus 2, as measured in the Zomba trial.[23]

Although structural interventions are targeted at clusters, the impact on HIV and related outcomes may be expected among a specific subpopulation within the clusters. For example, the implementation of an intervention targeting young women would be expected to have indirect effects on their male sexual partners. Once the target population for the evaluation has been defined, decisions need to be made on how to recruit a representative sample of this population and whether to follow up the same individuals over time (cohort) or conduct two independent surveys (cross-sections) before implementation of the intervention (baseline) and at the end of the study period. In IMAGE, three cohorts were followed up to measure the different outcomes of interest (Box 12.3). The primary outcome, experience of IPV, was measured among a cohort of women who applied for a loan, as the intervention was expected to reduce vulnerability to IPV among these women. In the pair-matched comparison villages, a household database was used to randomly select households that would have been eligible to apply for a loan had the intervention been available in the village. Eligible households were randomly selected until a household with an age- and sex-matched individual was identified. In SASA!, two independent surveys were conducted among a random sample of community members, one prior to intervention implementation and one 2.8 years after SASA! programming.[21,22]

Whether to recruit cohorts or conduct independent cross-sectional surveys requires consideration of the mobility of the population under study, the period of follow-up, and the target population for intervention delivery. In IMAGE, villages were randomized to the intervention but individual women were eligible to apply for a loan. If IMAGE had opted to conduct two *cross-sectional surveys* among randomly selected women, the study may have recruited a small sample of women who applied for a loan, such that few women would have been "exposed" to the intervention. The trial would likely have been underpowered to detect the effect on IPV. Conversely, in a CRT of community mobilization to change gender norms and reduce HIV risk in South Africa (Table 12.2), the target population for the intervention was men and women aged 18 to 35 although all adults were welcome to mobilization activities.[17] The CRT is estimating impact using two independent cross-sectional surveys with males and females aged 18 to 35 due to the high level of in- and out-migration in the trial communities.[17] Had the trial opted to recruit cohorts of men and women, the study may have failed to follow up all individuals initially recruited into the cohorts at the end of the two-year study period. If the individuals who could no longer be followed up were more (or less) likely to have the HIV outcomes, the individuals remaining in the study would not be representative of the wider population and the study would be biased. In SASA!, repeated cross-sectional surveys were conducted as the study aimed to measure community, rather than individual, level impact and, as the communities were high mobility settings, there were concerns that a cohort would be subject to selection bias from high levels of attrition.[21]

The IMAGE Process Evaluation[57]

Process evaluation aim: The mixed-methods process evaluation conducted of IMAGE was guided by a conceptual framework and explored the *feasibility* of delivering the intervention as planned, and how *accessible* and *acceptable* it was to its intended beneficiaries. The process evaluation intended to complement the impact evaluation by unpacking trial results and informing subsequent scale-up.

Focus of process evaluation: Delivery, uptake, and interaction with intervention components.

Timing of data collection: Process data was collected both during the trial (prospectively by exploring accessibility of the intervention, and implementers' and participants' perspectives on the intervention) and during scale-up (retrospective trial data and prospective scale-up data from several stakeholders).

Data sources and collection methods:

1. *Attendance registers:* Used during the trial to evaluate recruitment, dropout, and attendance of the intervention;
2. *Participant observations and diaries:* Used during trial to explore intervention feasibility and acceptability;
3. *Structured questionnaires:* Used during the trial to provide quantitative data on acceptability by evaluating participation and satisfaction;
4. *Focus group discussions and interviews with clients, drop-outs, managers, and field staff:* Used during trial and during scale-up to explore intervention feasibility and acceptability.

Key findings of the process evaluation were:

1. Microfinance and gender/HIV training were feasible to deliver during the time frame of the trial;
2. Both components were accessible and acceptable to most clients;
3. Participation in community mobilization was high for some clients, but others experienced barriers, and this may explain lack of intervention effect among some beneficiaries;
4. While the delivery was feasible in the short term, it was not considered sustainable for the long term.

Feasibility, Ethics, and Applicability

Where an adequate number of clusters are available, evaluation using a CRT design may, nonetheless, not be feasible, ethical, or applicable.[2,8] Feasibility may be an issue if randomization is considered unacceptable by individuals within the cluster or representatives of the cluster. In an RCT, individuals are asked for verbal or written informed consent to be randomized as part of the informed consent process.[28] In a CRT, obtaining informed consent from all members of a cluster prior to random allocation of the cluster is usually not possible. *Cluster representatives* are therefore asked for consent on behalf of cluster members for the cluster to participate in the randomization process. Within clusters, individuals who are randomly selected to be part of the evaluation of the intervention are asked for informed consent to participate in data collection processes. For example, in the CRT of community mobilization to change gender norms and reduce HIV risk in South Africa, community representatives and leaders agreed to participate in the study and participated in the randomization.[17] Within the 22 community clusters, individuals aged 18 to 35 were randomly selected and asked for informed consent to complete a survey.[17]

The feasibility of a CRT may be limited for logistical reasons. For example, if the intervention was implemented prior to designing the evaluation. Cost may also preclude the use of the CRT design, as randomization of an adequate number of clusters and implementation in each cluster simultaneously is costly. The feasibility of a CRT may be limited if stakeholders/participants do not adhere to allocation following randomization. This could happen either because they are not committed to implementing the intervention (if in the control cluster) or they are in a control cluster but perceive the intervention to be of value and therefore implement a similar programme in the cluster.

The use of the CRT design may be opposed for ethical reasons. In clinical trials, scientists adhere to principles of *clinical equipoise*, which allows experimentation involving humans only if there is clear uncertainty about the potential benefits, yet all available information indicates that there are no expected risks.[29] Or, if there are risks, then they are not life threatening and the potential benefits can be shown to far outweigh the risks. This principle is central to experimentation of structural interventions as well and includes ensuring that no standard of care is withheld from individuals. For structural interventions, which target distal determinants of health, the situation is more complicated because it is more difficult to anticipate all risks. Additionally, although the HIV prevention benefits of a structural intervention may not be known, its effects on other, non-health-related outcomes, may already be established. Where this is the case, it may be deemed unethical to randomly allocate the intervention.

Where randomization is feasible and ethical, a CRT may nonetheless not be necessary if the evidence arising from a trial is not considered pertinent to policymakers and programmers.[8] Decision-makers may not see the added value of evidence arising from a CRT depending on the evidence they require for decision-making. As such, evidence arising from *nonrandomized studies*, which are often less costly and less likely to raise complicated questions about ethics, may suffice for policymakers and programmers.

In summary, CRTs are the most credible study design for evaluating whether a structural intervention has a causal effect on HIV and related outcomes. The availability of an adequate number of clusters that are sufficiently spaced to minimize contamination can be difficult and costly, and encouraging stakeholders to participate in randomized allocation and adhering to this randomization, of an intervention can prove challenging. Where these challenges have been addressed, deciding whether to use a CRT design requires consideration of ethics and the applicability of the evidence arising from a CRT in light of the availability of alternate, rigorous quasi-experimental methods for evaluation.

Alternative Impact Evaluation Designs

To date, few structural HIV prevention interventions have been evaluated using a CRT design.[13] Limited use of the CRT design may be for reasons of feasibility, costs, or ethics, as described earlier, because the intervention has already been implemented, or because alternative designs are considered equally rigorous in providing evidence of the possible effect of the intervention on HIV.[16]

Numerous nonrandomized evaluation designs have been described in the literature,[30] ranging from weak designs with no comparison group, including the before-after study, to more rigorous designs that include measure(s) of the primary outcome taken before intervention implementation and a prospective comparison group. Nonrandomized designs use differences over time, place, or a combination of time and place to compare outcomes and assess whether any difference can be attributable to the intervention.[31,32] The main limitation of nonrandomized studies is confounding. Allocation of an intervention to the intervention group is not randomized but determined by other factors, for example disease burden. In nonrandomized designs that include a comparison group, the comparison group is selected by evaluators and this group is unlikely to be similar to the intervention in all potential confounding factors. Minimizing confounding requires measures of the outcome before the intervention was implemented to determine comparability of the intervention and control groups and for adjustment of any confounding factors at the analysis stage of an evaluation.

The Stepped-Wedge CRT

The *stepped-wedge CRT* is an alternative study design when a CRT is considered impractical due to the costs and logistics of implementing the intervention simultaneously in a number of clusters or where randomized allocation of the intervention to half the study clusters is unacceptable to cluster representatives.[33] In this design, all clusters receive the intervention but in phases, with the order in which clusters will receive the intervention determined randomly.[33] Confounding by changes over time in the outcome needs to be considered because data during the intervention period are collected at different time-points. In theory, outcomes can be compared over time (*"horizontal" comparison*), using measures of the outcome before and after the intervention was delivered in each cluster, or compared across places within the same timeframe (*"vertical" comparison*).[34] In practice, most analysis strategies for stepped-wedge CRTs include information from both horizontal and vertical comparisons.[35]

The Cambodia Integrated HIV and Drug Prevention Implementation study is a multicomponent intervention, which includes conditional cash transfers, to reduce HIV risk among FSW in Cambodia (Table 12.3).[36] The stepped-wedge design was used for ease of implementation by the core study team across 10 provinces (the study clusters), with ethical reasons also cited. As individual intervention components had known efficacy, phased implementation would allow everyone to receive the intervention within a framework of rigorous evaluation. The study will compare outcomes over the period before the intervention was implemented to outcomes after intervention implementation, including an assessment of short term impact at six months.[37]

Interrupted Time Series

A design that can be used where randomization is not feasible or ethical, or where the intervention has already been implemented is the *interrupted time series* (ITS). In the ITS design, changes in the outcome are compared over time. Multiple measures of the outcome taken among the population before intervention implementation are compared to measures taken after the date of intervention implementation. Measures of the outcome are taken among the same population at repeated time points, generally at equal intervals. This design assumes that the preintervention time trend in the outcome can be modeled from the data and, from this, that predictions can be made about what would happen in the future in the absence of the intervention.[38] The predicted trend in the outcome is then compared to measured postintervention trends to determine whether the intervention modified the trend observed before the intervention was implemented. A minimum of three to four preintervention time points is considered a requirement for establishing reliable and robust information about the preintervention trends: in practice, many more are often needed.[37]

For the ITS to provide robust evidence of impact, the intervention must be implemented at a well-defined time point, and there needs to be certainty that no other, related intervention was implemented at the same time point. Further, the design requires that there is no time lag between intervention implementation and changes in the outcome, or that the length of any lag is well understood. In considering whether to adopt the ITS design to evaluate the impact of a structural intervention, there must be reliable data on preintervention trends with the same data available after intervention implementation. Ruiz et al. used the ITS design to estimate the impact of a change in needle and syringe exchange programming policy in Washington, D.C (Table 12.3).[38] The authors found that a 2007 lift on a funding ban for needle and syringe exchange programming averted almost 300 new HIV infections. To estimate this impact, the authors used monthly observations of reported HIV cases between August 1996 and December 2011 that were attributed to injecting drug use (IDU), or IDU and/or among men who have sex with men. The policy change occurred in December 2007; however, as the policy change was only implemented in March 2008, the authors used the date of policy implementation as the date of "interruption" in time.

Table 12.3 Key Features of Nonrandomized Evaluations of Structural HIV Prevention Interventions

Study Name/Description	Intervention under Evaluation	Number and Type of Clusters Included	Evaluation Design	Primary Outcome(s)	Population for Outcome Measurement
Cambodia Integrated HIV and Drug Prevention Implementation Study[36]	12-week conditional cash transfer combined with four weeks of cognitive-behavioral group aftercare for FESW who use amphetamine-type stimulants, Cambodia	10 provinces included as the clusters	Stepped-wedge cluster randomized trial	Prostate-specific antigen test results (positive vs. negative); self-reported consistent condom use paying/nonpaying partners in past three months; self-reported number; and type of sex partners in past three months	Biologically female FESW aged ≥18 who report ≥2 different sex partners and/or transactional sex in the past month
Evaluation of a policy intervention on funding for syringe exchange programs[39]	Change in policy regarding funding for needle syringe exchange programs in Washington, DC	One city (Washington, DC)	Interrupted time series	Injecting drug use-associated cases of HIV	Data obtained from the Department of Health's HIV/AIDS, Hepatitis, Sexually Transmitted Diseases, & Tuberculosis Administration

SAGE4Health Study[40]	Community-based multilevel economic and food security program (Support to Able-Bodied Vulnerable Groups to Achieve Food Security), in Malawi; includes savings and loans groups and improved farming practices	Six traditional authority areas of rural central Malawi: three selected by CARE to receive SAFE and three receiving unrelated CARE programming (controls).	Nonequivalent-control group design	Uptake of HIV testing services, self-reported HIV infection, and perceived risk of infection	Individuals participating in the intervention and individuals matched on demographics and distance to urban center in control areas

Note. FESW = female entertainment and sex workers.

Nonequivalent Comparison Group

The *nonequivalent comparison group* study combines a comparison group with pre- and postintervention outcome measures.[30] Preintervention measures are used to determine whether the two groups are similar before intervention implementation, and postintervention outcomes are compared at the end of intervention period between the clusters that received the intervention and the comparison clusters. For this design to provide rigorous evidence of an intervention effect, the preintervention measures of the outcomes should be similar to those in the intervention group. Further, the selected comparison group should be similar to the intervention group in observable confounders. The latter is challenging, as it requires that the evaluator knows and measures all potential confounders. Further, in the absence of any intervention, the outcome should be expected to be similar in both groups at the end of the period of observation. As with the ITS design, the implementation of other interventions that may confound any observed effect need to be known to allow for adjustment of confounding effects.

An example is the SAGE4Health Study in rural Malawi (Table 12.3), which evaluated the impact of a community-based, multilevel economic and food security intervention on HIV vulnerability.[39] The study includes three traditional authority areas in central Malawi that received the SAGE4Health intervention and three areas that did not receive the intervention but received other, unrelated programming from the organization implementing SAGE4Health. To estimate the effect of the intervention, two cohorts are being followed over a 36-month period. In intervention sites, the cohort includes individuals participating in the intervention; in control areas, individuals matched on demographics and distance to an urban center were recruited.[39]

A specific analytic approach in this study is a *difference-in-difference analysis*. In this analytic approach, pre- and postintervention measures of the outcome must be measured in the same way. The differences in the outcomes before and after intervention implementation are measured in each group, and these differences are also compared between the two groups. Effectively, if there is a greater difference in the outcomes in the intervention group compared to the difference in the outcomes observed in the control group and potential biases and confounders are assessed as minimal, then it is plausible that the difference is attributable to the intervention.

Use of Process Evaluation to Evaluate Structural HIV Prevention Interventions

Structural interventions are often "complex interventions" as they involve numerous organizational levels and stakeholders and multiple interacting components and are highly influenced by contextual factors. These features challenge implementation and complicate the causal pathways through which structural interventions operate. Outcome data, often in the form of effect sizes, are important for establishing the effectiveness of structural interventions; however, these data alone are unable to explain how or why an intervention worked (or did not).[40]

Process evaluation plays an essential role in evaluating complex structural interventions and should be conducted alongside impact and economic evaluations of such interventions. Doing so adds understanding and depth to outcome data, including understanding why and how an intervention worked or did not, and provides valuable information to a range of stakeholders including policymakers, implementers, and evaluators and informs the extent to which findings are likely to be reproducible in other settings.[8] Process data accomplishes this by describing the broader social processes in which the intervention being studied occurs and the layers of interacting situations and circumstances that either lead to an effect or lack thereof.[41,42] Further, process evaluations can help distinguish between interventions that are based on flawed theory or are poorly designed versus those that are poorly or incompletely implemented.[43] Process evaluation has a particularly important role where the same intervention is being delivered at multiple sites and by numerous implementers,[41,42] which is often the case for structural interventions.

Several theories and frameworks for process evaluation, many of which are particularly relevant to the evaluation of structural interventions, are described in the literature.[18,20,44-49]

The recent UK Medical Research Council (MRC) guidance has drawn upon and consolidated these numerous approaches in an effort to provide extensive practical guidance on planning and operationalizing process evaluations of complex public health interventions.[50,51] It includes a framework that describes three key domains of process evaluation: studying implementation, mechanisms of impact, and context. These aspects can be incorporated in the design and operationalizing of process evaluations to support informing the interpretation of outcomes and providing practical information to stakeholders. These functions are not unique to the evaluation of structural interventions, in particular, but are critical components toward a comprehensive evaluation of structural interventions for HIV prevention.

Implementation: What Is Implemented and How

Process evaluation is necessary to assess *intervention fidelity*: if intervention delivery differed from what was planned, and how and why it may have varied, in order to understand impact evaluation outcomes. For example, variation in intervention delivery may occur across geographical areas or between implementers, and may be influenced by a range of contextual factors.[52] An intervention may have limited effects either because of weakness in its design or implementation.[48] Conversely, positive effects can sometimes be achieved even in the absence of an intervention being delivered with complete fidelity.[53] Being able to understand outcome data in light of implementation is important, particularly as structural interventions are likely to show variability in local implementation.[54] Within the domain of implementation, process evaluations aim to assess fidelity of implementation (whether the intervention and any facilitator training was delivered as intended), the quantity (dose) of intervention implemented, any adaptations that were made, and whether the intended beneficiaries were "contacted" by the intervention and how (reach).[50]

Mechanisms of Impact: How the Delivered Intervention Works to Produce Change

Although the primary aim of *impact evaluations* is to estimate the size of the effect of an intervention, evaluations of structural interventions should also investigate the complex, multiple, and extensive causal pathways through which structural interventions modify HIV risk and reduce HIV.[8] Exploring the mechanisms through which interventions are hypothesized to bring about change is important for understanding how the intervention produced the observed effect and how these effects might be replicated in other settings by similar interventions.[47] Mechanisms of impact may be assessed through quantitative or qualitative methods. Quantitative measures of satisfaction or acceptability can be collected, but data collection of this process domain most often focuses on exploring participant and facilitator responses to, and interactions with, the intervention as well as illuminating any unexpected pathways or unintended consequences. In the IMAGE process evaluation (Box 12.3), focus group discussions and interviews with clients, clients lost to follow-up, managers, and field staff were conducted during the trial and scaled up to explore intervention feasibility and acceptability.

How Does Context Affect Implementation and Outcomes?

Context can be defined as the conditions within which everyday lives are lived including "the social, cultural, economic, educational, and occupational as well as the physical and mental environment."[55] Structural interventions often work by interacting with, and altering the context within which, health is produced or reproduced.[8,9] It is important, therefore, that evaluations not only aim to understand this context, and how it varies across time and place, but also document how the intervention interacts with and affects or is affected by context. Understanding context is essential in interpreting the findings of a specific evaluation and generalizing beyond it.[50]

Planning, Designing, and Conducting a Process Evaluation

There are several steps to planning and operationalizing a process evaluation. It is important to note, however, that since complex interventions and the environments in which they operate are so diverse, there is no "one-size fits all" checklist that can be applied across process evaluations. Rather, we can provide some guidance that should be used to help think through some of the key considerations and inform decisions.[50] Further, although evaluations should aim to incorporate process evaluations from the outset, and as a component of the overall study design, process evaluations are often not linear and require a flexible and iterative approach.

Ahead of designing specific aspects of the process evaluation, several overarching considerations should be considered, and the general approach to the process evaluation decided in a transparent manner. This includes, but is not limited to the relationship between the process evaluation and intervention developers and implementers, as well as among the process evaluation and broader impact and economic evaluation study teams, resources available for data collection, and the timing of process evaluation.

Considerations for Planning

Achieving a productive and balanced relationship with stakeholders responsible for the development and implementation of the intervention is particularly important in process evaluations, where having a thorough understanding of how an intervention is intended to produce change and having access to intervention activities to observe its implementation is crucial. Achieving this relationship may be challenging, particularly where process evaluation may be viewed as threatening to individuals or an organization which has been closely involved in the intervention development or have an interest in showing its effectiveness. Further, the way in which findings emerging from the process evaluation will be communicated to stakeholders *during* the evaluation (if at all) should be agreed upon ahead of time. Maintaining good relationships with stakeholders, while remaining sufficiently independent, as not to introduce bias data collection or analysis, is an important consideration.

Similarly, relationships within evaluation teams, and the degree to which the process evaluation will be integrated with the impact and economic evaluation components, needs to be discussed. Process evaluations, which are usually conducted by a team separate to the impact and economic evaluation team, may be highly integrated into the overall study or kept relatively separate. They may also be conducted retrospectively (although not always ideal), due to practical or logistical constraints.

A further consideration in the overall design of the process evaluation is whether process data will be collected by those designing and/or implementing the intervention, by staff hired specifically to conduct the process evaluation, or by a combination of both. Although having intervention staff members also serve as data collectors can be a cost-effective method for gathering data, there is the potential of bias in the overlap of implementation and evaluation roles. As process evaluations usually draw on both routine intervention data, as well as data collected specifically for the evaluation, a compromise of having intervention staff collect routine monitoring and evaluation data, while evaluation staff collect process data can be a feasible approach.

Considerations for Design and Conduct

The first step in designing a process evaluation (including defining research questions and choosing appropriate methods and corresponding indicators) is developing a detailed description of the intervention through a logic model or theory of change, and in which causal assumptions underpinning the workings of the intervention are clarified. Defining the components of the intervention, and understanding how it is intended to produce change, will help guide which *domains of process evaluation* (implementation, mechanisms of impact, and context) require investigation and how evaluation resources should best be allocated. At this stage, it is also helpful to refer to the literature and review the aims and methods of process evaluations of similar interventions to help inform decisions about core research questions.

Once a comprehensive description of the intervention and its causal assumptions has been described and agreed with intervention staff, attention turns to defining research questions related to implementation, mechanisms of impact and contextual factors, and choosing corresponding methods for data collection. Research questions should emerge from examining the assumptions behind the intervention, from drawing on the empirical literature, and be framed in alignment with the areas of investigation described within each of the three process evaluation domains presented in the MRC framework. The nature of process evaluations often means that evaluators are faced with deciding from a wide range of important research questions and must make decisions regarding the depth and breadth of questions that the process evaluation will aim to answer. Because of the range of questions that a process evaluation can investigate, evaluators need to be cautious and plan carefully the amount of data to be collected; this is important to ensure that there is the capacity for analysis, and to avoid data collection burden on participants or influencing the intervention. Decisions regarding research questions can also be guided by discussions with the wider evaluation team and stakeholders who will be using findings generated by the process evaluation. Although process evaluations typically collect the majority of data from intervention clusters, it is advisable to consider collecting limited data from the control clusters to understand if any intervention spillover has occurred, if other similar interventions have been implemented, or if there may be factors previously unaccounted for which could affect the ability of the study to detect an effect in relation to the outcome.

Process evaluations draw on a range of both quantitative and qualitative methods and often apply a mixed methods approach. In IMAGE, data were collected through focus group discussions, attendance registers and through the questionnaire used as part of the impact evaluation.[56] Further, process evaluations can use a combination of intervention data routinely collected by implementers, together with data collected specifically for the process evaluation itself. It is useful to note that one method may be used to generate data toward answering more than one research question, while research questions may draw upon data from more than one method. Examples of these methods can include: surveys, reviews of routine data collected, in-depth interviews, focus group discussions, and structured or unstructured observations; however, details of each data collection methods is beyond the scope of this chapter.

Economic Evaluation Methods

Sound decisions in resource allocation require reliable evidence on the consequences of alternative investments. When decision-makers or funders determine how to spend their scarce resources, they need to know the costs, outcomes, and opportunity costs of their intervention options. Economic evaluation is a set of tools used to compare the costs and consequences of alternative investments, to inform a specific decision problem. In public health, economic evaluation is often used interchangeably with the term cost-effectiveness analysis (CEA), although strictly speaking, CEA is only one type of economic evaluation.

It is important to note that cost-effectiveness, or value for money, is a relative concept, not an absolute. An intervention is cost-effective compared to the next best use of available resources. This relates to the fundamental economic concept of *opportunity cost* whereby the value of an investment is measured by the foregone benefits of its alternative use. Stated differently, the opportunity cost to a funder that decides to invest in a structural intervention is the greatest benefit that could have been achieved by redeploying the invested resources.

Types of Economic Evaluation

There are four types of economic evaluation techniques, each responding to specific objectives, valuing different outcomes, and of relevance to different decision-makers (Table 12.4).[57,58] CEA considers "natural units" of

Table 12.4 Economic Evaluation Methods, Decision Rules, and Implications
for Structural Interventions

Method	Outcome Unit	Implications for Structural Interventions and Relevant Decision-Makers	Decision Rule to Guide How or to Which Intervention(s) to Allocate Resources
Cost-effectiveness analysis	Natural unit (e.g., HIV infection averted or AIDS death averted)	Considers variations in effectiveness between interventions But single outcome analysis impedes the incorporation of multiple outcomes within HIV (treatment and prevention interventions cannot be compared) and beyond HIV → *Relevant for an HIV payer (e.g., HIV program manager)*	Intervention with the lowest CER Rank interventions from lowest to highest CER in a league table and allocate fixed budget starting from the lowest CER until the budget is spent
Cost-utility analysis	Disability-adjusted life year, quality-adjusted life year	Allows for HIV-wide and health-sector-wide comparisons But single health outcome precludes the consideration of non-health outcomes → *Relevant for a health payer (e.g., Ministry of Health)*	Intervention(s) with the lowest CERs in league tables (see above) Interventions with CERs below the cost-effectiveness threshold
Cost-benefit analysis	Monetized outcome	Benefits from all sectors (e.g., health, education, agriculture) can be accounted for and monetized → *Relevant for a supra-ministerial payer (e.g., Ministry of Finance)*	Every intervention option where Benefits > Costs (or Benefit-Cost Ratio>1) In a ranking, interventions with the largest net benefit should be prioritized

(continued)

Table 12.4   Continued

Method	Outcome Unit	Implications for Structural Interventions and Relevant Decision-Makers	Decision Rule to Guide How or to Which Intervention(s) to Allocate Resources
Cost-consequence analysis	Multiple natural units	Used to present multiple outcomes, where CBA is not feasible Does not combine measures of benefit into a single measure so cannot be used to rank	No rule

Note. CER = cost-effectiveness ratio; CBA = cost-benefit analysis.

outcome, such as HIV infections averted, while *cost-utility analysis* (CUA) uses a summary health measure, such as the *disability-adjusted life year* (DALY) averted or the *quality-adjusted life year* (QALY) gained. Both measures combine dimensions of quantity and quality of life but have different theoretical underpinnings.[59] CEA and CUA are often used interchangeably. *Cost-benefit analysis* (CBA) is distinct in that it compares costs and benefits in the same monetary metric. In a *cost-consequence analysis* (CCA), multiple outcomes are presented in natural units and are not combined with costs. This method provides the most flexibility in what information is factored into decision-making but does not offer any decision rule or possibility to rank interventions, based on an objective measure of efficiency. The usefulness of each method depends on the decision-maker's specific problem and the social value judgements that prevail in each setting or sector. For example, the health sector is predominantly geared towards CEA/CUA, whereas the environmental sector typically uses CBA.[60]

Designing an Economic Evaluation for a Structural Intervention

Certain features of structural interventions have implications for their economic evaluation, including context-dependent consequences, and their upstream and multisectoral nature. Given the indivisibility of interventions, it is not possible to fund a discrete part of a structural intervention with multi-sectoral outcomes, just to yield the HIV-specific benefit.[61,62] The repercussion when assessing value for money is that the analysis will end up comparing the full intervention costs to its HIV-specific consequences alone, thereby undervaluing it. For example, extending access to secondary schooling may appear prohibitively expensive when comparing its costs to its HIV prevention impact, despite its large educational benefits.[63] Indeed, economic evaluation in health tends to focus on single health outcomes, but interventions with multiple outcomes of interest to multiple decision-makers require a different decision frame.

Numerous *design elements* are to be considered when defining the decision problem that the economic evaluation seeks to inform. First, the decision-maker(s) and their budget constraint(s) need to be identified, including which payer(s) has an interest in the expected outcome(s) of the intervention, and what budget(s) they are optimizing. Second, the *comparator* that the intervention is to be assessed against must be defined and should reflect the alternative use of resources that the decision-maker faces. It would typically be the same as the comparator in the impact evaluation. Third, the scope and perspective of the analysis needs to be aligned with the decision problem. If it concerns the best use of a health provider's budget, then a healthcare provider perspective should be taken. If the decision relates to the societal value of the intervention, a societal perspective should be adopted that considers client/patient costs, healthcare provider costs, and non-health sector costs and effects.[64,65]

The decision frame will clearly depend on the type of structural intervention under consideration. Structural interventions that are designed to prevent HIV are more likely to be funded from an HIV or health budget. Their single outcome and single-payer characteristics make them suitable for a CEA or CUA. Another set of structural interventions have multiple objectives beyond HIV and health, are typically funded by non-health budgets, and require approaches that can factor in multiple outcomes, such as CBA. However, this would only be appropriate if the funding decision is being made by a payer with multiple objectives, or a single objective with multiple components, such as social welfare or well-being. In the case where various funders or government sectors with single objectives are deciding whether to fund such interventions, another approach would be needed that combines the inclusiveness of CCA, with decision rules that reflect the investment alternatives that each payer is deciding against. A novel cofinancing approach is proposed in this regard.

Cost-Effectiveness Analysis for Structural Interventions with Mainly Health Outcomes

CUA is recommended for structural interventions that are delivered with the intention of having primarily a single outcome, such as preventing HIV infections, or that are expected to have health outcomes alone. In practice, this requires an element of costing or cost modeling, as well as a trial- or model-based analysis of health outcomes. Standardized guidance is available on how to design, conduct, and report costing analyses and economic evaluations in global health.[61,62]

IMAGE was costed and evaluated from the perspective of a public payer who was interested in reducing IPV (Box 12.4).[66] Jan and colleagues adopted a provider perspective in costing, excluding the costs incurred by beneficiaries to participate in the training sessions.[66] Although the impact observed was a result of the combined microfinance and gender/ HIV training, the microfinance component was found to be cost-neutral following loan repayments and development and delivery of the training the only incremental costs. The authors conducted a CEA to estimate the cost per woman with an IPV-free year gained, comparing the incremental intervention costs to the incremental effect on reduced past-year experience of IPV. Based on an estimated number of DALYs per year lived with violence, from national South African burden of disease data, this was then translated into a cost per DALY averted in a CUA. Although this was a trial-based economic evaluation, it involved further modeling to explore the scale effect. Intervention costs and cost-effectiveness were estimated during the scale-up phase (when the number of clients tripled), by assuming the effect observed during the trial was maintained. IMAGE was found to be cost-effective in its trial phase and highly cost-effective in its scale-up phase.

IMAGE was evaluated against a "do-nothing" comparator (Box 12.2). If the intervention had cost less than the comparator but achieved the same or better outcomes, then it would clearly dominate the alternative and should replace it. In the opposite case, it should not be funded. However, as in most cases, IMAGE had an incremental cost, as well as an incremental effect. The question then becomes whether that benefit gained is worth the cost. Cost-effectiveness is assessed with reference to the decision-makers' willingness to pay (WTP) for the outcome, or the cost-effectiveness threshold (CET).

BOX 12.4

The IMAGE Economic Evaluation[67]

The aim of the economic evaluation was to determine the cost-effectiveness of the IMAGE combined microfinance and gender/HIV training intervention.

Economic evaluation methods: Cost-effectiveness analysis and cost utility analysis. The intervention was evaluated from the perspective of a public payer interested in reducing IPV and therefore excluded costs incurred by beneficiaries to participate in the trainings. Costs were measured during the trial and collected over two years after trial completion, during scale-up.

Outcome unit: Cost per woman with an IPV-free year gained (CEA); cost per DALY averted (CUA).

Alternative investment that IMAGE was compared against: "Do nothing" comparator as described in Box 2.

Key findings of the economic evaluation: IMAGE was cost-effective in the trial phase and very cost-effective in the scale-up phase. The incremental cost of delivering IMAGE during the trial phase was $42.93/client. The evaluation included modeling to estimate costs in the scale-up phase, in which the effects of the intervention observed during the trial were expected to be constant. In the scale-up phase, when coverage of the intervention extended to more than 2,000 additional clients, the incremental cost was $12.88/client, and a cost per DALY averted of $2,307.

There has been substantial debate in the literature about what this CET represents, and much of it stems from the different theoretical frameworks of CBA and CEA.[67-69] For IMAGE, the incremental CER was assessed against a proxy measure of the health sector's opportunity cost, or WTP for a DALY averted. The standard at the time was to use the WHO recommended threshold of one to three times a country's gross domestic product (GDP) per capita, which was set to roughly reflect the human capital productivity value of a healthy year of life.[70] More recently, there is consensus that this threshold is an empirical measure of supply-side opportunity costs and needs to be estimated by measuring how much health gain the health budget is currently achieving at the margin.[71] However, this is a data-intensive and complex exercise that has only been thoroughly done in the UK.[72] Extrapolations have been used to estimate CETs in low and middle-income countries and suggest that they are likely to be considerably lower than previous figures (closer to 0.5 times GDP per capita).[73]

Cost-Benefit Analysis for Structural Interventions with Health and Non-Health Benefits

For structural interventions with multiple consequences within and beyond health, CBA is conventionally considered the most appropriate method. However, it is critiqued for placing a monetary value on life and health. Although there are some clear ethical controversies surrounding this, it is also implicitly done in CEA, when using CETs as decision rules. Nonetheless, this overt monetization can preclude the acceptability of CBA in practice. There are two main approaches to monetizing health outcomes, like DALYs: the human capital approach mentioned earlier, whereby DALYs averted are valued in relation to averted economic productivity losses, and the value of a statistical life approach, which uses an individual's rate of substitution between wealth and small changes in life expectancy.[74–76]

In a CBA, the *valuation of utility*, an economic concept of the "satisfaction" an individual derives from the consumption of a good or a service, is determined by individuals' preferences, because individuals are viewed as the best (or most legitimate) judges of their own well-being. Intervention outcomes are therefore monetized based on individuals' WTP for interventions or their intermediate outputs, which is typically measured with stated or revealed preferences methods.[77] By using monetary values to make interpersonal comparisons, an important systematic bias is introduced whereby benefits and harms are valued more when accrued to rich individuals than poor individuals. In practice, however, CBA tends to apply a population average or representative value to all individuals.[75]

Another key tenet of CBA is that it asserts that a policy or intervention is worthwhile if the monetary value of the benefits accrued to some individuals outweighs the monetary value of the costs borne by others. The reasoning behind this is that those benefitting could, in principle, compensate those who are made worse off. Clearly, this exacerbates the equity concerns mentioned earlier. Moreover, CBA does not question the initial distribution of societal resources, meaning that if a policy improves the well-being of the poor and increases equity, it is likely to be evaluated negatively, unless the overall monetary gains to the poor are greater than the losses to those with higher incomes.[78] Nonetheless, CBA has the advantage of evaluating interventions in a broader context, where multiple objectives are being pursued and have valid claim to scarce societal resources. Conducting a CBA for a structural intervention would imply that the evaluation could inform a central decision-maker with multisectoral objectives, and one budget constraint; or a health decision-maker with health and non-health objectives, subject to a health budget constraint.

In 2011, the Copenhagen Consensus Centre commissioned CBAs for 19 HIV interventions to identify the most cost-effective way to spend a hypothetical additional US$10 billion in sub-Saharan Africa over five years.[79] This is one of the few efforts to evaluate HIV interventions using CBA, which included four structural interventions (i.e., cash transfers for girls, microfinance and gender/HIV training, increased alcohol taxation, and agricultural livelihoods training).[79,80]

Cofinancing Analysis for Structural Interventions with Multiple Payers Across Sectors

The *compensation test* or a cofinancing analysis has been proposed as an alternative approach for structural interventions with multiple outcomes that cut across sectors.[81] As with CCA or CBA, it starts from disaggregated estimates of all costs and consequences of intervention options, but it differs in its valuation of outcomes and the decision rules applied. First, it posits that any payer or sector can cofinance an intervention with other interested (benefitting) payers. Second, it suggests that it is efficient for an HIV payer (for example) to do so, where a non-HIV intervention achieves HIV gains more efficiently than the next best HIV investment, when costs are shared. Each sector's CET is used to value outcomes, as it reflects its WTP per unit of outcome given its current resource allocation.

This approach was illustrated with the example of the Zomba CRT (Table 12.2). In addition to reductions in HIV and herpes simplex virus type 2, the evaluation found impacts on school drop-out rates, teenage pregnancy, and early marriage.[23] The primary effectiveness study suggested that the intervention was not cost-effective for the HIV budget, based on its HIV outcome alone. In a cofinancing analysis, the other intervention outcomes were valued at the CER of each (sub)sector's alternative intervention, which would have hypothetically led to the intervention being funded and efficiency gains for each sector.[82]

The Future of Evaluations of Structural HIV Prevention Interventions

The complexity of structural interventions and their dependency on context has caused debate on methods to evaluate their impact. This debate has centered on the utility and suitability of trials, whose design elements are founded in methods to determine the efficacy of drugs and vaccines. Critics of the trials argue that these methods should not be used in the evaluation of complex interventions that aim to modify behavior. We argue that a well-designed CRT provides the most credible evidence of intervention effectiveness precisely by including a comparison group that is similar with regard to social and economic contexts that influence whether an intervention works. A strong logic model, quantitative and qualitative enquiry into this logic, and an economic evaluation that explores value for money is key to providing a comprehensive evidence base to support decision-making.

With declines in investments in HIV prevention research in recent years, the CRT design has become increasingly challenging to implement. A key challenge for evaluators of complex structural HIV prevention interventions is therefore how to provide rigorous evidence of effectiveness with fewer resources. Rigorous nonrandomized designs are available to support our understanding of what works to prevent HIV and, in some scenarios, may prove the most applicable designs to evaluate a structural intervention. Like the CRT design, nonrandomized designs need to be bolstered by theory and process data. The absence of such data fails to provide an understanding of the complex causal pathways inherent to structural interventions. Numerous evaluations of structural HIV prevention interventions have been conducted.[13] How to translate this available evidence base into programs and policies that are effective and cost-effective across time and place is a critical question as we move toward ending HIV by 2030.[83]

A key challenge in this translation of evidence is how the intervention worked, or why it did not, and what elements of context are critical to effectiveness. Process evaluation supports further understanding of whether the intervention is applicable in other settings. To date, integration of findings from impact, particularly CRTs, and process evaluation has been limited. Better integration of these evaluations to gain greater insight into what works, for whom, and in what context is a topic of current debate and would support the translation of the evidence into action across settings.

Although it is critical to determine what interventions work, evidence of impact and process are not sufficient to ascertain whether to invest HIV resources in them. Economic evaluation is required to compare the costs and benefits of intervention options and guide decisions on whether to allocate scarce HIV resources to a structural intervention or its next best alternative. Any economic evaluation is intended as an aid to thought for decision-makers and by no means a replacement for the value-laden priority-setting process. As such, it requires clarity and transparency to ensure its findings are well understood and can even be partly transferred across settings. There are different economic evaluation techniques available, depending on the decision-maker, the objective being optimized, and the budget constraint faced. The design of an economic evaluation should align to the decision-makers' funding decision and their social value judgments, as well as being pragmatic enough to incorporate multiple decision-makers when considering multisectoral interventions with multiple funding streams.

References

1. Pronyk PM, Hargreaves JR, Kim JC, et al. Effect of a structural intervention for the prevention of intimate-partner violence and HIV in rural South Africa: a cluster randomised trial. *Lancet.* 2006;368(9551):1973–1983. doi:10.1016/S0140-6736(06)69744-4.
2. Hennekens CH, Buring J. *Epidemiology in Medicine.* Philadelphia: Lippincott Williams and Wilkins; 1987.
3. Hayes R, Moulton LH. *Cluster Randomised Trials.* Boca Raton, FL: CRC Press; 2009.
4. World Health Organization. Metrics: Disability-Adjusted Life Year (DALY): Quantifying the Burden of Disease from Mortality and Morbidity. http://www.who.int/healthinfo/global_burden_disease/metrics_daly/en/.
5. National Institute for Health and Care Excellence: Glossary. https://www.nice.org.uk/glossary?letter=q. Accessed September 20, 2017.
6. Adimora AA, Auerbach JD. Structural interventions for HIV prevention in the United States. *J Acquir Immune Defic Syndr.* 2010;55(2):S132–S135. doi:10.1097/QAI.obo13e3181fbcb38.
7. Gupta GR, Parkhurst JO, Ogden JA, Aggleton P, Mahal A. Structural approaches to HIV prevention. *Lancet.* 2017;372(9640):764–775. doi:10.1016/S0140-6736(08)60887-9.
8. Bonell C, Hargreaves J, Strange V, Pronyk P, Porter J. Should structural interventions be evaluated using RCTs? The case of HIV prevention. *Soc Sci Med.* 2006;63(5):1135–1142. doi:10.1016/j.socscimed.2006.03.026.

9. Blankenship KM, Friedman SR, Dworkin S, Mantell JE. Structural interventions: concepts, challenges and opportunities for research. *J Urban Health*. 2006;83(1):59–72. doi:10.1007/s11524-005-9007-4.

10. Shannon K, Strathdee SA, Goldenberg SM, et al. Global epidemiology of HIV among female sex workers: influence of structural determinants. *Lancet*. 2015;385(9962):55–71. http://dx.doi.org/10.1016/S0140-6736(14)60931-4.

11. Chersich MF, Luchters S, Ntaganira I, et al. Priority interventions to reduce HIV transmission in sex work settings in sub-Saharan Africa and delivery of these services. *J Int AIDS Soc*. 2013;16(1):17980. doi:10.7448/IAS.16.1.17980.

12. Boerma JT, Weir SS. Integrating demographic and epidemiological approaches to research on HIV/AIDS: the proximate-determinants framework. *J Infect Dis*. 2005;191(Suppl 1):S61–S67. http://dx.doi.org/10.1086/425282.

13. Krishnaratne S, Hensen B, Cordes J, Enstone J, Hargreaves JR. Interventions to strengthen the HIV prevention cascade: a systematic review of reviews. *Lancet HIV*. 2016;3(7):e307–e317. doi:10.1016/S2352-3018(16)30038-8.

14. Remme M, Siapka M, Vassall A, et al. The cost and cost-effectiveness of gender-responsive interventions for HIV: a systematic review. *J Int AIDS Soc*. 2014;17. http://www.jiasociety.org/index.php/jias/article/view/19228.

15. Victora CG, Habicht J-P, Bryce J. Evidence-based public health: moving beyond randomized trials. *Am J Public Health*. 2004;94(3):400–405. doi:10.2105/AJPH.94.3.400.

16. Habicht JP, Victora CG, Vaughan JP. Evaluation designs for adequacy, plausibility and probability of public health programme performance and impact. *Int J Epidemiol*. 1999;28(1):10–18. http://dx.doi.org/10.1093/ije/28.1.10.

17. Pettifor A, Lippman SA, Selin AM, et al. A cluster randomized-controlled trial of a community mobilization intervention to change gender norms and reduce HIV risk in rural South Africa: study design and intervention. *BMC Public Health*. 2015;15(1):752. doi:10.1186/s12889-015-2048-z.

18. Pawson R, Tilley N. *Realistic Evaluation*. London: SAGE; 1997.

19. Kippax S. Sexual health interventions are unsuitable for experimental evaluation. In: Stephenson JM, Bonell C, Imrie J, eds. *Effective Sexual Health Interventions: Issues in Experimental Evaluation*. Oxford: Oxford University Press; 2002:17–34.

20. Bonell C, Fletcher A, Morton M, Lorenc T, Moore L. Realist randomised controlled trials: a new approach to evaluating complex public health interventions. *Soc Sci Med*. 2012;75:2299–2306.

21. Abramsky T, Devries K, Kiss L, et al. A community mobilisation intervention to prevent violence against women and reduce HIV/AIDS risk in Kampala, Uganda (the SASA! Study): study protocol for a cluster randomised controlled trial. *Trials*. 2012;13. doi:10.1186/1745-6215-13-96.

22. Abramsky T, Devries K, Kiss L, et al. Findings from the SASA! Study: a cluster randomized controlled trial to assess the impact of a community mobilization

intervention to prevent violence against women and reduce HIV risk in Kampala, Uganda. *BMC Med.* 2014;12(1):122. doi:10.1186/s12916-014-0122-5.

23. Baird SJ, Garfein RS, McIntosh CT, Ozler B. Effect of a cash transfer programme for schooling on prevalence of HIV and herpes simplex type 2 in Malawi: a cluster randomised trial. *Lancet.* 2012;379(9823):1320–1329. http://dx.doi.org/10.1016/S0140-6736%2811%2961709-1

24. Hayes R, Moulton L. Cluster randomised trials: basic principles of analysis. Dordrecht, The Netherlands: Chapman and Hall/CRC Biostatistics Series; 2009.

25. Hayes R, Bennett S. Simple sample size calculation for cluster-randomized trials. *Int J Epidemiol.* 1999;28. doi:10.1093/ije/28.2.319.

26. Beattie TS, Isac S, Bhattacharjee P, et al. Reducing violence and increasing condom use in the intimate partnerships of female sex workers: study protocol for Samvedana Plus, a cluster randomised controlled trial in Karnataka state, south India. *BMC Public Health.* 2016;16(1):660. doi:10.1186/s12889-016-3356-7.

27. Beattie TS, Bhattacharjee P, Isac S, et al. Supporting adolescent girls to stay in school, reduce child marriage and reduce entry into sex work as HIV risk prevention in north Karnataka, India: protocol for a cluster randomised controlled trial. *BMC Public Health.* 2015;15(1):292. doi:10.1186/s12889-015-1623-7.

28. Guidance for Industry E6 Good Clinical Practice: Consolidated Guidance. Rockville, MD: Center for Biologics Evaluation and Research; 1996.

29. Freedman B. Equipoise and the ethics of clinical research. *N Engl J Med.* 1987;317(3):141–145. doi:10.1056/NEJM198707163170304.

30. Shadish WR, Cook TD, Campbell DT. *Experimental and Quasi-Experimental Designs for Generalized Causal Inference.* New York: Houghton Mifflin; 2002.

31. Davey C, Boulay M, Hargreaves JR. Strengthening nonrandomized studies of health communication strategies for HIV prevention. *JAIDS J Acquir Immune Defic Syndr.* 2014;66. http://journals.lww.com/jaids/Fulltext/2014/08151/Strengthening_Nonrandomized_Studies_of_Health.5.aspx.

32. Davey C, Hargreaves J. *Designing an Evaluation of a HIV Prevention Program* (Unpublished manuscript).

33. Prost A, Binik A, Abubakar I, et al. Logistic, ethical, and political dimensions of stepped wedge trials: critical review and case studies. *Trials.* 2015;16:351. doi:10.1186/s13063-015-0837-4.

34. Hargreaves JR, Copas AJ, Beard E, et al. Five questions to consider before conducting a stepped wedge trial. *Trials.* 2015;16:350. doi:10.1186/s13063-015-0841-8.

35. Davey C, Hargreaves J, Thompson JA, et al. Analysis and reporting of stepped-wedge randomised-controlled trials: synthesis and critical appraisal of published studies. *Trials.* 2015;16:358.

36. Page K, Stein ES, Carrico AW, et al. Protocol of a cluster randomised stepped-wedge trial of behavioural interventions targeting amphetamine-type stimulant

use and sexual risk among female entertainment and sex workers in Cambodia. *BMJ Open*. 2016;6(5). http://bmjopen.bmj.com/content/6/5/e010854.abstract.

37. Kontopantelis E, Doran T, Springate DA, Buchan I, Reeves D. Regression based quasi-experimental approach when randomisation is not an option: interrupted time series analysis. *BMJ*. 2015;350. doi:10.1136/bmj.h2750.

38. Ruiz MS, O'Rourke A, Allen ST. Impact evaluation of a policy intervention for HIV prevention in Washington, DC. *AIDS Behav*. 2016;20(1):22–28. doi:10.1007/s10461-015-1143-6.

39. Weinhardt LS, Galvao LW, Mwenyekonde T, et al. Methods and protocol of a mixed method quasi-experiment to evaluate the effects of a structural economic and food security intervention on HIV vulnerability in rural Malawi: The SAGE4Health Study. *Springerplus*. 2014;3:296. doi:10.1186/2193-1801-3-296.

40. Munro A, Bloor M. Process evaluation: the new miracle ingredient in public health research? *Qual Res*. 2010;10(6):699–713. doi:10.1177/1468794110380522.

41. Oakley A, Strange V, Bonell C, Allen E, Stephenson J. Process evaluation in randomised controlled trials of complex interventions. *BMJ*. 2006;332(7538):413–416. http://www.bmj.com/content/332/7538/413.abstract.

42. Oakley A, Strange V, Stephenson J, Forrest S, Monteiro H. Evaluating processes: a case study of a randomized controlled trial of sex education. *Evaluation*. 2004;10(4):440–462.

43. Rychetnik L, Frommer M, Hawe P, Shiell A. Criteria for evaluating evidence on public health interventions. *J Epidemiol Community Health*. 2002;56(2):119–127. http://jech.bmj.com/content/56/2/119.abstract.

44. Hawe P, Shiell A, Riley T. Theorising interventions as events in systems. *Am J Community Psychol*. 2009;43(3–4):267–276. doi:10.1007/s10464-009-9229-9.

45. Rogers EM. *Diffusion of Innovations*. 5th ed. New York: Free Press; 2003.

46. Carroll C, Patterson M, Wood S, Booth A, Rick J, Balain S. A conceptual framework for implementation fidelity. *Implement Sci*. 2007;2(1):40. doi:10.1186/1748-5908-2-40.

47. Grant A, Treweek S, Dreischulte T, Foy R, Guthrie B. Process evaluations for cluster-randomised trials of complex interventions: a proposed framework for design and reporting. *Trials*. 2013;14:15. doi:10.1186/1745-6215-14-15.

48. Steckler A, Linnan LA. *Process Evaluation for Public Health Interventions and Research*. San Francisco: Jossey-Bass; 2002.

49. Weiss CH. Theory-based evaluation: past, present, and future. *New Dir Eval*. 1997; 76:41–55. doi:10.1002/ev.1086.

50. Moore G, Audrey S, Barker M, Bond L, Bonell C, Hardeman W. *Process Evaluation of Complex Interventions: Medical Research Council Guidance*. London: MRC Population Health Science Research Network; 2014.

51. Moore GF, Audrey S, Barker M, et al. Process evaluation of complex interventions: Medical Research Council guidance. *BMJ Br Med J*. 2015;350.

52. Wight D, Obasi A. Unpacking the "black box": the importance of process data to explain outcomes. In: *Effective Sexual Health Interventions*. Oxford: Oxford University Press; 2003. doi:10.1093/acprof:oso/9780198508496.003.0010.

53. Moore GF, Raisanen L, Moore L, Din NU, Murphy S. Mixed-method process evaluation of the Welsh National Exercise Referral Scheme. *Health Educ.* 2013;113(6):476–501. doi:10.1108/HE-08-2012-0046.

54. Bonell C, Oakley A, Hargreaves J, Strange V, Rees R. Assessment of generalisability in trials of health interventions: suggested framework and systematic review. *BMJ.* 2006;333(7563):346–349.

55. Dorner TE. Public health: social context and action. *Int J Integr Care.* 2012;12:e41. http://www.ncbi.nlm.nih.gov/pmc/articles/PMC3440253/.

56. Hargreaves J, Hatcher A, Strange V, et al. Process evaluation of the Intervention with Microfinance for AIDS and Gender Equity (IMAGE) in rural South Africa. *Health Educ Res.* 2010;25(1):27–40. doi:10.1093/her/cyp054.

57. Greco G, Lorgelly P, Yamabhai I. Outcomes in economic evaluations of public health interventions in low- and middle-income countries: health, capabilities and subjective wellbeing. *Health Econ.* 2016;25(Suppl 1):83–94. doi:10.1002/hec.3302.

58. Drummond M. *Methods for the Economic Evaluation of Health Care Programmes.* Oxford; New York: Oxford University Press; 2005.

59. Gold MR, Stevenson D, Fryback DG. HALYS and QALYS and DALYS, oh my: similarities and differences in summary measures of population Health. *Annu Rev Public Health.* 2002;23:115–134. doi:10.1146/annurev. publhealth.23.100901.140513.

60. Johannesson M, Jönsson B. Economic evaluation in health care: is there a role for cost-benefit analysis? *Health Policy.* 1991;17(1):1–23. http://dx.doi.org/ 10.1016/0168-8510(91)90114-D.

61. Vassall A, Sweeney S, Kahn J, et al. *Reference Case for Global Health Costing (Version 3);* 2017.

62. Wilkinson T, Sculpher MJ, Claxton K, et al. The international decision support initiative reference case for economic evaluation: an aid to thought. *Value Heal.* 2016;19(8):921–928. http://dx.doi.org/10.1016/j.jval.2016.04.015.

63. Remme M, Watts C, Heise L, Vassall A. Secondary schooling might be as good an HIV investment as male circumcision. *Lancet Glob Health.* 2017;3(10):e591. doi:10.1016/S2214-109X(15)00167-9.

64. Drummond M, Sculpher M, Torrance GW, Stoddart GL. Methods for the economic evaluation of health care programmes, 3rd ed. *J Epidemiol Community Health.* 2006;60(9):822–823. http://www.ncbi.nlm.nih.gov/pmc/articles/ PMC2566038/.

65. Garrison LPJ, Mansley EC, Abbott TA 3rd, Bresnahan BW, Hay JW, Smeeding J. Good research practices for measuring drug costs in cost-effectiveness analyses: a societal perspective: the ISPOR Drug Cost Task Force report—part

II. *Value Heal J Int Soc Pharmacoeconomics Outcomes Res.* 2010;13(1):8–13. doi:10.1111/j.1524-4733.2009.00660.x.

66. Jan S, Ferrari G, Watts CH, et al. Economic evaluation of a combined microfinance and gender training intervention for the prevention of intimate partner violence in rural South Africa. *Health Policy Plan.* 2011;26(5):366–372. doi:10.1093/heapol/czq071.

67. Bertram MY, Lauer JA, De Joncheere K, et al. Cost-effectiveness thresholds: pros and cons. *Bull World Health Organ.* 2016;94(12):925–930. doi:10.2471/BLT.15.164418.

68. Shillcutt SD, Walker DG, Goodman CA, Mills AJ. Cost effectiveness in low- and middle-income countries: a review of the debates surrounding decision rules. *Pharmacoeconomics.* 2009;27(11):903–917. doi:10.2165/10899580-000000000-00000.

69. Kahn JG, Marseille E, Larson B, Kazi DS, Kahn JG, Rosen S. Thresholds for the cost–effectiveness of interventions: alternative approaches. *Bull World Heal Organ.* 2015;93(2):118–124. http://www.escholarship.org/uc/item/1r25d1nr.

70. Robinson LA, Hammitt JK, Chang AY, Resch S. Understanding and improving the one and three times GDP per capita cost-effectiveness thresholds. *Health Policy Plan.* 2017;32(1):141–145. http://dx.doi.org/10.1093/heapol/czw096.

71. Culyer AJ. Cost-effectiveness thresholds in health care: a bookshelf guide to their meaning and use. *Heal Econ Policy Law.* 2016;11(4):415–432.

72. Claxton K, Martin S, Soares MO, et al. *Methods for the Estimation of the NICE Cost Effectiveness Threshold.* York, UK: University of York, Centre for Health Economics; 2013.

73. Woods B, Revill P, Sculpher M, Claxton K. Country-level cost-effectiveness thresholds: initial estimates and the need for further research. *Value Health.* 2016;19(8):929–935. https://doi.org/10.1016/j.jval.2016.02.017.

74. Brent RJ. A social cost-benefit criterion for evaluating voluntary counseling and testing with an application to Tanzania. *Health Econ.* 2010;19(2):154–172.

75. Robinson LA, Hammitt JK, O'Keeffe L, et al. *Benefit-Cost Analysis in Global Health and Development: Current Practices and Opportunities for Improvement Scoping Report.* Cambridge, MA: Harvard University.

76. Chang AY, Robinson LA, Hammitt JK, Resch SC. Economics in "Global Health 2035": a sensitivity analysis of the value of a life year estimates. *J Glob Health.* 2017;7(1):10401. doi:10.7189/jogh.07.010401.

77. Cookson R. Willingness to pay methods in health care: a sceptical view. *Health Econ.* 2003;12(11):891–894. doi:10.1002/hec.847.

78. Brouwer WBF, Culyer AJ, van Exel NJA, Rutten FFH. Welfarism vs. extra-welfarism. *J Health Econ.* 2008;27(2):325–338. doi:10.1016/j.jhealeco.2007.07.003.

79. Lomborg B. *Rethink HIV: Smarter Ways to Invest in Ending HIV in Sub-Saharan Africa.* Cambridge, UK: Cambridge University Press; 2012.

80. Vassall A, Remme M, Watts C. Social policy interventions to enhance the HIV/ AIDS response in sub-Saharan Africa. In: Lomborg B, ed. *Rethink HIV: Smarter Ways to Invest in Ending HIV in Sub-Saharan Africa.* Cambridge: Cambridge University Press; 2012.

81. Claxton K, Schulpher M, Culyer A. *Mark versus Luke? Appropriate Methods for the Evaluation of Public Health Interventions.* York, UK: Centre For Health Economics, Alcuin College, University of York; 2007. https://ideas.repec.org/p/ chy/respap/31cherp.html.

82. Remme M, Vassall A, Lutz B, Luna J, Watts C. Financing structural interventions: going beyond HIV-only value for money assessments. *AIDS.* 2014;28(3):425–434. doi:10.1097/QAD.0000000000000076.

83. Dehne KL, Dallabetta G, Wilson D, et al. HIV Prevention 2020: a framework for delivery and a call for action. *Lancet HIV.* 2017;3(7):e323–e332. doi:10.1016/ S2352-3018(16)30035-2.

13

Enhancing Theory of Structural-Level Interventions for HIV Prevention and Care

Kim M. Blankenship

Overview

Theories provide a means of systematically organizing and approaching inquiry for purposes of explanation—suggesting the conditions under which we can expect certain outcomes and not others—as well as a foundation from which to interpret and act on findings based on inquiry. These findings, in turn, may confirm a theory, direct its modification, or cause it to be abandoned or replaced altogether. In this way, the process of theoretically driven inquiry is simultaneously one of theory-testing and both theory- and knowledge-building. It is a process valuable in and of itself, but even more significant for our purposes are the possibilities it offers for revealing harm and injustice and directing efforts to create a healthier world. For, arguably, it is those efforts built on the soundest of theories that have the greatest potential for ensuring public health.

There are numerous theories across and within fields, subfields, and academic disciplines that have been, or could be used, to understand and direct public health efforts. Although sharing some general features, theories vary considerably in terms of what they mean by "explanation," what they seek to explain, and how they conceive of and the methods they employ in the process of theory-driven inquiry. To promote health, some may look to theories about the workings of the cells, tissues, or immune systems of the human body, while others may find answers in theories about the human psyche or individual motivation, and still others may be guided by theories that focus on what social institutions stand to gain or lose from practices with implications for health. Ultimately, knowledge gained in all of these realms has the potential to impact public health; indeed, it is often likely that knowledge gained in all of these realms is *necessary* to impact health.

Before proceeding with the question of where theory fits in the context of structural interventions and HIV/AIDS specifically, and without diving too deeply into the philosophy and sociology of science, it is important to acknowledge three additional features of the process of theory-driven inquiry. First, this process takes place within a social world that partially dictates, among other things, what theories and questions gain prominence, what data is considered relevant for theory testing, when findings will be acted on, and what form those actions will take. This means that the process partly reflects such issues as what kinds, amounts, and sources of funding are available for conducting theory-driven inquiry. It also means that attention should be devoted to determining whether certain theories and forms of inquiry better fit with the reward structures of universities, the economics of journal publication, or the priorities of politicians or the public. Finally, it means that added determination is important as to what groups, organizations, or institutions benefit the most from the interventions that derive from these inquiries.

Second, given its ongoing nature, it is rarely the case that theoretically driven inquiry produces a final and definitive answer to the questions it raises. This may not be of great significance if we are, for instance, trying to understand the conditions under which peasant revolutions have historically arisen; the consequences of continuing to explore this question through further theory-testing and -building may be relatively minor. Conversely, many health-related questions—including those involving HIV/AIDS—are of considerable urgency, asked specifically for purposes of identifying interventions or strategies with the greatest potential for reducing vulnerability to or minimizing the consequences of disease. Ideally, the theories that drive health-related inquiries and the research they inspire should be particularly robust. Invariably, however, it also means that interventions derived from this research will be based on knowledge that is incomplete at best. To be sure, there are established standards to help determine when it is more or less appropriate to intervene based on incomplete information, but these are subject to interpretation and leave room for doubt. It may not be surprising then, that interventions to address health can come with "unintended consequences"—consequences not anticipated by our theories even if (sometimes) they might have been anticipated had some other theory been applied instead, or if a different question was asked altogether.

Third, whatever interventions are used and however many unintended consequences they produce, once they are introduced they become a part of our history and, as such, may change the direction of future theory, inquiry, and interventions. This must be recognized in subsequent theoretically driven inquiry. Some interventions may impact on human biology, or human psyche, or social institutions in ways that must be accounted for moving forward. They may alter priorities and make some lines of inquiry less relevant and others more relevant.

It is within the changing and interconnected history of the science and sociology of HIV/AIDS that this chapter locates a discussion of theory and structural interventions. First, it briefly situates the emergence of the concept and pursuit of research related to structural interventions within the convergence of concerns to highlight, on the one hand, the relevance of social science theory for understanding the emerging HIV epidemic and, on the other hand, the growing recognition of the limitations of behavioral theories that predominated in discussions of how to curb the epidemic. The chapter then suggests that while social science theory is particularly relevant to the concept of structural interventions, it has not always been explicitly or consistently invoked in the structural interventions literature, nor has it always explicitly guided understanding of the epidemic or, accordingly, the development of structural interventions. In this regard, the chapter next discusses frameworks that have often driven research related to the social determinants of HIV/AIDS and critiques of these frameworks that derive from social science theory. Finally, the chapter argues that moving forward in addressing HIV/AIDS generally and in developing structural interventions in particular, the critical question for theory-guided inquiry is how to understand and, subsequently, address *persistent inequities in HIV/AIDS*—including the likelihood of acquiring, being diagnosed with, and receiving and responding to treatment for the virus, as well as dying from HIV/AIDS-related causes. Accordingly, the chapter discusses a theory-driven research agenda for moving our understanding and application of interventions forward.

The Emergence of "Structural Interventions" in HIV/AIDS

Arguably, a foundation for the developing attention to structural interventions in HIV/AIDS can be traced to a workshop convened by the Institute of Medicine (IOM) in June 1995.[1] According to the summary that begins the workshop's published report, it was convened by the IOM (and supported by the Office of AIDS Research at the National Institute of Health) to "consider the contributions of the social and behavioral sciences to AIDS prevention."[1(p.1)] But the summary quickly noted that its primary interest is the *social* sciences: "The workshop extend[s] the review of preventive interventions targeted at individual behavior change found in the 1994 IOM report, *AIDS and Behavior: An Integrated Approach.* Thus focused on more social-level analyses, this workshop summary and the accompanying background papers are useful companion documents to the earlier IOM report."[1(p.1)] The introduction also noted the limitations of both "biomedical developments" and "behaviorally based AIDS prevention research . . . focused on the individual" for slowing or eliminating the HIV/AIDS epidemic, and highlights that "broader social forces such as economics, politics, and international affairs" are critical to these purposes as wel.[1(pp.4–5)] Beyond an academic commitment to social science perspectives, the report demonstrates recognition of the social nature of scientific priority setting and theory-driven inquiry.[1] Accordingly, it noted: "This summary is targeted primarily to policy-makers who will be making the decisions for the HIV/AIDS research agenda in the next decade . . . a major theme of the workshop for policymakers is that programs to encourage and bolster use of social and behavioral methods in research supported by the National Institutes of Health, the Centers for Disease Control and Prevention, and other agencies will be good investments in the future."[1(p.5)]

The specific language of "structural interventions" does not appear in the 1995 IOM report. But one of the background papers discussed at the workshop, written by Samuel Friedman and Christina Wypijewska, was titled "Social Science Intervention Models for Reducing HIV Transmission" and formed the basis for a chapter.[1] That chapter discussed "basic social science research" (read: theoretically driven social science research) that has enhanced understanding of the epidemic, and it described existing development of new interventions based on these social science theories.[1(pp.29-40)] In this way, it anticipated growing attention to structural interventions.

The language of "structural interventions" is also relatively absent from the HIV/AIDS literature of the 1990s. A Google Scholar search of the string "'structural interventions' HIV" (conducted November 15, 2017) for the period from 1990 to 1995 brought up only three relevant citations.[2-4] From 1996 to 2000 the same search uncovered 50 relevant articles; a fifth (10) appeared in a 2000 supplement of *JAIDS* comprised of papers stemming from a February 1999 interdisciplinary meeting of researchers and policymakers organized by the Division of HIV/AIDS Prevention at the National Center of HIV, STD, and TB Prevention of the Centers for Disease Control and Prevention (CDC).[5-14]

Unlike the IOM meeting, the CDC meeting was not motivated by a desire to showcase the critical relevance of the theories and methods of the social sciences per se. Rather, its purpose was "to identify structural factors associated with HIV, and to assist the CDC in identifying priority areas for research and implementation."[15] One of the papers analyzed existing structural interventions across a range of public health areas and, based on that, proposed a framework for classifying structural interventions in terms of the kinds of contextual factors they focus on as determinants of health and the level at which they are targeted, suggested the conditions under which different types of structural interventions were likely to be more or less successful, and then discussed the implications for structural interventions for HIV prevention generally.[6] Another paper drew lessons from structural interventions in various domains of adolescent health for potential interventions to address HIV risk among adolescents.[8] But most of the papers in the issue identified different "structural factors," conceptualized as "barriers to" or "facilitators of" HIV prevention generally, or among particular subgroups—including women, drug users, adolescents, gay men, and HIV-positive individuals—and discussed interventions (or potential interventions) for addressing them. Neither these factors nor the interventions derived from them were explicitly based on social science theories. The one exception was a case study of the Family-to-Family intervention in Harlem, which was not specifically aimed at HIV/AIDS but instead was developed as a community-organizing project to increase social capital available to families and children living in Harlem.[13] In this sense, it could be argued to represent a structural intervention informed directly by social science theory.

Whether starting from structural interventions or from structural factors, many of the authors in the special issue acknowledged that they preferred to avoid defining structural interventions altogether, other than to describe them as interventions aimed either at modifying the environments in which HIV risk behaviors occur or, somewhat tautologically, at addressing the structural factors that they had identified as barriers to HIV prevention. Indeed, Sumartojo, in the first paragraph of the lead article to the issue, wrote: "The broad term 'structural' is used in this paper, with the assumption that its meaning will become clearer and more differentiated as work in this area progresses."[5(p.3)]

Moving Toward Theoretically Informed Structural Interventions

Although not explicitly invoking *social* theory in their papers, most authors in the 2000 *JAIDS* issue, and many since, refer to the limitations of theories rooted in social psychology invoked to explain health behavior and associated health outcomes (e.g., the health belief model,[16] theory of planned behavior,[17] theory of reasoned action[17]) and the interventions based on them. They look instead to "social factors" or "social context" or "risk environments" to understand such things as potential for acquisition or transmission of, or extent of access to treatments for HIV/AIDS. Accordingly, they propose structural interventions as alternatives to the individually targeted interventions produced by behavioral theories. Indeed, the structural interventions literature greatly expanded after the year 2000. The same Google Scholar search referred to previously revealed almost 90 relevant citations between 2001 and 2005 and over 500 between 2006 and 2010 (from 2011 to 2015 that number was over 1,100, though since 2016 there have been about 350 relevant citations, perhaps signifying some decline). Still, even by 2006, a review article published in the *Journal of Urban Health* as part of a special section entitled "HIV Perspectives after 25 Years" begins discussion of the state of research related to structural interventions in HIV/AIDS by noting that while they imply a theoretical understanding of HIV/AIDS as socially determined, specific structural interventions are rarely linked back to social science theories related to health, nor do such theories often give rise to specific interventions.[18]

Without the direction provided by theory, the identification of structural factors associated with HIV can proceed like a descriptive listing of laws, policies, norms, institutions (e.g., schools, media), health and social services (e.g., availability, accessibility, types, location), and characteristics of physical spaces, among others, thought to be part of the "social context" or "risk environment" that impacts HIV/AIDS. To account for the large number of potential factors that can influence HIV/AIDS generally, or among specific populations, some scholars have followed an ecological systems approach similar to that developed by Bronfenbrenner[19] whereby different levels at which factors may operate to produce risk are identified.[20–22] Rhodes[23(p.88)] developed an adaptation of this ecological framing in conceptualizing a "risk environment" as "the space—whether social or physical—in which a variety of factors interact to increase the chances of drug-related harm." He distinguished two dimensions characterizing this environment—types of environment (physical, social, economic, and policy) and level of environmental influences (micro-environment and macro-environment). This framework has subsequently been modified or expanded to characterize HIV risk environments among, for example, drug users,[24,25] women,[26,27] and sex workers.[28] Another variation of this approach distinguishes between "proximal" and "distal" causal factors[29] or processes,[30] with the more distal factors typically seen to be "further" from desired outcomes in terms of time or levels of impact, or more distal causal processes seen to involve longer causal chains or more diffuse impacts.

In general, critiques of such approaches have centered around three related issues: (a) their failure to attend to, or inadequate representation of, *the relationship among* different levels or groups of "social factors" and, subsequently, (b) their explanatory power (or lack thereof), and (c) their implications for the structure/agency dichotomy.

Although ecological approaches may capture aspects of the complexity of the social world by identifying multiple components (levels, factors, domains) of that world that can constrain or facilitate HIV-AIDS related behavior, they tend to conceptualize these different components as independent of one another and of the behaviors they are meant to explain. Causality in this framework is viewed as independent forces pushing on each other to produce outcomes. Like a set of different-colored billiard balls on a pool table, hitting one may bring about a response in another, either directly or indirectly via a second ball. One ball may even be hit by multiple others coming from different directions. But none of the balls are substantively changed by their interaction. Take them off the pool table and they are still billiard balls, and the pool table remains a pool table whether the balls are removed, remain idle, or are moving around on it.

An alternative, *relational approach* to structure recognizes individual behaviors as deriving their very meaning from the social world in which they occur; specifically, they are seen to embody patterned social relations of inequality (e.g., gender, race, class) that structure that world and when they are enacted, they are reflecting and reproducing those structures, sometimes reinforcing them but sometimes modifying them in ways that may in turn, affect the meaning and operation of both. As an extension, individual behavior is reconceptualized as *social practice*.[31–33] Further, those same patterned social relations are reflected and reproduced in multiple contexts or along multiple dimensions (not just at the level of individual behavior). For example, Risman[34] identified three levels at which gender is deeply embedded and for which it has consequences: individual (personalities), cultural rules, and institutions. According to relational theory, causality is recursive, not linear.[34,35] It makes little sense to discuss "proximal" and "distal" levels of analysis or causal relations from this perspective. Indeed, Krieger[36] argued that maintaining such distinctions obscures relations of power operating simultaneously, even if in distinctly distinguishable ways, at multiple levels and time points, and ultimately, can produce public health interventions that do not hold accountable those who benefit from the status quo.

In regard to HIV/AIDS in particular, both Connell[31] and Friedman and colleagues[35,37,38] have elaborated relational theories that are representative of alternative ways of conceptualizing social "context" that capture the dynamic and multilayered complexity of the social world, make room for agency, and provide a guide for theory-driven explanations for outcomes ranging from individual risk for HIV to whether an HIV epidemic emerges in a given population. For example, in her work, Connell[31(p.1677)] elaborates a relational theory of gender and power in which gender represents a social structure that derives from patterned relations between and among women and men. Gender as social structure is embedded in multiple relations (e.g., economic, political, affective, symbolic) and operates in multiple dimensions (e.g., intrapersonal, interpersonal, institutional). Furthermore, it may manifest itself and operate differently across relations and dimensions, changing rapidly in some and more slowly in others, for example, or taking one form in a given historical moment and another at a different moment. From this perspective, health outcomes are analyzed not as an effect or consequence of gender but as they are produced in the processes through which gender is made.[31(p.1678)]

Applying this framework to HIV/AIDS, Connell[31] considers how sexual practices that are "risky" for HIV may emerge from gender dynamics that characterize a particular historical moment as they intersect with economic and political relations that are themselves not independent of gender relations. Although the process of applying a relational gender analysis to explain HIV-related outcomes (or any health outcomes) is not a standardized one, and in fact may be quite complex, it does involve a set of common concerns. According to Connell,[31(p.1679)] it must "consider simultaneously the shape of the gender order and its historical transformations, the pattern of institutional and interpersonal relations, and the body-reflective practices in which health consequences are produced." In this way, she provides a focal point for theoretically-driven inquiry to understand the production of risk or the context that produces risk and subsequently, potential intervention points and strategies, as well as potential consequences of intervening.

In a series of articles, Friedman and colleagues[35,37] elaborate a different relational theory, namely a dialectical theory, to account for how "big events" such as wars and political-economic transitions may produce the conditions in which an HIV epidemic emerges, and, more specifically, may precipitate increases both in the numbers of people engaging in behaviors that are risky and in the riskiness of those behaviors. In a 2009 article, Friedman, Rossi, and Braine[37] critique explanations of how big events may sometimes lead to increases in HIV transmission that are based on ecological frameworks. They argue that such approaches fail to adequately theorize the *mechanisms* through which environmental factors influence one another and, as a consequence, convey the sense that change is produced by "external variables pushing people and communities towards outcomes."[37(p.288)] Their primary concern is with the lack of attention to agency in these models, and they propose instead conceptualizing the relationship of environment to outcomes as "pathways." Understanding pathways as mechanisms of change is seen as a less passive alternative insofar as it credits individuals and collectivities with enacting change.

In subsequent articles, Friedman and Rossi[38] and Friedman et al.[35] expanded on this further by describing pathways in terms of dialectical theory. In accordance with relational theory, a dialectical approach views social structures of inequality (typically the focus has been on class and capitalism), characterized by oppression and exploitation, as deeply embedded in social institutions (e.g., the economy, politics, the work-place) and social processes. As such, "large-scale" social structures and processes are viewed as mutually constitutive of one another and of their parts; what may seem to be independent variables (characteristics of the social environment) may actually be co-defining one another as parts of larger processes.[35(p.1916)]

Furthermore, dialectical theory conceptualizes change as emerging from contradictions embedded within structures and processes, at multiple levels, that are resolved in ways eventually leading to new contradictions. But the form these contradictions and their resolutions take are shaped as much by human actions, both individual and collective, as they are by the contradictory operations of structures and processes. Indeed, each is constitutive in some ways, of the other. In this way, dialectical theory has the potential to explain how the present state of the HIV epidemic came to be, as well as to suggest both how and where to intervene to change its direction and from where and in what forms potential reactions to those changes may occur (perhaps anticipating what otherwise might be considered "unintended consequences"). Finally, while dialectical theory has tended to focus in particular on the structures of capitalism as they unfold through contradictory processes shaped by human agency, the exchange that followed publication of Friedman and Rossi's article outlining a dialectical theory of HIV/AIDS[39–42] and their response[43] suggests the possibility for expanding the analysis to include attention to other structures of oppression beyond capitalism, including gender, sexuality, and place.

In sum, relational theories applied to explain how social context produces HIV-related outcomes, whether measured for particular individuals or distinct subpopulations or in epidemic patterns more generally, provide a more complex and dynamic representation of the social world than ecological approaches that understand social context as a distinct set of factors operating at multiple levels, independent of one another. Insofar as they capture the complexity of that world, they provide a robust framework for unraveling the history of HIV/AIDS and related interventions, one that includes an understanding of the interaction between structure and agency at multiple levels and at specific times and locations in history. They can suggest the conditions under which we might expect to see HIV epidemics emerge or not,[35,37] or particular gendered patterns of HIV/AIDS,[31(p.1679)] or increases in the behaviors of men that put women at risk,[44] or under what conditions women engaged in sex work will practice condom use with both paid and intimate partners.[45]

They also have the potential both to suggest the forms that structural interventions may take in the future and to anticipate likely reactions to such interventions and thereby, perhaps, to reduce or avoid what might once have been considered their "unintended consequences."

A Theoretically Informed Agenda for a New Generation of Structural Interventions

There is much more work to be done to elaborate the implications of relational theories of structure for the development of structural interventions addressing HIV/AIDS. In this last section, I suggest a research agenda that can move us forward in this direction. This agenda is based on three additional characteristics of relational theories that are implied by but have not been explicitly identified in the previous discussion. First, in part, movement forward in understanding HIV/AIDS is like movement forward in the development of theoretically driven research on any topic, achieved by asking the "right questions." And the "right questions" are themselves a product of particular historical moments. In this regard, I argue that the important question at this point in the history of HIV/AIDS is how to understand and what to do about the *persistence of inequities in HIV/AIDS based on race* (and to a somewhat lesser degree ethnicity) both across and within gender and sexuality. Globally, as well, the important questions relate to understanding and addressing tremendous inequities across and within nations.

Second, the structured relations that are the focus of relational theory are social relations of inequality; conceived of as relations that express and perpetuate oppression and exploitation and through which some stand to gain while others are harmed. Relational theories of gender focus on gender inequality, and dialectical theory has tended to focus on class inequality, but there is room in each for incorporating attention to other axes of social inequality. Indeed, intersectionality theory, whereby the social world is viewed as comprised of multiple axes of oppression (e.g., race, class, gender, sexuality) operating simultaneously, but distinctly, mutually constituting one another on micro and macro levels, represents a robust and important contemporary relational theory of gender.[46,47] Intersectionality is receiving growing attention in the context of health research generally[48,49] and HIV research in particular.[50,51] Across all of these approaches, a major project for theoretically driven research is to reveal how relations of oppression are expressed and reproduced in the present moment in space and time and to demonstrate the ways they are actively maintained to the benefit of some and challenged through the resistance of others. As such, research driven by relational theory is itself, arguably, a form of intervention.

Third, one implication of a relational theory is that individuals from oppressed groups (e.g., women, blacks, black women, gay Latinos) are rarely, if ever, "similarly situated" to those in privileged groups.[34] Even if they occupy the same level within the same institution—for example, consider two professors in a prestigious department at a prestigious university—they are likely to experience these institutions and their positions differently. This is because individuals embody structured relations of inequality within their own self-understandings, just as the institutions they occupy are reflective of these same structures of inequality. Any intervention aimed at enhancing their quality of life or improving their experience of the institution or outcomes related to their position in it must recognize and attend to these differences. Otherwise, they may not only lack an effect, but they may also run the risk of exacerbating inequities.

Answering the question of how best to explain and address persistent race inequalities in HIV/AIDS, then, requires conducting theoretically informed research aimed at revealing contemporary structures and expressions of racism—how they operate, who benefits from them, and how they are differentially experienced both by individuals and across other dimensions of social inequality (e.g., gender, sexuality) in ways that create vulnerability to HIV/AIDS. The question also requires identifying opportunities and possibilities that exist for resisting and transforming these structures. A good place to start is with mass incarceration. It is an often-repeated fact that the United States incarcerates more people than any other country in the world,[52] and at a higher rate than all but one.[52] It is also clear that Blacks, both across and within gender, are disproportionately affected.[53] Indeed, sociologist Loic Wacquant[54] argues that "mass incarceration" is a misnomer insofar as it suggests that incarceration is experienced en masse when it is, rather, concentrated by class, race, and place. Michelle Alexander[55] has referred to mass incarceration as the "new Jim Crow," a contemporary mechanism of racial control that has replaced explicit race-based exclusionary policies with exclusions based on criminal record and that is enforced through a wide range of policies and practices that ensure Black men in particular have a high likelihood of ending up with a criminal record.[55] She attributes the rise of mass incarceration to the war on drugs. Others dispute the role of drug policies in producing high rates of incarceration and their disproportionate burden on Black/African Americans.[56] But they do not dispute the importance of mass incarceration as a modern system of racial control. Alexander's book[55] stands as an indication of the transformative power of theoretically informed research in and of itself, insofar as the widespread public attention it has received has not only raised awareness of the extent of incarceration in the United States but also has exposed the structural relations of race inequality and race-based power that it hides, revealed multiple mechanisms through which it does this, and identified beneficiaries of this system. Indeed, the book was banned in the New Jersey State Prison and Southern State Correctional Facility until the American Civil Liberties Union intervened.[57] At the same time, there is more work to be done to understand the multiple levels at which, and mechanisms through which, mass incarceration operates to produce race-based and likely other specific forms of social inequality.

In the context of HIV/AIDS, much of the research related to mass incarceration has focused on understanding the impacts of personal incarceration on sexual risk behaviors. At the population level, research suggests an association between incarceration and HIV and other sexually transmitted infections (STIs) as well as race disparities in both.[58] A number of mostly cross-sectional studies, with either national samples[59-61] or convenience samples[62-64] indicate that a history of personal incarceration is associated with STIs and HIV-related risk behaviors, including multiple partnerships, inconsistent condom use, concurrent partnerships, and sex with risky partners. Little research explicitly analyzes incarceration's impact on race disparities in HIV, but there is evidence that a history of incarceration affects HIV risk among blacks, including condom use among young black men;[65] concurrent partnerships among Black women;[63] and multiple partners and sex trade among rural Black men and women.[67] Such research only begins to skim the surface. Moving forward, it will be important to extend the conceptualization of mass incarceration beyond personal incarceration to include attention to the ways that the criminal justice system reaches into the lives of individuals, families, and communities through, for example, community supervision and policing practices[68,69] and the subsequent implications of this for HIV/AIDS.

Also critical will be to understand better how the experiences of mass incarceration are fundamentally distinct by race and by gender and, within race, by gender and sexuality. Even those who are "similarly situated" in terms of having been incarcerated are likely to have very different experiences depending on race, gender, and sexuality configurations. With an understanding of mass incarceration as a mechanism through which race inequality is reproduced in the United States, and its implications for HIV at multiple levels, will come greater potential to develop structural interventions with the possibility of challenging these inequities.

Conclusion

Whether the emphasis is on mass incarceration or other structural mechanisms through which race (and other social) inequities are produced, the more general point is that the structural interventions most likely to be successful at addressing persistent, and potentially growing inequities in HIV/AIDS are those that reflect a relational understanding of social context. Such interventions might be based on an understanding of what relational theory tells us about the various ways affected groups have resisted oppressive social relations and, subsequently, targeted to fostering collective energy to address them. In this regard, there is much to be learned from community mobilization strategies that have been implemented to address HIV among female sex workers,[70-72] drug users,[73,74] and gay communities in Australia,[32] and the national response in Brazil.[32] Or, such interventions may be targeted to the policies that institutionalize and perpetuate social inequities. Guided by a relational perspective, these policy-focused interventions would reflect an understanding of who benefits from and is harmed by current policies, as well as how those benefits and harms may vary. Accordingly, they would be developed in ways that address the experiences of various oppressed race/sex/sexuality groups and not just the most privileged among them.

Relational theories might also suggest strategies for successfully navigating the consensus-building process required for ensuring policy adoption.[18] Or, such strategies might lead to intervention programs aimed at alleviating the harms associated with structures of social oppression. Even if they do not take on the structures that have produced those harms per se, relational theory can provide insight into specific ways those harms are experienced along different axes of inequality and guide the development of interventions.

To be sure, relational theory offers a complex conceptualization of the social context that produces inequities in HIV/AIDS. But the virus itself is extremely complicated, and this has not deterred us from seeking to understand it in all of its complexity for purposes of developing effective biomedical interventions. Similarly, the complexity of the social world should not deter our efforts to develop effective structural interventions.

References

1. Institute of Medicine. Assessing the social and behavioral science base for HIV/AIDS prevention and intervention: workshop summary. Washington, DC: National Academy Press; 1995. doi:10.17226/9207

2. Tawil O, Verster A, O'Reilly KR. Enabling approaches for HIV/AIDS prevention. *AIDS.* 1995;9(12):1299–1306. doi:10.1097/00002030-199512000-00001.

3. Lachenicht L. A skeptical argument concerning the value of a behavioural solution for AIDS. *South African Journal of Psychology.* 1993;23(1):15–20. doi:10.1177/008124639302300103

4. Sweat MD, Denison JA. Reducing HIV incidence in developing countries with structural and environmental interventions. *AIDS.* 1995;9(Suppl A):S251–S257.

5. Sumartojo E. Structural factors in HIV prevention: concepts, examples, and implications for research. *AIDS.* 2000;14. doi:10.1097/00002030-200006001-00002

6. Blankenship KM, Bray SJ, Merson MH. Structural interventions in public health. *AIDS.* 2000;14. doi:10.1097/00002030-200006001-00003

7. Parker RG, Easton D, Klein CH. Structural barriers and facilitators in HIV prevention: a review of international research. *AIDS.* 2000;14. doi:10.1097/00002030-200006001-00004

8. Rotheram-Borus MJ. Expanding the range of interventions to reduce HIV among adolescents. *AIDS.* 2000;14. doi:10.1097/00002030-200006001-00005

9. Jarlais DCD. Structural interventions to reduce HIV transmission among injecting drug users. *AIDS.* 2000;14. doi:10.1097/00002030-200006001-00006

10. Taussig JA, Weinstein B, Burris S, Jones TS. Syringe laws and pharmacy regulations are structural constraints on HIV prevention in the US. *AIDS.* 2000;14. doi:10.1097/00002030-200006001-00007

11. Wohlfeiler D. Structural and environmental HIV prevention for gay and bisexual men. *AIDS.* 2000;14. doi:10.1097/00002030-200006001-00008

12. Shriver MD, Everett C, Morin SF. Structural interventions to encourage primary HIV prevention among people living with HIV. *AIDS.* 2000;14. doi:10.1097/00002030-200006001-00009

13. Fullilove RE, Green L, Fullilove MT. The family to family program: a structural intervention with implications for the prevention of HIV/AIDS and other community epidemics. *AIDS.* 2000;14. doi:10.1097/00002030-200006001-00010

14. Oleary A, Martins P. Structural factors affecting women's HIV risk: a life-course example. *AIDS.* 2000;14. doi:10.1097/00002030-200006001-00011

15. Sumartojo E, Doll L, Holtgrave D, Gayle H, Merson M. Enriching the mix: incorporating structural factors into HIV prevention. *AIDS.* 2000;14. doi:10.1097/00002030-200006001-00001

16. Rosenstock IM. The health belief model and preventive health behavior. *Health Education Monographs.* 1974;2(4):354–386. doi:10.1177/109019817400200405

17. Fishbein M, Ajzen I. *Belief, Attitude, Intention, and Behavior: An Introduction to Theory and Research.* Reading, MA: Addison-Wesley; 1975.

18. Blankenship KM, Friedman SR, Dworkin S, Mantell JE. Structural interventions: concepts, challenges and opportunities for research. *Journal of Urban Health.* 2006;83(1):59–72. doi:10.1007/s11524-005-9007-4

19. Bronfenbrenner U. Toward an experimental ecology of human development. *American Psychologist.* 1977;32(7):513–531. doi:10.1037//0003-066x.32.7.513

20. Prado G, Huang S, Maldonado-Molina M, et al. An empirical test of ecodevelopmental theory in predicting HIV risk behaviors among Hispanic youth. *Health Education & Behavior.* 2010;37(1):97–114. doi:10.1177/1090198109349218

21. Diclemente RJ, Salazar LF, Crosby RA. A review of STD/HIV preventive interventions for adolescents: sustaining effects using an ecological approach. *Journal of Pediatric Psychology.* 2007;32(8):888–906. doi:10.1093/jpepsy/jsm056

22. Larios SE, Lozada R, Strathdee SA, et al. An exploration of contextual factors that influence HIV risk in female sex workers in Mexico: the social ecological model applied to HIV risk behaviors. *AIDS Care.* 2009;21(10):1335–1342. doi:10.1080/09540120902803190

23. Rhodes T. The "risk environment": a framework for understanding and reducing drug-related harm. *International Journal of Drug Policy.* 2002;13(2):85–94. doi:10.1016/s0955-3959(02)00007-5

24. Rhodes T, Singer M, Bourgois P, Friedman SR, Strathdee SA. The social structural production of HIV risk among injecting drug users. *Social Science & Medicine.* 2005;61(5):1026–1044. doi:10.1016/j.socscimed.2004.12.024

25. Strathdee SA, Hallett TB, Bobrova N, et al. HIV and risk environment for injecting drug users: the past, present, and future. *The Lancet.* 2010;376(9737):268–284. doi:10.1016/s0140-6736(10)60743-x

26. Gupta GR, Ogden J, Warner A. Moving forward on women's gender-related HIV vulnerability: the good news, the bad news and what to do about it. *Global Public Health.* 2011;6(Suppl 3). doi:10.1080/17441692.2011.617381

27. Blankenship KM, Reinhard E, Sherman SG, El-Bassel N. Structural interventions for HIV prevention among women who use drugs. *JAIDS Journal of Acquired Immune Deficiency Syndromes.* 2015;69. doi:10.1097/qai.0000000000000638

28. Shannon K, Strathdee SA, Goldenberg SM, et al. Global epidemiology of HIV among female sex workers: influence of structural determinants. *The Lancet.* 2015;385(9962):55–71. doi:10.1016/s0140-6736(14)60931-4

29. Boerma JCAT, Weir SS. Integrating demographic and epidemiological approaches to research on HIV/AIDS: the proximate- determinants framework. *The Journal of Infectious Diseases.* 2005;191(s1). doi:10.1086/425282

30. Auerbach JD, Parkhurst JO, Cáceres CF. Addressing social drivers of HIV/AIDS for the long-term response: conceptual and methodological considerations. *Global Public Health.* 2011;6(Suppl 3). doi:10.1080/17441692.2011.594451

31. Connell R. Gender, health and theory: conceptualizing the issue, in local and world perspective. *Social Science & Medicine.* 2012;74(11):1675–1683. doi:10.1016/j.socscimed.2011.06.006

32. Kippax S, Stephenson N, Parker RG, Aggleton P. Between individual agency and structure in HIV prevention: understanding the middle ground of social practice. *American Journal of Public Health.* 2013;103(8):1367–1375. doi:10.2105/ajph.2013.301301

33. Parker R, Aggleton P. HIV and AIDS-related stigma and discrimination: a conceptual framework and implications for action. *Social Science & Medicine.* 2003;57(1):13–24. doi:10.1016/s0277-9536(02)00304-0

34. Risman BJ. Gender as a social structure. *Gender & Society.* 2004;18(4):429–450. doi:10.1177/0891243204265349

35. Friedman SR, Sandoval M, Mateu-Gelabert P, et al. Theory, measurement and hard times: some issues for HIV/AIDS research. *AIDS and Behavior.* 2013;17(6):1915–1925. doi:10.1007/s10461-013-0475-3

36. Krieger N. Proximal, distal, and the politics of causation: what's level got to do with it? *American Journal of Public Health.* 2008;98(2):221–230. doi:10.2105/ajph.2007.111278

37. Friedman SR, Rossi D, Braine N. Theorizing "big events" as a potential risk environment for drug use, drug-related harm and HIV epidemic outbreaks. *International Journal of Drug Policy.* 2009;20(3):283–291. doi:10.1016/j.drugpo.2008.10.006

38. Friedman SR, Rossi D. Dialectical theory and the study of HIV/AIDS and other epidemics. *Dialectical Anthropology.* 2011;35(4):403–427. doi:10.1007/s10624-011-9222-1

39. Palmer BD. A comment on Friedman and Rossi's dialectical theory and the study of HIV/AIDS: dialectical correctness. *Dialectical Anthropology.* 2011;35(4):429–433. doi:10.1007/s10624-011-9246-6

40. Susser I. A comment on Friedman and Rossi's dialectics of HIV: agency, resistance and gender for dialectical anthropology. *Dialectical Anthropology.* 2011;35(4):435–441. doi:10.1007/s10624-011-9251-9

41. Bongmba EK. A comment on Friedman and Rossi's dialectical theory and the study of HIV/AIDS: a broad Marxist critique. *Dialectical Anthropology.* 2011;35(4):443–447. doi:10.1007/s10624-011-9245-7

42. Floyd K. A comment on Friedman and Rossi's dialectical theory and the study of HIV/AIDS: thought to the second power. *Dialectical Anthropology.* 2011;35(4):449–452. doi:10.1007/s10624-011-9255-5

43. Friedman SR, Rossi D. A reply to Bongmba, Floyd, Palmer, and Susser: an invitation to dialectics. *Dialectical Anthropology.* 2011;35(4):453–457. doi:10.1007/s10624-011-9257-3

44. Silberschmidt M. Men, male sexuality and HIV/AIDS: reflections from studies in rural and urban East Africa. *Transformation: Critical Perspectives on Southern Africa.* 2004;54(1):42–58. doi:10.1353/trn.2004.0026

45. Young G, Danner M, Fort L, Blankenship KM. Sexual practice in structural context: condom use among women doing sex work in southern India. Manuscript under review. 2018.

46. Crenshaw K. Mapping the margins: intersectionality, identity politics, and violence against women of color. *Stanford Law Review.* 1991;43(6):1241. doi:10.2307/1229039

47. Collins PH. *Black Feminist Thought: Knowledge, Consciousness, and the Politics of Empowerment.* New York: Routledge; 2015.

48. Bowleg L. The problem with the phrase women and minorities: intersectionality—an important theoretical framework for public health. *American Journal of Public Health.* 2012;102(7):1267–1273. doi:10.2105/ajph.2012.300750

49. Hankivsky O. Women's health, men's health, and gender and health: implications of intersectionality. *Social Science & Medicine.* 2012;74(11):1712–1720. doi:10.1016/j.socscimed.2011.11.029

50. Bowleg L, Teti M, Malebranche DJ, Tschann JM. "It's an uphill battle everyday": intersectionality, low-income black heterosexual men, and implications for HIV prevention research and interventions. *Psychology of Men & Masculinity.* 2013;14(1):25–34. doi:10.1037/a0028392

51. Doyal L. Challenges in researching life with HIV/AIDS: an intersectional analysis of black African migrants in London. *Culture, Health & Sexuality.* 2009;11(2):173–188. doi:10.1080/13691050802560336

52. Highest to Lowest—Prison Population Total. World Prison Brief. London: Institute for Criminal Policy Research. http://www.prisonstudies.org/highest-to-lowest/prison-population-total. Accessed August 8, 2017.

53. Carsen EA. Prisoners in 2013. Washington, DC: US Bureau of Justice Statistics; 2014. http://www.bjs.gov/content/pub/pdf/p13.pdf. Accessed August 4, 2017.

54. Wacquant LCAF. Class, race & hyperincarceration in revanchist America. *Daedalus.* 2010;139(3):74–90. doi:10.1162/daed_a_00024

55. Alexander M. *The New Jim Crow: Mass Incarceration in the Age of Colorblindness.* New York: New Press, 2012.

56. Pfaff JF. *Locked In: The True Causes of Mass Incarceration—and How to Achieve Real Reform.* New York: Basic Books; 2017.

57. Bromwhich JE, Mueller B. Ban on book about mass incarceration lifted in New Jersey prisons after A.C.L.U. protest. *The New York Times;* January 8, 2018. https://www.nytimes.com/2018/01/08/nyregion/new-jim-crow-nj-jails.html. Accessed January 12, 2018.

58. Wildeman C. Imprisonment and (inequality in) population health. *Social Science Research.* 2012;41(1):74–91. doi:10.1016/j.ssresearch.2011.07.006

59. Khan MR, Rosen DL, Epperson MW, et al. Adolescent criminal justice involvement and adulthood sexually transmitted infection in a nationally representative US sample. *Journal of Urban Health.* 2012;90(4):717–728. doi:10.1007/s11524-012-9742-2

60. Knittel AK, Snow RC, Griffith DM, Morenoff J. Incarceration and sexual risk: examining the relationship between men's involvement in the criminal justice system and risky sexual behavior. *AIDS and Behavior.* 2013;17(8):2703–2714. doi:10.1007/s10461-013-0421-4

61. Khan MR, Doherty IA, Schoenbach VJ, Taylor EM, Epperson MW, Adimora AA. Incarceration and high-risk sex partnerships among men in the United States. *Journal of Urban Health.* 2009;86(4):584–601. doi:10.1007/s11524-009-9348-5

62. Epperson MW, Khan MR, El-Bassel N, Wu E, Gilbert L. A longitudinal study of incarceration and HIV risk among methadone maintained men and their primary female partners. *AIDS and Behavior.* 2010;15(2):347–355. doi:10.1007/s10461-009-9660-9

63. Epperson MW, Khan MR, Miller DP, Perron BE, El-Bassel N, Gilbert L. Assessing criminal justice involvement as an indicator of human immunodeficiency virus risk among women in methadone treatment. *Journal of Substance Abuse Treatment.* 2010;38(4):375–383. doi:10.1016/j.jsat.2010.03.004

64. Khan MR, Wohl DA, Weir SS, et al. Incarceration and risky sexual partnerships in a southern US city. *Journal of Urban Health.* 2007;85(1):100–113. doi:10.1007/s11524-007-9237-8

65. Ricks JM, Crosby RA, Terrell I. Elevated sexual risk behaviors among postincarcerated young African American males in the south. *American Journal of Men's Health.* 2014;9(2):132–138. doi:10.1177/1557988314532680

66. Nunn A, Dickman S, Cornwall A, et al. Concurrent sexual partnerships among African American women in Philadelphia: results from a qualitative study. *Sexual Health.* 2012;9(3):288. doi:10.1071/sh11099

67. Khan MR, Miller WC, Schoenbach VJ, et al. Timing and duration of incarceration and high-risk sexual partnerships among African Americans in North Carolina. *Annals of Epidemiology.* 2008;18(5):403–410. doi:10.1016/j.annepidem.2007.12.003

68. Cooper H, Moore L, Gruskin S, Krieger N. Characterizing perceived police violence: implications for public health. *American Journal of Public Health.* 2004;94(7):1109–1118. doi:10.2105/ajph.94.7.1109

69. Cooper HL. War on drugs policing and police brutality. *Substance Use & Misuse.* 2015;50(8–9):1188–1194. doi:10.3109/10826084.2015.1007669

70. Kerrigan D, Kennedy CE, Morgan-Thomas R, et al. A community empowerment approach to the HIV response among sex workers: effectiveness, challenges, and considerations for implementation and scale-up. *The Lancet.* 2015;385(9963):172–185. doi:10.1016/s0140-6736(14)60973-9

71. Dhungana N, Blankenship KM, Biradavolu MR, Tankasala N, George A. No-one-size-fits-all: addressing the social and structural dimensions of sex worker vulnerability to HIV through community mobilization in Avahan. In: Kerrigan D, Barrington C, eds. *Structural Dynamics of HIV.* Cham, Switzerland: Springer; 2017:67–96. doi:10.1007/978-3-319-63522-4_4

72. Cornish F, Priego-Hernandez J, Campbell C, Mburu G, Mclean S. The impact of community mobilization on HIV prevention in middle and low income countries: a systematic review and critique. *AIDS and Behavior.* 2014;18(11):2110–2134. doi:10.1007/s10461-014-0748-5

73. Latkin C, Friedman S. Drug use research: drug users as subjects or agents of change. *Substance Use & Misuse.* 2012;47(5):598–599. doi:10.3109/10826084.2012.644177

74. Friedman SR, Schneider E, Latkin C. What we do not know about organizations of people who use drugs. *Substance Use & Misuse.* 2012;47(5):568–572. doi:10.3109/10826084.2011.629707

14

Social Conditions and the AIDS Pandemic

A PROPOSED FRAMEWORK FOR STRUCTURAL-LEVEL
INTERVENTIONS

Richard A. Crosby, Ralph J. DiClemente, and Jacqueline P. Sims

Introduction

The now widespread use of Treatment as Prevention (TasP) and pre-exposure prophylaxis (PrEP) represents a milestone in the global quest to end AIDS. Despite this great progress, the social and economic conditions underlying the pandemic remain largely intractable. As the late Jonathan Mann passionately argued, AIDS is a social disease—one that is fueled by income inequality, oppression of minority members (including sexual and gender minorities), gender inequity, urbanization, and violence against women and sexual/gender minorities. Had he lived into the new millennium, Mann would surely be quick to note that many of the culprit social conditions have gone largely unabated.

The preceding chapters in this volume have provided a wealth of options that can be applied as "stop-gap solutions" to these social conditions. Unfortunately, structural-level intervention programs have not advanced to the level of actually rectifying the social conditions that Mann, and so many others since his time, described as "drivers" of the epidemic (see Chapter 2).

A fundamental aspect of public health practice may have become "lost" in the excitement of the recent biomedical revolution in antiretroviral

---

BOX 14.1

Types of Interventions Contained in the World Health Organization Guidelines

"There comes a point where we need to stop just pulling people out of the river. We need to go upstream and find out why they are falling in."

—Bishop Desmond Tutu[1]

---

therapy (ART) to end AIDS. That aspect involves the recognition that socioeconomic conditions are the foundation of health and health behaviors. Applying this concept to sexual health, former US surgeon general David Stacher (and colleagues) advocated a five-tier pyramid model, with the bottom tier being socioeconomic drivers of the conditions that lead to risk of HIV/sexually transmitted infections (STIs) and other risks to sexual health and well-being.[2] The subsequent tiers are best summarized as (1) making strategic changes to systems and the sociopolitical environment that enable people to easily adopt sexual health protective behaviors, (2) the widespread implementation of intervention programs that produce long-term maintenance of sexual health protective behaviors, (3) clinical interventions, and (4) education programs, including one-to-one counseling. In this paradigm, sole reliance on a smaller tier (i.e., tier 3) approach is considered suboptimal. Thus, although the global vision of 90-90-90 has been widely embraced, it is nonetheless only a small part of what can and should be done to truly end AIDS.

Global Incidence Is Not Declining

Optimism about ending AIDS requires a corresponding commitment to monitoring the pandemic and increasing the intensity of prevention efforts as suggested by surveillance data. Global declines in HIV incidence have *not* occurred since 2011. In 2016, Michel Sidibé, executive director of UNAIDS, stated, "We are sounding the alarm. The power of prevention is not being realized. If there is a resurgence in new HIV infections now, the epidemic will become impossible to control. The world needs to take urgent and immediate action to close the prevention gap." The *Prevention Gap Report* issued by UNAIDS in 2016 provided a sobering set of statistics that are of direct relevance to anyone with an investment in ending AIDS.[3] These include:

- Between 1990 and 2015, an estimated 45 million new infections were averted due to condom use, yet nations such as South Africa lack adequate resources to provide condoms to all of those at risk of HIV acquisition/transmission.
- Two-thirds of all young people do not have adequate knowledge about HIV and its prevention.
- PrEP coverage is less than 5% of the 2020 target goal.
- Only 38% of persons living with HIV are virally suppressed.

The fact that global incidence of HIV has not declined since 2011 does not imply a lack of change. Without question, some populations have experienced declines, while others have experienced escalations. It is likely that the escalations occurred in nations poorly resourced and ill-prepared politically to confront HIV-related stigma and gay-related stigma. The *Prevention Gap Report*, for instance, estimated the HIV-related costs of homophobia in western/central Europe and North America at US$49.7 billion. The proportion of the global spending on HIV prevention that was dedicated specifically to men who have sex with men was 2.1%. This meager allocation also applies to people who inject drugs (3.3%) and commercial sex workers (3.8%). Homophobia, however, is only one of many social conditions driving the HIV/AIDS pandemic. Transphobia, misogyny, racism, stigmatization of people who inject drugs, and a general social disdain for the poor are equally strong drivers of the pandemic. Clearly, none of these conditions will be altered by a purely biomedical approach to the AIDS pandemic.

Social Drivers of the Pandemic

HIV continues to be a "disease of marginalized populations"— particularly women residing in highly patriarchal cultures. Despite great progress in treating women with antiretrovirals during pregnancy, women still comprise 51% of the global burden of HIV/AIDS.[4] The social conditions that placed women at a disadvantage relative to HIV acquisition 30 years ago are still as prevalent today. For example, based on reports from 32 countries, intimate partner violence is extremely common among girls 15 to 19 years of age as well as women over the age of 19.[3] In many countries women continue to lack legal protections regarding property rights and rights to divorce, to have bank accounts, to enter into contracts, and to inherit money/property.[5] Female genital mutilation—a common source of blood-to-blood transmission of HIV—is perhaps one of most extreme demonstrations of the social subordination of women. Despite "zero tolerance" campaigns mounted by the World Health Organization, recent estimates indicate at least 30 countries continue this form of subordination, with more than 200 million being affected and an estimated 3 million girls each year likely to undergo this mutilation.[6]

That social conditions are the true cause of HIV transmission is especially clear when considering the enormous levels of gender inequality that exist in almost all nations. Many countries actually legislate this inequality through laws and policies that favor men over women.[7] From the start of the AIDS pandemic it has been characterized as one of women. Michel Sidibé (executive director of UNAIDS) stated this succinctly by saying, "The epidemic unfortunately remains an epidemic of women."[8] The etiology of this point cannot be understated—it is a reflection of marginalization. Unequal treatment of girls/women culturally, socially, and economically clearly translates into greatly elevated HIV risk for females. Sadly, that risk is especially great for those who are the youngest. For instance, globally, young girls/women who are 10 to 24 years of age are twice as likely to become infected with HIV compared to their same-age male counterparts.[8] For young girls/women living in east and southern Africa, HIV infection occurs five to seven years earlier in life compared to males.[9] In Russia (where injection drug use is a key driver of the HIV epidemic), young girls/women who are 15 to 24 years of age have an incidence rate of HIV infection that is more than twice as high as that for same-age males.[10]

The extreme disparities in social conditions for girls/women span a range from a "sugar daddy" culture, to widespread practices of transactional sex with young girls/women, to lack of sexual health services/lack of provider willingness to provide these services to unmarried females, to the inequitable education provided to females and the corresponding lack of economic opportunity. In a purely biomedical approach to HIV prevention (i.e., TasP, PrEP, and voluntary male circumcision) it is difficult, at best, to imagine any changes occurring to these underlying causes of the epidemic.

The most pervasive driving factor in the HIV/AIDS pandemic is poverty. Tied to homelessness, engaging in commercial sex work, and a lack of access to healthcare, poverty has not changed greatly since the first cases of HIV were reported in 1981. Recent heightened attention to food insecurity (see Chapter 5), microfinance programs (see Chapters 6 and 7), and stable housing (see Chapter 4) represents encouraging trends in both preventing HIV acquisition and transmission. Highly encouraging, for example, is a report from UNAIDS noting that many nations have incorporated nutritional assistance programs into HIV care, and many have reallocated a portion of their funding for ART to food assistance.[11] Ample evidence suggests that, compared to HIV-infected people with adequate caloric intake, food-insecure persons living with HIV are likely to fare poorly relative to treatment.[4–6, 11–13] Food assistance programs are also valuable as a method of preventing HIV acquisition, given that food insecurity is a clear risk factor for engaging in behaviors that lead to HIV acquisition.[11–18]

Ultimately, it is most likely that the prevailing social conditions that have been driving HIV/AIDS for decades are the primary barriers to stalled progress. As described in Chapter 2, the global goal of 90-90-90 is a dominating force in the public health response to the pandemic. Yet, in 2016 UNAIDS reported progress at the level of 60-46-38.[3] This observation begs the question of whether 90-90-90 (a vision focused solely on TasP) should be re-evaluated as a "center-stage" strategy for the investment of already scarce resources into the prevention and control of HIV/AIDS.

A clear and present danger regarding sole reliance on the 90-90-90 paradigm is that it may exacerbate already existing health disparities. For example, in 2017 the Joint United Nations Programme on AIDS reported

---

BOX 14.2

Words to Guide Future Action in the AIDS Pandemic

"Like slavery and apartheid, poverty is not natural. It is man-made and it can be overcome and eradicated with the actions of human beings."

—Nelson Mandela[19]

that 25 nations had met the 90% goal regarding viral suppression.[20] The vast majority of these 25 are developed nations, and none of the 25 nations were in Africa. The very real risk that the Joint United Nations Programme report does *not* address is that TasP will become a socioeconomic condition that leads to polarized progress in the effort to end AIDS.

A Prevention Paradigm

As opposed to the current paradigm of TasP with the corresponding goals of 90-90-90, a far more upstream approach—and one that also addresses underlying social conditions—has been advanced by the United Nations General Assembly (see Figure 14.1).[3] The "five pillars of prevention" is an approach suggesting that provision of comprehensive HIV prevention services to young women, adolescent girls, and their male partners is paramount. These same comprehensive HIV prevention services are also advocated for all at-risk populations (e.g., men who have sex with men, transgender women, prison populations, sex workers, homeless and unstably housed persons). Harm reduction programs and services are

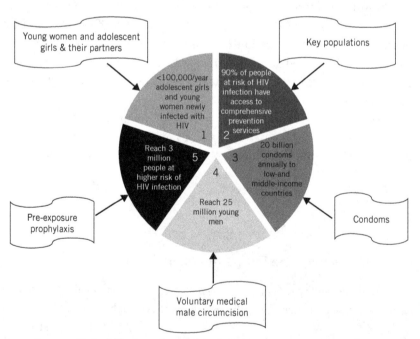

FIGURE 14.1 United Nations General Assembly prevention targets: five prevention pillars

specifically mentioned as being a key aspect of these comprehensive HIV prevention services. It is these first two pillars that acknowledge social conditions as barriers to prevention, and thus the corresponding actions will require navigation and at least partial solutions to these conditions. The pillars further include the goal of providing 20 billion condoms to persons at risk of HIV acquisition or transmission by the year 2020, providing voluntary male circumcision to 25 million men, and providing PrEP to 3 million men by the year 2020.

For persons highly dedicated to ending AIDS, an easily overlooked advantage of the five-pillar approach is that the pillars do far more than prevent HIV. For instance, syringe and needle exchange programs avert untold millions of cases of hepatitis B and C, staphylococcus aureus (a common cause of endocarditis), and a host of other blood-borne infections. Condom use averts millions of cases of STIs, including those with highly devastating effects regarding pregnancy and neonatal outcomes (e.g., Zika virus, syphilis, and genital herpes), as well as gonorrhea (an especially important public health concern given the ever-expanding prevalence of drug-resistant strains). Further, the relatively modest goal regarding PrEP in the five-pillar approach is respectful of the fact that PrEP is a resource-intensive prevention method that can (as was suggested early in the movement to advance PrEP as a prevention method[21]) greatly detract from the resources available for the array of other, less expensive prevention approaches. Finally, it is vital to bear in mind that the five-pillar prevention approach is ecologically responsible relative to the very real threat of drug resistance to HIV.[22]

A Proposed Framework for Structural-Level Interventions

Often practiced at local levels, public health relies on the use of creative solutions to otherwise seemingly intractable social conditions. This is particularly the case with the AIDS pandemic. We propose a framework that can become a simplified planning tool for public health professionals charged with HIV prevention. A framework is simply a method of applying multiple, interlocking strategies designed to achieve goals (such as those comprising the five-pillar approach). For from being a definitive framework, this initial model (see Figure 14.2) is also an invitation for researchers and scholars, devoted to HIV prevention, to refine, test, and apply the model in an iterative fashion.

The model begins with the premise that differences exist between drivers of HIV-risk behavior (whether this is risk of acquisition or risk of transmission) and HIV-preventive behaviors. Because it is the prevention behavior that will actually lead to decreased incidence, this is the focal point of the framework. The framework suggests that identification of the one driver that is most influential in enabling the preventive behavior is the starting point for change. Once that driver is identified and clearly understood, the next step is to determine the corresponding intervention options. Based on the chapters in this volume, the framework offers two distinct lists of options—one or both lists can be used. List A provides options focused around poverty. For instance, as was exemplified in Chapters 6 and 7, micro-lending and micro-enterprise programs can be highly effective stop-gap solutions to poverty. Similarly, food security programs, housing assistance, and providing access to a public education for female students are potential structural-level "tools" that can be used to address the first selected driver. List B provides systems-based options, such as those described in Chapters 8, 9, and 10 of this volume. Although many other options exist, Figure 14.2 simply displays those described in this volume. These options are more systemic than purely structural, but each exemplifies a method of addressing the drivers of prevention behaviors.

As Figure 14.2 displays, after selecting options to address the first selected driver, the process may be repeated in the event that a second driver is considered to be valuable and thus important to address. Because structural-level interventions are often a massive undertaking, the decision to select a second driver should be made with caution and great consideration as to the expected benefit. Finally, as shown, the framework suggests that attention to community mobilization (Chapter 11), evaluation for program improvement (Chapter 12), and using the program findings to inform theory and to be improved by theory (Chapter 13) are vital steps in the overall process of ending AIDS.

Practice-Based Research

A long acknowledged but seldom addressed problem in public health research (including HIV prevention research) is the tremendous lag time that occurs between the inception of a prevention program and its ultimate "readiness" for widespread dissemination and implementation. That this lag time is generally estimated at 17 years[23] does not bode well for the

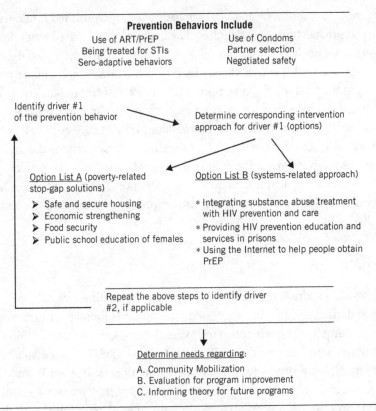

Prevention Behaviors Include

Use of ART/PrEP	Use of Condoms
Being treated for STIs	Partner selection
Sero-adaptive behaviors	Negotiated safety

Identify driver #1
of the prevention behavior

Determine corresponding intervention
approach for driver #1 (options)

Option List A (poverty-related
stop-gap solutions)

➤ Safe and secure housing
➤ Economic strengthening
➤ Food security
➤ Public school education of females

Option List B (systems-related approach)

∗ Integrating substance abuse treatment
  with HIV prevention and care
∗ Providing HIV prevention education and
  services in prisons
∗ Using the Internet to help people obtain
  PrEP

Repeat the above steps to identify driver
#2, if applicable

Determine needs regarding:

A. Community Mobilization
B. Evaluation for program improvement
C. Informing theory for future programs

FIGURE 14.2 A proposed framework for structural-level intervention planning

prospect of ending AIDS in the near future. The protracted length of time, however, is largely a consequence of the process of translating evidence-based practice (i.e., findings from randomized controlled trials) into real-world settings. Fortunately, structural-level interventions can forego this step because these are not tested in the context of randomized trials (see Chapter 12). Instead, structural-level approaches are inherently amenable to being tested in real-world settings—thus creating practice-based evidence from the start. It is this practice-based evidence that circumvents the protracted lag time in translation.[24] In essence, structural-level approaches are tested in the same context in which their eventual application will occur—at the community level or as applied to an entire population.

That only practice-based research occurs at the population level is a critically important point to consider. Ultimately, the value of any intervention approach (or combination of intervention approaches) must be judged on the degree of positive change in a defined population. This criterion of success is very different than that applied to tightly controlled randomized trials or prospective cohort studies. For instance, a US-based study found strong evidence for the efficacy of PrEP, but this was among established patients in a highly efficient managed care organization.[25] This is much different than asking the question of whether the introduction and use of PrEP in a given geographic location (e.g., an entire city, state, province, territory, etc.) has an overall effect on reducing HIV incidence for all people in that area. As of the date when this chapter was written, the authors were not aware of any published evaluation showing population declines in HIV incidence attributable to the introduction/use of PrEP. This level of evidence is needed to justify future emphasis on PrEP as a prevention method.

Conclusion

The World Health Organization consolidated guidelines for HIV prevention and care and included suggested interventions for (a) the health sector and (b) "an enabling environment." Clearly both sets of interventions are distinct and thus can (and should) be used in parallel. Box 14.1 displays the primary types of interventions included in both sets. It is set B that is of keen interest in this volume. The structural-level interventions examples in this volume do not exhaust the broad range of possibilities. Without question, the future will bring other examples to the surface. As shown in set B of Box 14.1, this range of possibilities can and should include expanded approaches to community empowerment, clearer methods of garnering the all-so-critical financial support for structural-level intervention efforts, and programs designed to reduce violence against women, racial minorities, sexual minorities, and gender minorities. Most importantly in set B is the ongoing challenge of how to best leverage legislative support designed to reduce the drivers of HIV-risk behavior and augment the drivers of HIV-protective behaviors (Box 14.2 and Box 14.3).

We conclude this chapter, and this volume, by suggesting that the AIDS pandemic requires, even demands, creative solutions to the chronic social problems of all nations, regardless of per capita gross national product and irrespective of the current and past impact of HIV/AIDS on a nation. Viewing the AIDS pandemic in a void—one separated from public health and its tenets—is a paradigm that will produce sub-optimal success in ending AIDS and one that will lack value in terms of improving the human condition as it exists in the much larger realm of health and

---

BOX 14.3

Words to Guide Future Action in the AIDS Pandemic

SET A: HEALTH SECTOR INTERVENTIONS

- Programs promoting use of condoms and lubricants
- Harm-reduction programs for persons abusing substances
- Behavioral interventions for at-risk populations
- HIV testing and counseling
- HIV treatment and care
- Prevention and management of HIV coinfections and comorbidities
- Sexual and reproductive health interventions

SET B: STRATEGIES FOR AN ENABLING ENVIRONMENT

- Supportive legislation, policy, and financial commitment
- Addressing stigma and discrimination
- Community empowerment
- Addressing violence against key populations

---

well-being. Again, with the words and work of Jonathan Mann in mind, ending AIDS must involve changing the underlying social conditions that provide the current pandemic with an ecological advantage. Ultimately, a socially responsible approach to ending AIDS will need to have ensuring human rights and equitable social conditions as the primary features of coordinated global efforts.

References

1. Nathaniel M. Human trafficking—Prevention is better than a cure. *AsianAID.* April 24, 2018. https://www.asianaid.org.au/news/human-trafficking-prevention-is-better-than-a-cure/
2. Satcher D, Hook EW, Coleman E. Sexual health in America: Improving patient care and public health. *JAMA.* 2015;314:765–766.
3. UNAIDS. Prevention Gap Report. Available at: http://www.unaids.org/en/resources/documents/2016/prevention-gap
4. World Health Organization. Global Health Observatory Data: Number of women living with HIV. Available at: http://www.who.int/gho/hiv/epidemic_status/cases_adults_women_children_text/en/

5. UN Women. Facts and Figures: HIV and AIDS. Available at http://www. unwomen.org/en/what-we-do/hiv-and-aids/facts-and-figures

6. World Health Organization. Female Genital Mutilation. Fact Sheet. Available at: http://www.who.int/mediacentre/factsheets/fs241/en/

7. Kristof N, WuDunn ND. *Half the sky: Turning oppression into opportunity for women worldwide.* New York: Alfred A. Knopf, 2009.

8. United Nations News Centre. Noting progress to date, ban urges greater efforts against HIV/AIDS. June 9, 2010.

9. AVERT. Women and Girls, HIV and AIDS. Available at: https://www.avert.org/ professionals/hiv-social-issues/key-affected-populations/women

10. UNAIDS. Feature story: HIV increasingly threatens women in eastern Europe and central Asia. March 12, 2012.

11. UNAIDS. HIV, Food Security, and Nutrition. Policy Brief. Available at: http:// www.unaids.org/sites/default/files/media_asset/jc1565_policy_brief_nutrition_long_en_1.pdf

12. Gillespie S, Kadiyala S. *HIV/AIDS and food and nutrition security: from evidence to action.* (Food Policy Review No. 7. Washington, DC: International Food Policy Research Institute, 2005.

13. Scrimshaw N, SanGiovanni JP. Synergies of nutrition, infection and immunity: an overview. *Am J Clin Nutr.* 1997;66:464S–477S.

14. Paton NI, Sangeetha S, Earnest A, Bellamy R. The impact of malnutrition on survival and the CD4 count response in HIV-infected patients starting antiretroviral therapy. *HIV Med.* 2006;7(5), 323–330.

15. Weiser SD, Frongillo EA, Ragland K, et al. Food insecurity is associated with incomplete HIV RNS suppression among homeless and marginally-housed HIV-infected individuals in San Francisco. *J Gen Intern Med.* 2008;24:14–20.

16. Weiser SD, Fernnades KA, Brandson EK, et al. The association between food insecurity and mortality among HIV-infected individuals on HAART. *J Acquir Immune Defic Syndr.* 2009;52:342–349.

17. Ivers LC, Cullen KA, Freedberg KA, et al. HIV/AIDS, undernutrition and food insecurity. *Clin Infect Dis.* 2009;49:1096–1102.

18. Mena L, Crosby RA, Geter A. A novel measure of poverty and its association with sexual risk among young Black MSM. *Int J STD AIDS.* 2017;28:602–607.

19. In full: Mandela's poverty speech. *BBC News.* February 3, 2005. Available at: http://news.bbc.co.uk/2/hi/uk_news/politics/4232603.stm

20. Joint United Nations Programme on AIDS. Ending AIDS: Progress toward the 90-90-90 targets. Available at: http://www.unaids.org/sites/default/files/media_ asset/Global_AIDS_update_2017_en.pdf

21. Curran JW, Crosby RA. Preexposure prophylaxis (PrEP): Who will benefit and what are the challenges? *Am J Prev Med.* 2013;44:S163–S166.

22. Wensing AM, Calvez V, Guinthard H, et al. Updates on the drug resistant mutations in HIV-1. *Topics Antiviral Med.* 2016;24:132–141.

23. Morris SZ, Wooding S, Grant J. The answer is 17 years, what is the question? Understanding time lags in translational research. *J Res Soc Med.* 2011;104:510–520.

24. Swisher AK. Practice based evidence. *Cardiopulm Phys Ther J.* 2010;21:4–5.

25. Volk JE, Marcus JL, Pengrasamy T, et al. No new HIV infections with increasing use of HIV preexposure prophylaxis in a clinical practice setting. *Clin Infect Dis.* 2015;61:1601–1603. doi:10.1093/cid/civ778

Index